MONSTROUS CONCEPTIONS

Race, Inequality, and Health

COLUMBIA UNIVERSITY PRESS

RIH

RACE, INEQUALITY, AND HEALTH

RACE, INEQUALITY, AND HEALTH

Edited by Samuel Kelton Roberts Jr. and Michael Yudell

The Race, Inequality, and Health series explores how forms of racialization have created a wide range of phenomena, from producing inequities in health and health care to inspiring social movements around health. The goal of this series is to publish field-defining works across history, the social sciences, the biological sciences, and public health that deepen our understanding of how claims about race and race difference have affected health and society.

Jay S. Kaufman, *The Race Variable: How Statistical Practices Reinforce Inequality*

Diana Martha Louis, *Colored Insane: Slavery, Asylums, and Mental Illness in the Nineteenth Century*

Jonathan Kahn, *The Uses of Diversity: How Race Has Become Entangled in Law, Politics, and Biology*

Eram Alam, Dorothy Roberts, and Natalie Shibley, editors, *Ordering the Human: The Global Spread of Racial Science*

Sebastián Gil-Riaño, *The Remnants of Race Science: UNESCO and Economic Development in the Global South*

Rob DeSalle and Ian Tattersall, *Troublesome Science: The Misuse of Genetics and Genomics in Understanding Race*

Michael Yudell, *Race Unmasked: Biology and Race in the Twentieth Century*

For a complete list of books in the series, please see the Columbia University Press website.

Monstrous Conceptions

A History of Race, Disability, and Reproductive Medicine in the United States

Miriam Rich

Columbia University Press New York

Columbia University Press
Publishers Since 1893
New York Chichester, West Sussex
cup.columbia.edu

Cataloging-in-Publication Data is available from the Library of Congress.

ISBN 9780231200325 (hardback)
ISBN 9780231200332 (trade paperback)
ISBN 9780231553551 (EPUB)
ISBN 9780231567510 (PDF)

LCCN 2026001084

Printed and bound by CPI Group (UK) Ltd, Croydon, CR0 4YY

Cover design: Elliott S. Cairns
Cover image: Egon Schiele, *Schwangere Frau und Tod* (*Mutter und Tod*), 1911 (detail).
Photo: Ablakok / Wikimedia Commons / CC BY-SA 4.0.

GPSR Authorized Representative: Easy Access System Europe, Mustamäe tee 50, 10621 Tallinn, Estonia, gpsr.requests@easproject.com

To Bernie, Esther, June, and Samuel

Contents

Introduction

In 1868, a young Anglo-American woman anxiously prepared to give birth. She lived in Somerville, Massachusetts, an area recently transformed from colonized rural farmland into an urbanizing, densely populated industrial township. She had lost her second pregnancy, and now a vague but persistent sense of foreboding seemed to suffuse this third one. She worried that, compared to the vigorous fetal movements she remembered preceding the birth of her "well-formed" first child, the motions this time felt "very feeble." She described the feeling as a "fluttering sensation" inside her womb.[1]

She gave birth at home on a cold December day, attended by her private physician and likely also by female friends and family. The tiny infant, born with a rare congenital condition involving complete fusion of the lower limbs, weighed less than three pounds. Upon laying a hand on the infant's chest, the little heart could be felt "beating strongly."[2] The newborn seemed to gasp for air for some fifteen or twenty minutes. Then, the breathing ceased. What did the woman think and feel during this time? How did she make sense of all that happened? Her experiences following the birth, never entered into the historical record, are left for us to imagine.

The extant record is more forthcoming on the fate of her infant. Following the child's death, practitioners transformed the newborn body into a medical specimen of monstrosity. An account titled "Case of Monstrosity—(Siren)" appeared in a leading American medical journal in 1869, authored by the former dean of Harvard Medical School. The preserved bones and organs of the infant, mounted on bent glass rods and suspended in glass jars filled with alcohol, joined the Monstrosities Division in the Anatomical Cabinet of the Boston Society for Medical Improvement, an elite professional association of male Anglo-American physicians. Cataloged alongside the "national skulls" and "phrenological collection" also included within the remit of professional nineteenth-century specimen acquisition, these monsters of medical science served to produce knowledge not just about the formations but also about the imagined value of different kinds of human bodies.[3]

Almost one hundred years after this infant's transformation into a specimen of "siren monstrosity," Dr. Hulda Thelander was shocked to encounter a nearly identical term in the pages of a major medical journal. The 1963 issue of the *Journal of the American Medical Association* teemed with news of innovation in medical science, touting cutting-edge surgical and pharmaceutical developments. Yet Thelander found her attention lingering on a photograph of two newborn babies in a brief, unassuming case report tucked near the back. The image legend identified the infants as "sireniform monsters."[4]

Troubled by the captioning of this photograph, Thelander turned to her bookshelf. In a letter to *JAMA*'s editor, she explained that she first consulted *Dorland's Illustrated Medical Dictionary,* where she found the following definition of *monster*: "An infant born with an anomaly so pronounced that it interferes with the general or local development of the body." Reluctantly, she conceded that *JAMA*'s use of the term was "technically correct." But then she provided a second definition of *monster,* this time quoted from Webster's: "[Orig., a divine omen, indicating misfortune.] 1/ An animal or plant departing greatly in form or structure from the usual type of species, a monstrosity. . . . Anything monstrous, esp. a person of unnatural ugliness, cruelty, etc." This last entry, she argued, expressed the "usual connotation" of the word. "Is it not, therefore, rather monstrous for physicians to call infants, no matter how greatly deformed, 'monsters'?" she queried.[5]

To Thelander, the inclusion of the term *monster* in clinical literature seemed to be a shocking and inexplicable oversight, a crude holdover of prescientific thought that medical professionals had somehow diverse media into medical specimens, some remain to this day. They persist in fluid-filled jars housed in the storerooms of an Ivy League medical school in New England; clustered along sliding shelves in the museum collections of a US Army installation outside Washington, DC; and maintained in a red-brick and sandstone medical building on an island off the Texas Gulf Coast. Others exist as skeletal specimens, boxed away in pieces or mounted whole for exhibition: lever-shaped skull perched atop a tiny fetal body posed fully upright, the climax position of the iconic "Descent of Man" series rendered in monstrous miniature. And still others endure as images in woodcuts, copper engravings, and photographic prints.

Historical practitioners elaborated the category of monstrosity within the expanding activities and knowledge systems of "medical science" and "scientific medicine"—terms they used to refer to an emerging assemblage of practices, institutions, and epistemologies that treated the human body as an anatomical/physiological entity and linked a healing profession to the ideals and authority of scientific knowledge making.[10] Starting in the nineteenth century, US practitioners collected and classified anomalous births in accordance with the transatlantic field of *teratology*, formalized as "the modern scientific study of monstrosity" by the French scientist Isidore Geoffroy Saint-Hilaire in the early 1830s.[11] Invoked in its teratological sense, the term *monster* routinely appeared in US medical literature throughout the nineteenth and early twentieth centuries. Although its usage waned in the mid- and later twentieth century, the term occasionally still surfaced in leading medical journals as late as the 1980s.[12]

Attention to this history offers a new focus in the rich and wide-ranging scholarship on monstrosity. Existing scholarship on monstrous births in the history of science and medicine tends to concentrate on early modern Europe, while a largely separate literature in disability studies examines the lives and experiences of individuals positioned as "freaks" in histories of popular exhibition and display.[13] Overlapping both these literatures, a multidisciplinary body of scholarship examines representations of monsters in the literary, visual, popular, commercial, religious, and political cultures of numerous eras and regions.[14]

Monstrous Conceptions provides a different perspective by exploring the processes that constituted material bodies as monsters in

These contradictions, far from dissolving or destabilizing the category of monstrosity, instead gave it structure and salience. As conceptualized in antiquity, the monster embodied a central paradox of human relation, entailing simultaneous kinship and alienation: the offspring of human parents but not recognizable as the type of the human species.[9] It was this centrality of contradiction—the impossible yet emphatic existence of a being simultaneously family and stranger, human and not human, same and other—that long sustained the monster as a figure of cultural resonance and fascination. Translated and remade through the variegated activities of modern US medical science, the resonant contradictions of monstrosity were never resolved. Rather, they gained new social and political significance. In this new biomedical iteration, the paradoxes of monstrosity became a way to negotiate the contradictions of racial imaginaries and to define the stakes of women's childbearing as an aspirational site of eugenic control. Refigured as a transfer point between the social and biological meanings of human difference, the monster anchored unstable conceptions of race, sex, and disability in the materiality of development and reproduction.

THE BIRTH OF MONSTERS IN MODERN AMERICAN MEDICINE

The history of American medicine is marked by monsters. Their bodies and likenesses lined the display cases and cabinets of medical museums, the dissection rooms of medical schools, and the pages of medical journals and monographs. They were monsters not in a phantasmal or metaphorical sense but rather in a historical one: the corporeal referents of what once was a formally designated category within medical science.

These monsters were conceived, gestated, and birthed by human parents, and they had an undeniably material existence that could not be ignored by those who encountered them. Sometimes they were living newborn babies to be cleaned and clothed; nursed or given sugared milk from a finger, sop, or spoon; and swaddled when they cried. In many cases, they were also biological tissues to be molded in plaster, mounted on plates, or sealed in clear glass canisters of formalin, preserved in various forms for the interest and education of generations to come. Passed through sundry hands and across state borders, transformed through biologically monstrous. Despite the appellation "monstrous birth," these bodies were not *born* monstrous. Rather, they were made into monstrosities through specific historical practices. *Monstrous Conceptions* traces how a diffuse array of medical and scientific activities turned newborns into specimens of monstrosity, covering a period of US history that extends from the 1830s to the 1930s.

This book is centrally concerned with what we might call *medical meaning making*: the constellation of material, relational, and intellectual practices that together define and constitute bodily attributes, events, and experiences as legible biomedical phenomena.[8] It examines "medical monster making" as a multisited, multisensory, densely interactive process that ineluctably engaged the ideas and experiences of historical lay patients as well as formally credentialed medical practitioners—even as primarily white, male professionals increasingly sought to assert control over women's reproduction across this period. The meanings of monstrosity took form when, for instance, childbearing women and physicians negotiated narratives of causality; when families and birth attendants touched, cared for, or turned away from living newborns; when medical professors prepared and exhibited specimens in jars of clear liquid; when clinicians photographed infant bodies in sharp profile against featureless black backgrounds; when eugenicists labeled monsters on cautionary pedigree charts; and when laywomen sought and applied biomedical advice to manage and interpret their own experiences of reproduction and disability. At diverse sites of medical and scientific practice, which shaped both the physical and conceptual configuration of bodies, the monster became meaningful.

This is not to suggest that these processes materialized the body of a monster as a single, coherent object. They patently did not. Across arenas of medical meaning making, multimodal practices constructed the category of biological monstrosity in contradictory ways. Monstrosity signified a difference of relational degree and a difference of categorical separation; a creature within a taxonomy of animal kinds and a pathology within a taxonomy of human disease; a spectacle to display and a secret to conceal. The monster seemed at once to displace, affirm, and revise the logics of human racial hierarchy that pervaded nineteenth- and early twentieth-century American medical science.

forgotten to expunge from their modern lexicon. But as the story of the unnamed Somerville woman suggests, the term's presence in prominent medical literature was no accident. Rather, *monster* denoted a formal category produced and reproduced for generations in the activities, institutions, and epistemologies of modern American medical science. In this context, practitioners applied the term to infants born with major and usually fatal differences of anatomical development. In later periods, many of these conditions would be described using terms such as *major birth defects*, *congenital anomalies*, and *congenital disabilities*.

Histories of monstrous birth typically focus on medieval and early modern Europe, often treating the scientific Enlightenment as the natural cutoff point for this topic. In these earlier periods, popular and elite discourse frequently cast anomalous births as portents of divine intention, signs of social and political disorder, or reflections of moral transgression. Sometimes, such births also inspired awe and wonder.[6] In traditional accounts of this history, the rise of scientific teratology in the early nineteenth century jettisoned the old category of "the monstrous," replacing the fraught cultural connotations of "monstrous birth" with a modern medical understanding of congenital anomaly as a defect of embryological development.[7]

But, in fact, the category of monstrous birth persisted for the duration of the nineteenth century and well into the twentieth, its salience charged rather than extinguished by the rising authority of medical science. When nineteenth-century practitioners redefined monstrosity in scientific terms, they claimed to be dispelling the category's cultural meanings. By contrast, *Monstrous Conceptions* argues that the modern medical engagement with monstrosity instead produced new cultural meanings of human difference. As a category that simultaneously indexed the boundaries of bodily normalcy and the human species, locating bodies within a developmental hierarchy of kinds, the monster materialized and linked shifting concepts of racial, reproductive, and corporeal deviance. Embodying both the genesis of human difference and the mechanism of human degeneration, monstrosity theorized a relational order of race that was at once grounded in and perpetually imperiled by imaginaries of disability and women's reproduction.

This history illuminates not only the concepts that monstrous bodies came to signify but also the processes that rendered bodies relation to biological reproduction, examining multisensory practices and experiences linked to pregnancy, childbirth, postpartum care, obstetrics, embryology, and eugenics in the modern United States.[15] The book draws on historical documentation of more than five hundred cases of "monstrous" birth, all involving newborns formally classified as teratological "monstrosities" within US medical and scientific institutions.

This book covers the period when teratological monstrosity constituted an accepted and ubiquitous category in US medical science, spanning roughly from the 1830s to the 1930s. Teratology during this time represented a markedly transnational field that also engaged medical and scientific practitioners in many countries outside the United States, including France, Mexico, and Britain.[16] However, by tailoring its focus to the US context, *Monstrous Conceptions* explores how formations of monstrosity illuminate nationally specific (if not nationally bounded) histories of race, reproduction, and medicine. Elite nineteenth-century physicians discussed and imagined "American medicine" as a distinctive national enterprise; early twentieth-century eugenicists explicitly framed their agenda as a project of national American salvage.[17] And while local variations existed within the US medical collection and study of monstrosity, the circulation of teratological specimens and knowledge regularly exceeded intranational boundaries. This book draws on reports of births in thirty-seven US states as well as in a few sites of formal or informal US imperialism overseas, attended by medical practitioners who frequently called upon, collaborated with, sent specimens to, and cited colleagues in other regions of the nation and empire.[18]

The interest in scientific monstrosity engaged broad institutional and cultural shifts in the modern history of US medicine. Practitioners' uptake of teratology began in the early nineteenth century, a time when the sparse institutional apparatus of US medicine was concentrated largely in cities such as Philadelphia, Boston, and New York and the emerging medical profession, despite emphatically professed aspirations, could claim little actual authority over US childbearing. The collection of monstrous specimens burgeoned in regional and institutional scope in the later nineteenth century, a period characterized by the growth and elaboration of medical institutions and specialties, the widespread linkage of physician identity to ideals of scientific knowledge production, and the increasing assertion of (largely white, male) medical authority over biological bodies and birth.[19] And biomedical discourses of monstrosity persisted in the early twentieth century as the ascendant American eugenics movement deployed monstrous new imaginaries of deviance to exert control over reproduction. The book's periodization thus reveals continuities between nineteenth-century interest in medical monstrosity and later eugenic projects as the locus of interest in "defective" development shifted to a larger and larger set of smaller and smaller deviations from a projected normality. Far from a vestige of a prescientific past, the medical engagement with monstrosity instead illuminates an enduring modern investment in interpreting, configuring, and managing human difference and reproduction.

US medical practitioners, of course, did not invent the term *monstrosity*. By the nineteenth century, *monster* already constituted a capacious word layered with centuries of meaning. In the Aristotelian tradition, the monster was a being unlike its progenitor, an offspring who strayed so far from type that they were no longer recognizable as a human being.[20] An insistent specter of bodily alterity and transgression, the figure of the monster has long troubled the boundaries of that which is human, natural, normal, familiar—which kinds of bodies are recognized and cared for as kin and which are cast out of the family in fear or revulsion.[21] By embodying that which is definitively "Other," the monster shores up the status of the centered self. In marking what lies beyond its limits, it secures the position of the normative human subject, body, and species.[22] Yet, paradoxically, the monster destabilizes the very categories it structures, blurring and upending the distinctions between human and beast, kin and stranger, self and other, recognition and denial, affection and repulsion, the living and the nonviable.[23]

In the medieval and early modern periods, the term *monster* denoted a broad array of anomalous and sometimes fantastical beings.[24] However, in its codified use within the "modern medical nomenclature" of the nineteenth and early twentieth centuries, it denoted something considerably more specific.[25] As the proper object of scientific teratology, *monstrosity* described a specific biological phenomenon that arose exclusively during the early stages of gestation through an arrest or departure in the course of embryological development. The term appeared as an expansively fearsome symbol, sign, or portent; now, in the realm of medical science, the monster could be contained and seen for what it really was—its neutral and objective biological reality.[41] The elite nineteenth-century physician and author Oliver Wendell Holmes Sr. exclaimed that "people used always to be terribly frightened by those irregular vital products which we now call 'interesting specimens' and carefully preserve in jars of alcohol." Deriding the prescientific understandings of his predecessors in colonial America, he recounted how a seventeenth-century monstrous birth "was enough to scare the colonists from their propriety, and suggest the gravest fears of portended disaster." By contrast, for Holmes and his nineteenth-century peers, this kind of birth now constituted a specimen for "our Professor of Pathological Anatomy" to "imprison in one of his immortalizing jars of alcohol."[42] Embedded in a network of practitioners who claimed authority to define, administer, and contain such specimens, Holmes lauded the transformation of monstrosities from objects of superstition into objects of medical science.

A key part of this narrative was that in becoming a scientific object, the monster ceased to be a cultural one. Science, in asserting its mastery—"imprisoning" and "immortalizing"—effectively neutralized the fearsome cultural imaginary of the monstrous. To contain this "irregular vital product" was to strip it of its capacity to evoke "terrible fright," to remove the weight of its portentous signifiers. Medical science had quelled those "gravest fears of portended disaster," successfully turning cultural portent into scientific specimen. This narrative of scientific demystification persists unquestioned in much of the later scholarship on this history. These accounts present the emergence of scientific teratology as a pivotal moment in the "domestication of monstrosities," ushering in a new scientific worldview that supplanted and "defanged" the cultural and symbolic meanings of monstrous birth.[43]

As this book reveals, however, medical attention to "monstrosity" did not actually scrub the term of cultural signification. In fact, it did the opposite. Rendered as biological specimens, monstrosities remained freighted with social and political meanings—both through the retention of older meanings and through the active generation of new ones, produced within and specific to the shifting material, institutional, and knowledge-making practices of nineteenth- and early twentieth-century medical science. A scientific specimen of monstrosity was both product and producer of a distinct cultural epistemology of the body: a way of knowing that could confer differential value on human bodies, locate them within relational orders of species and kin, and construct their social legibility. By offering a biological developmental framework to address questions of bodily variation and human descent, the scientific study of monstrosity linked it powerfully to shifting scientific concepts of race as well as to aspirations toward the medical and scientific management of women's reproduction. In this new teratological discourse, monstrosity came to embody the production of racial difference, the danger of racial degeneration, and the volatility of women's procreative bodies, fusing cultural imaginaries of racial and reproductive deviance under the sign of disability.

For the historical actors discussed in this book, *race* could refer to both a broad designation of the entire species—the singular "human race"—and to the putatively natural distinctions between populations within the species, defined in relation to geographic region, ancestry, or phenotype. These multiple significations of race suggest the intimate relationship between historical logics of classifying animal kinds and of classifying human variation. In each case, "race" denoted a way to mark category differences between putatively separate kinds of beings. Across this period of US history, sundry and often contradictory concepts of human racial difference coexisted, from early nineteenth-century ideas about the climatic and environmental malleability of racial traits to the assorted notions of immutable biological difference that predominated later on.[44]

Abstract imaginaries of race affected historical lives, practices, and institutions in very concrete and real ways. Social and legal hierarchies of race conditioned access to medical care and the development of professional medical practice. They also shaped the production of medical-scientific knowledge—from providing an epistemology of human variation that guided how data were gathered and interpreted to establishing who could be recognized as a producer of authoritative knowledge and to rendering certain research methods imaginable and others unimaginable.[45] And just as racial inequality shaped the practices of medical science, practices of medical science shaped racial inequality. Histories of discriminatory public-health practices, medical abuse and neglect, and segregated health-care systems engendered distinctive lived experiences of racial injustice.[46] Further, medical and scientific practitioners played a central role in theorizing and circulating concepts of biological race, variously positing anatomical, physiological, developmental, evolutionary, biogeographical, or genetic bases for supposedly fixed racial categories.[47]

Concepts of biological race proved contradictory and ever changing in their particulars. Proponents disagreed on the number of racial groups, their characteristic features, their origins, and where the boundaries between them lay—questions that scientific experts and judicial court systems alike proved unable to adjudicate consistently. Medical-scientific sources from this period contain references to a dizzying array of different human "races," some of which roughly map onto racial categories used today and others that decidedly do not. Yet despite its patent failures of coherence, the idea of biological race remained powerful and durable in its political applications. Shifting, unstable, and contested schematics of race scaffolded nineteenth-century histories of slavery, segregation, settler colonialism, immigration, and the expansion of US imperialism overseas. American institutions invoked concepts of innate racial difference to structure and justify codified discrimination in systems of governance, citizenship, labor, education, housing, marriage, and the production and generational inheritance of wealth.[48]

In this period, reproductive medicine emerged as a prominent site where unstable concepts of race were mobilized and given form.[49] Anglo-American physicians advocated for increased medical intervention by invoking the allegedly greater suffering and difficulties of "civilized" upper-class white women in childbirth. At the same time, they exploited the supposedly insensate bodies of Black and immigrant women to develop procedures and train practitioners in the expanding fields of obstetrics and, later, gynecology. In teaching and professional practice, physicians theorized and grounded conceptions of racial and sexual difference in the anatomy and physiology of gendered reproductive bodies.[50]

Analyzing the medical engagement with monstrous birth illuminates how historical practices reflected, reproduced, and refigured discourses of race in tandem with discourses of sex and disability.[51] Teratological taxonomy ostensibly positioned monstrosity as a "race apart," existing in a separate and incommensurable classificatory universe from categories of human division. Monstrous offspring received their own genus, species, and subspecies designations, separate from and regardless of their parents' racial classification, and their sex was frequently assigned outside of a male/female binary. In these respects, monstrosity appeared able to overwrite or elide nineteenth-century categories of human race and sex.

Yet at the same time teratological monstrosity became densely enrolled in Anglo-American imaginaries of human difference. In this period, a pervasive discourse posited a hierarchical continuum of animal species and races, positioning human beings as the pinnacle of animal development and Western Europeans as the pinnacle of human racial development. This cast the "lower" human races as temporal dislocations: imperfect versions of humanity arrested in an earlier stage of developmental time, stuck in a "primitive" order of being characterized by closer proximity to bestial animal kinds.[52] Practitioners invoked a recapitulation of developmental timescales—the embryological development of the individual and later in the nineteenth century the explicitly Darwinian evolutionary development of the species—to cast a teratological condition of "arrested development" as a state of racial-biological regression, a slide back down the scale of racial and animal forms. Framing a sharply distinguished sex binary as an attainment of advanced racial evolution, practitioners presented the often sexually ambiguous body of the monster as further evidence of racial primitivism.[53]

In this way, medical-scientific discourse on monstrosity concretized an understanding of racial difference intimately linked to imaginaries of sex and disability. Practitioners invoked monstrosity to theorize a biological racial order that was developmental, hierarchical, temporalized, and fraught with reproductive danger. Monstrous birth became a warning about the vulnerability of racial inheritance and the liabilities of women's reproductive bodies, positioning pregnancy as a critical window in which racial heritage could be perfectly realized or radically degraded in the offspring's physical form. This interpretation of monstrosity grew increasingly charged in the later nineteenth century during a period of rising cultural anxieties about Anglo-American racial decline.[54] Cast as an extremity of racial-sexual degeneration, the figure of the monster suggested and affirmed a nascent biomedical imperative to intervene on reproduction for the protection of the racial order.

This imperative later animated the early twentieth-century American eugenics movement, a hugely influential political, popular, and scientific undertaking that called for "race improvement" through "better breeding."[55] As eugenicists redirected attention away from "major monstrosities" and toward subtler but far more common conditions of "hereditary defect," they simultaneously conferred monstrous meanings onto a far more sweeping range of variant human bodies. Leading eugenic scientists invoked concepts of teratological development to theorize the origins and nature of defect and racial difference, to conflate moral and biological deviance, and to specify a bodily developmental basis for constructs of social hierarchy. Moreover, some laypeople came to understand their own reproductive bodies in ways that reproduced the frameworks and significations of biological monstrosity.

CONCEPTIONS OF HUMAN DIFFERENCE

Monstrous Conceptions explores how multisited, multimodal practices of medical science linked and materialized concepts of race, sex, and disability in the body of the biological monster. *Race*, *sex*, and *disability* are complex and politically potent terms. At the time of this book's writing, all three appear on the "list of discouraged words" flagged by US federal agencies to limit or avoid.[56] Yet ongoing attempts to purge and suppress discussion of these terms only underscore the importance of more clearly and robustly understanding what they signify.

Feminist historians of health and medicine note both the centrality and the inextricable entwinement of race and sex/gender as concepts in emerging biomedical discourse.[57] Nineteenth-century practitioners used the word *sex* alone to signify a gendered division of both biological bodies and social roles into a binary of *man* and *woman*, anchored by invocations of imputed reproductive capacity. These conceptions of sex difference were heavily racialized as well as gendered, linking aspirational categories of "true" womanhood and manhood to ideals of middle- and upper-class Anglo-American whiteness.[58] Of note, although this book frequently refers to "women" or "laywomen" to indicate a gendered historical population of childbearing people, the category of *woman* in the nineteenth-century United States was messy, contested, and polysemous in ways that belied the construct of a simple binary of sex.

Race and *sex* in this book are both actors' categories—concepts and words used verbatim in the historical sources—and terms of analysis. Following scholars such as Dorothy Roberts, Evelynn Hammonds, and Nancy Stepan, this book understands *race* and *sex* as "political categories" that serve to naturalize arrangements of power through reference to the "givenness" of the physical order, legitimizing social hierarchies of difference through an invocation of nature and human biology.[59] In this function, race and sex operate in tandem with intersecting categories such as disability, which, in the words of the disability theorist Rosemarie Garland-Thomson, "legitimate a system of social, economic, and political empowerment" that is "justified by physiological differences."[60] This book considers race, sex/gender, and disability as categories of historical analysis and as mutually defining discourses that structured social relations of power, configured cultural difference, and grounded political hierarchy in renderings of biological embodiment.

The word *disability* rarely appears in historical medical sources on monstrosity. Although today the broadly inclusive term *congenital disabilities* can apply to most of the conditions formerly classified as monstrosities, nineteenth-century practitioners did not characterize differences of anatomical development in this way. They referred to "congenital malformations," "congenital anomalies," "congenital abnormities," "congenital aberrations," "congenital deformities," "congenital deviations," and "congenital defects"—but not to *congenital disabilities*.[61] When nineteenth-century sources used the word *disability,* it denoted an individual's incapacity to perform certain kinds of labor, especially military service, rather than their bodily morphology per se.[62]

In this context, a too-sweeping application of the term *disabled* to nineteenth-century individuals with variations of physical form, if done in an uncritical or unreflective manner, can risk essentializing and flattening the historical specificity of disability as a contingent rather than predetermined way of ordering and signifying bodily difference.[63] This book, then, does not use *disability* as an exact synonym for *monstrosity*, the historical actor's category. Instead, informed by scholarship in disability studies, it invokes disability as an analytic concept to refer to the social and cultural construction of "othered" embodiment.[64] Understood in this broader interpretive sense, *Monstrous Conceptions* contributes to a burgeoning literature that explores multifaceted intersections of disability with race and gender.[65]

On the surface, a focus on medical discourse might initially seem to sit uneasily with the concerns of disability studies. After all, a founding scholar of the field writes that disability studies is concerned with "cultural understandings of disability," positioned as fundamentally separate from and oppositional to "medical understandings of disability."[66] However, *Monstrous Conceptions* approaches medical understanding as itself a *form* of contingent cultural understanding. In doing so, it draws on a foundational precept of disability studies—that is, the understanding of disability as a contingent "cultural interpretation of human variation" rather than an inherent "property of bodies"—to analyze the modern medical configuration of monstrosity.[67] The medical and scientific practices that constructed the category of biological monstrosity were simultaneously social and cultural practices. They included interpersonal negotiations of knowledge making between medical practitioners and patients, affective relations of touch and caregiving, material routines of tissue preparation and display, and social and political theorizations of difference. Attention to these meaning-making practices highlights the multisited, multisensory, densely relational processes through which an experience of childbearing became legible as a medical case of monstrous birth and an infant body became legible as a scientific specimen of monstrosity.

Monstrous Conceptions focuses on biomedical discourse not because it represents the only or most important way of making sense of bodies but rather because it represents a complex historical development of critical social and cultural significance with urgent relevance to the present day. In the period covered by this book, biomedical discourse began to play an increasingly prominent role in explaining and adjudicating human difference, reproduction, and bodies, rendering them knowable and governable within particular social and political institutions.[68] By the mid–twentieth century, biomedical cosmologies of the body had become some of the most widely available frameworks through which not only experts but also many laypeople could interpret and make sense of their own bodies and reproductive experiences. Today, biomedical understandings of bodies and health continue to circulate far beyond the formal practice and pedagogy of professional medicine: They suffuse aspects of private self-understanding, popular public discourse, contemporary social movements, and even political claims to citizenship.[69] In this context, then, understanding how bodies were configured through biomedical discourse is not just about better understanding the ideas of physicians for their own sake—it is also important for understanding how a great number of people and communities have experienced and interpreted embodiment.

Recognizing this contingent historical entanglement of biomedical discourse with everyday lived experience, the books' chapters attend carefully to the ideas and embodied experiences of both laypeople and professional medical practitioners. *Monstrous Conceptions* is simultaneously a social history of women and childbirth, a material history of medical practice, an intellectual history of scientific knowledge production, and a cultural history of bodies and disability in the modern United States. It refuses an imposed dichotomy between the medical/scientific and the social/cultural as areas of historical inquiry, instead revealing medical meaning making as itself a dynamic social and cultural process that engaged multiple kinds of people, practices, sites, and sensorial registers.

By exploring medical understanding as a type of cultural understanding, this approach can also help to denaturalize and contest historically embedded frameworks of human difference that might otherwise present themselves as immutable or inevitable. Efforts to robustly understand and historicize biomedical discourses of disability, race, and sex play a vital role within larger projects of recognizing and challenging harmful legacies of these discourses and ultimately of opening up space to think beyond them.

SOURCES AND METHODS

This book engages a range of sources and methods to attend to varied historical experiences (both lay and professional) and to explore multisensory, multimodal dimensions of medical knowledge making. It draws on primary sources such as medical illustrations and photography; extant historical anatomical collections; organizational records of medical and scientific research institutions; textbooks and treatises in obstetrics, teratology, embryology, and eugenics; popular medical advice manuals and newspapers; and personal writing and correspondence by laywomen, physicians, and scientists. The book relies in largest part on a voluminous nineteenth- and early twentieth-century US medical case literature on monstrous birth, which comprises published reports in medical journals, medical museum catalogs and accession notes, transcripts of professional society presentations, and patient case records.

Although this medical case literature is abundant in quantity, it also presents notable challenges. Most conspicuously, it is reported heavily (though not exclusively) by male Anglo-American professionals, tending to conceal or elide the experiences and perspectives of childbearing women, families, and communities, especially non-Anglo-American ones. To work more richly and generatively with historical medical sources, I use creative readings informed by analytic frameworks from multiple fields of study, foregrounding what Carolyn Roberts calls the "integral, yet-underappreciated, role that imaginative labor represents in the craft of academic history."[70] Each chapter opens with one or more narrative vignettes focused on individual birth stories, with shorter vignettes woven throughout. These vignettes are imaginatively reconstructed from medical case reports and renarrated to center the lives and experiences of childbearing women. If part of producing monstrous specimens involved decontextualizing bodies from their social and familial worlds, then the method used here strives to make those contexts evident again.

To create these vignettes, I search for "fragmentary details" in the case histories that reflect or offer clues into patients' physical and sensory experiences, their kinship ties and networks of social relation, their subject positionality, the array of institutions and interpretive frameworks that scaffolded their daily worlds. Informed by the historian Marisa Fuentes's method for reading "along the bias grain," I contextualize and elaborate on these documented details in order to amplify the "spectral" presence of those excluded from more direct archival representation, while still remaining grounded in and taking care to "retain the historical integrity of the documents."[71] In addition to engaging methods developed by African American studies scholars such as Fuentes, this approach engages methods from feminist historians of medicine, who read physician-authored texts against the grain for insight into lay perspective and social relations of power. It also engages methods from disability studies scholars, who explore "alternate meanings" by narratively centering the "ghostly presences" that "haunt" the margins of texts.[72] These methods further direct attention to texts' revelatory absences and omissions, taking up Evelynn Hammonds's insight that hidden presences may be detected in the "distorting and productive effects" that they create on surrounding fields.[73]

I also employ interdisciplinary methods to explore the making of monstrous bodies across multiple sensory, affective, and symbolic registers. *Monstrous Conceptions* seeks to understand how material aspects of bodily phenomena are semiotically configured and, reciprocally, how meaning is materialized through configurations of embodiment. In other words, it explores both how bodies are made into meanings and how meanings are made into bodies. It traces how biological events and attributes are constituted through the sensory interfaces, affective relations, physical practices, social institutions, political economies, and interpretive frameworks that together structure the perception and experience of day-to-day living. It also examines how, in a related process, abstracted concepts of difference and relations of power take form in the anatomized human body. This conceptual framing draws on multidisciplinary scholarship that theorizes the meaning and materiality of bodies as mutually constituted and that elaborates the social and experiential dimensions of knowledge creation.[74]

To center the multimodal materialization of monstrous bodies in nineteenth-century medical science, I attend closely and creatively to the ways in which emotional, sensory, and embodied practices and experiences are described or implied in sources: the semantic clusters used to characterize maternal feelings, the conventions of sensory reveal in the dramaturgy of the case narrative, the contrasting modes of touch in settings of postpartum care, the olfactory terrains of the dissecting room, the postural arrangements of monstrous bodies in artistic representation, the visualization of category relations in taxonomic charts. Drawing on theorizations of affect from queer, feminist, and disability studies scholarship, I consider how embodied interactions and emotions worked to locate individual subjects within frameworks of social difference and relation.[75]

STRUCTURE OF THE BOOK

Using these varied sources and methods, *Monstrous Conceptions* charts the multisited transformation of newborn bodies into medical specimens of monstrosity. The chapters are organized to follow this trajectory, revealing how nineteenth-century medical practices configured bodies as monstrous across successive and overlapping domains: experiences of pregnancy, childbearing, and postpartum care; the material preparation, institutional collection, and visual representation of bodies as specimens; and the conceptual classification and theorization of monstrosity in the medical and scientific press. Together, the chapters show how these multiple practices reflected, negotiated, and merged shifting conceptions of racial, reproductive, and bodily defect in the nineteenth-century United States, laying groundwork for the ascendant eugenic discourses of the early twentieth century.

The book's first four chapters examine the affective and material configuration of monsters in nineteenth-century medical science, exploring how an array of practices gave form to the embodied category of monstrosity. Chapter 1 analyzes how narratives of diverse women's pregnancies located the genesis of monstrosity in disruptions of social, racial, and human–animal orders. Chapter 2 focuses on the postpartum period, showing how physicians and family members affectively configured the ambivalent subjecthood and alienated kinship of the monster through emotional and physical interactions with living but "nonviable" infants. Chapter 3 reveals how the production and circulation of anatomical specimens engaged a multisensory process of making monsters visible on both material and symbolic levels, which positioned them as a form of biological information that only the authoritative eyes of a (white, male) professional could read. Chapter 4 considers the representation of monsters in medical illustrations and photographs, showing how these images alternately visualized the familiarity and alterity of newborn bodies by locating or displacing them within signified orders of familial, racial, and species kinds.

The book's final two chapters explore the conceptual configuration of monstrosity, examining the theorization and classification of monstrous bodies within nineteenth- and early twentieth-century fields of obstetrics, embryology/teratology, and eugenics. Chapter 5 analyzes how the production and circulation of teratological knowledge in the medical press drew on and refigured unstable nineteenth-century discourses of race, sex, and disability. American physicians engaged teratological monstrosity to theorize and navigate the contradictions of shifting racial imaginaries, grounding constructions of racial-sexual order in conceptions of disability and women's reproductive bodies. Finally, chapter 6 traces the uptake and eugenic afterlives of medical monstrosity in the early twentieth-century United States. Even as the locus of scientific interest in this era shifted toward the subtler "hereditary defects" of greatest interest to US eugenicists, the logics and significations of biomedical monstrosity continued to haunt American imaginaries of racial, reproductive, and embodied human difference.

CHAPTER ONE

Monstrous Pregnancies

Women's Narratives and Medical Knowledge Making

1834: BOSTON, MASSACHUSETTS

The pregnancy, as the woman would later recall it, was a strange one. It would be impossible, of course, to untangle her memories of this period—recorded only in retrospect—from her knowledge of its "monstrous" culmination. But, as transcribed by the prominent Boston physician Charles Hildreth in an 1834 case report, the woman's sense of unease began long before the night of her disquieting delivery.[1]

Though Hildreth attributed to her a "delicate frame" and a "very excitable temperament," the woman's prior experience with pregnancy and childbearing gave her reason for nothing but confidence. She had two sons, two and four years old, at the time of this third pregnancy, both of them "stout" and in good health. She had never experienced an infant death, a stillbirth, or, to her knowledge, a miscarriage—a notable circumstance for a married thirty-five-year-old woman in early nineteenth-century New England. She and her family were longtime private patients of Hildreth, suggesting, along with other details of the case history, that they belonged to a social class of wealthy, white, Anglo-American Protestants in Boston. She could expect to receive attentive care from her doctor and his assistants as well as from a robust cadre of relatives, friends, neighbors, and attendants.[2]

Yet this third pregnancy had been marked by uneasy experiences that, in light of the delivery, now seemed to assume a certain premonitory significance. Throughout the pregnancy, she had cared for an aged relative who was confined to a second-story chamber of the house. Over the strenuous objections of her friends, she would often bring her younger son with her, balancing the robust two-year-old child on her growing belly as she climbed up and down the stairs. Then, several months before her delivery, while riding back to town after an outing with her husband, their horse took a fright and began to run away with them. Though they managed to stop and calm the agitated animal, she remembered experiencing a brief but marked surge of fear.[3] She had thought little of these incidents at the time, but now, after the birth, she felt compelled to recount them—perhaps at the doctor's urging but relayed nonetheless in clear and granular detail. These kinds of remembrances held particular significance during an era of widespread belief in "maternal impression": the concept that a woman's thoughts, feelings, and experiences during pregnancy could physically imprint themselves upon her developing offspring.[4]

In this instance, the woman did not give any indication that she assigned causality in retrospect to any particular incident during her pregnancy. Yet she could not deny that this period had been a discomfiting one, filled with strange sensations and pains that appeared to her to establish a vague aura of menace around her pregnancy—a nebulous sense of foreboding that seemed to seep into the edges of her thought. At no point, she said, did she explicitly suspect a malformation, yet she did describe a despondent premonition that the child would be a sickly one, destined to "die young."[5]

The quality of the fetal movement concerned her the most. There was a delay in feeling the first "decided motion" of the child in her womb—by her attentive calculations, this moment of quickening came fully five months into the pregnancy, later than she had expected. She felt some anxiousness at this, which soon turned to alarm at "the infrequency and imperfection, or rather singularity of the child's motions." She felt them only once or twice a week, and she found the internal sensation odd and unsettling. Unlike the sensation of her previous children's "rigorous movements in utero," this one felt "more as if it fell, or impinged on some intervening substance between the child and the uterus, than as if it moved its limbs or body." When she touched her distended belly from the outside, something also seemed amiss: Her belly felt tense and uniformly rigid under her hand, with no suggestive gradations "either of surface or solidity" to suggest the shape of the fetus within.[6]

Toward the end of the seventh month, her uneasy experience intensified into acute misery. Her belly swelled to nearly double in size quite suddenly, overwhelming her with discomfort and pain. After rising one night in this state to attend to her youngest child, who had taken ill, she described "a very remarkable subsidence" of the mass in her womb; she told Hildreth that she "felt the child fall." This sudden descent was marked by wracking spasms of pain that coursed through her left hip, suffusing the tense joining where her hipbone connected to the base of her spine and persisting in acute form for nearly a week. She received a variety of medical treatments intended to relax this spasmed state, mainly by effecting the release of bodily fluids, which included bloodletting, blistering, laxatives, and enemas.[7] Nineteenth-century patients did often find subjective relief from such measures; for both patients and physicians, they made sense in the context of a shared cosmology of health that centered flow and equilibrium and conceptualized healing as a restoration of the body's balance of fluid exchange with its environment.[8]

In this case, however, comfort proved elusive: The woman remained tense and wracked with nausea, her flesh tender to the touch, her pulse racing. The intensity of her discomfort eventually diminished but did not resolve. Two weeks before the delivery, she finally got some respite in the form of a tremendous discharge of water, which ran "in a broad stream across the floor from her chair, a large cushion on which she sat," overflowing the floor "to the amount of half a pailful" and leaving her clothes "completely drenched." She experienced an enormous feeling of relief after this immense release of fluid, grateful to be "relieved from the load which had oppressed her." It left her feeling "more light and comfortable than for a long time before," and for the first time in a while she was "rather disposed to be cheerful." The fetal motion remained weak and infrequent but could still be felt every day or two leading up to the birth. The labor began in the dead of night; two female friends came immediately to attend her, and Hildreth was summoned from a mile away.[9]

Calling a male physician to a birthing room in the early nineteenth century was unusual but certainly not unheard of. Across the course of the nineteenth century, the United States underwent a massive transition in the customary conventions of childbirth, from an earlier model of "social childbirth"—typically a home event attended by female relatives, friends, neighbors, and lay midwives—to one increasingly conceptualized and administered in medical terms. Although most nineteenth-century women continued to give birth in homes rather than in hospitals, it became more and more common for them to employ professional male physicians as childbirth attendants, usually as an addition to rather than a replacement for female midwives, relations, and friends. In the early nineteenth century, those who did so were most often wealthy Anglo-American women in the densely populated cities of the Northeast, who paid physicians such as Hildreth to attend them in their own homes.[10]

Nineteenth-century physicians claimed that upper-class white women were in special need of medical aid to make it through the ordeals of childbirth, thus amplifying a pervasive nineteenth-century theory that the "excesses and artifices of civilization" rendered these women fragile, nervous, and overly sensitive to pain.[11] In this period, when affluent urban women might choose between multiple kinds of birth attendants, Hildreth and other physicians advertised a distinct set of therapeutics and instruments that most other attendants did not use, initially including interventions such as opium and bloodletting. Later in the century, physicians employed anesthetic technologies, such as chloroform and ether, as well as obstetric instruments, including the forceps.[12]

In this case, though Hildreth was summoned to the birth, he arrived too late to attend the actual delivery. Initially, all had seemed to go well. The woman described "the conscious happiness she experienced on the birth of the child": She perceived a "sensation at that moment as if [the infant] were moving its arms and body in endeavoring to crawl" and rejoiced to know her child lived. But this happiness turned out to be bitterly fleeting. The child was born *en caul*, still encased in the amniotic membranes, and appeared to have suffocated by the time Hildreth arrived some half an hour after the birth. Hildreth thought there might still be a chance of resuscitation; however, upon clearly viewing the infant for the first time, he summarily abandoned this idea.[13]

Drawing on the new transatlantic field of teratology, recently defined as the "modern scientific study of monstrosity," Hildreth classified the child as a "case of *notencephale*": a major anomaly of fetal head development in which the cranial vault remains open and the brain forms outside the skull. "Upon discovering the monstrosity," Hildreth wrote, "we concluded not to attempt the inflation of the lungs." He and his assistants instead turned their attention to extracting the placenta through manual techniques and the administration of ergot. A commissioned medical illustration suggests that at some point the newborn's body was cleaned and carefully nestled on a pile of bedding. Hildreth and others attended the woman for two weeks after the birth, at one point providing ample opium to relieve a migrainelike headache, before she was "discharged cured."[14]

Hildreth went on to document the case in an extended published report, accompanied by a colored drawing, a lithographic print, and several commissioned engravings depicting the infant. He enlisted the help of his eminent colleagues John Barnard Swett Jackson, later dean of Harvard Medical School, and Walter Channing, Harvard's first professor of obstetrics and a founder of the Boston Lying-In Hospital, to dissect the infant's body. The physicians produced multiple anatomical specimens: a "dry" preparation of the skeleton as well as "wet" preparations of the kidneys and renal capsules suspended in preservative fluid, which they added to the Monstrosities Division of the Boston Society for Medical Improvement's Anatomical Cabinet.[15] A Boston medical journal reprinted Hildreth's report, and the case was cited in the second volume of the French scientist Isidore Geoffroy Saint-Hilaire's seminal treatises on teratology.[16]

The study and collection of "monstrous births"—infants born with major and usually fatal congenital conditions such as anencephaly—were widespread in nineteenth-century American medical practice. Drawing on the tenets of scientific teratology, physicians transformed anomalous newborn bodies into anatomical specimens, presented them before medical and scientific societies, published on them in the burgeoning American medical press, and added them to the collections of medical schools and museums.[17]

Many of the "monstrous specimens" produced and circulated through nineteenth-century medical practices were birthed by women like Hildreth's patient. The contingent history of US physicians' involvement in childbearing tended to facilitate collection of infant bodies birthed by white, Protestant, US-born women, who were far likelier in the nineteenth century to be attended by professional physicians during childbearing. However, several distinct nineteenth-century institutions also facilitated interactions between physicians and childbearing women in far more socially and economically vulnerable positions, forming conduits by which their "monstrous births" might also be exposed to medical attention. Within these institutions, socially marginalized women were frequently exploited as sources of "experimental 'material'" and clinical training experience for students and practitioners in the expanding professional fields of obstetrics and, later, gynecology. In populous cities, women who did not have the social and material resources to give birth at home—often impoverished and unmarried women or immigrants without local family ties—might give birth in maternity wards, dispensaries, and "lying-in hospitals" designed to serve the poor and friendless.[18] In the antebellum South, physicians also encountered and exercised authority over childbearing women within the institution of racial slavery—as occurred in another account of "monstrous" birth published in the medical press just a few years after Hildreth's report.[19]

1837: SAVANNAH, GEORGIA

By the time she was around thirty, the enslaved Black woman in Savannah, Georgia, had given birth eight times before—never, it was reported to the doctors, with any significant trouble. This time initially seemed to her no different. The gestation had been "nothing peculiar." Indeed, the woman had felt her child move "sensibly" inside the womb up until the birth. Labor began slightly early, in the eighth month; however, she remembered that two of her older children had also been born before full term, and at first nothing seemed awry with the delivery. The attendants noticed a greater quantity of amniotic fluid than expected, but "nothing to lead to a suspicion of anything unusual"—that is, until the stillborn child was "fairly exposed to the light." To someone familiar with the condition, the infant showed a classical presentation of anencephaly: the round, prominent eyes atop the upturned face; the steeply angled crown, sloping back from the brow ridge in the absence of a cranial vault; broad, low-set ears projecting out to the sides; and an open lesion at the back of the head, where the scalp had never formed or closed.[20]

Unlike Hildreth's upper-class Anglo-American patient, whose matronly "respectability" was emphasized against any judgments that might arise from the appearance of her offspring, the birth of this child immediately raised suspicions. Were the missing skull and scalp evidence of violent mutilation? Was the open lesion at the back of the head an inflicted wound? Unspecified birth attendants eventually summoned local physicians Alexander Nicoll and Richard Arnold to render a professional medical judgment on "whether violence had been used or not, which in consequence of the singular appearance [the child] presented, was supposed by those who attended at the delivery."[21] An incident rendered as personal tragedy in the case of Hildreth's patient was readily interpreted here as grounds for probable wrongdoing. Nicoll and Arnold encountered the mother not as a patient to be treated but as a potential criminal to be investigated.[22]

The woman's treatment was contextualized most immediately by the imperatives of racial slavery, an institution sustained by the violent requisition of Black women's reproductive labor for white men's financial gain. Within the brutal racial, sexual, and capitalist logics of this system, an enslaved woman's failure to produce a live, healthy child constituted a direct economic affront to the man who claimed her as property, preventing him from "realizing a profit on the birth" by increasing the amount of capital he owned.[23]

This was not the only systemic aspect of slavery that conditioned the ease and rapidity with which an enslaved Black mother was accused of killing her child. On the level of moral imaginary, the tenability of racial slavery rested on the vicious fiction that enslaved mothers birthed and reared offspring without forming bonds of kinship with them—the forced reproduction of what the scholar Hortense Spillers terms "kinlessness."[24] Finally, in addition to their economic dependance on Black women's childbearing and their moral dependence on the negation of Black kinship bonds, white plantation authorities were eager to displace blame for enormously high infant-mortality rates onto enslaved women rather than themselves.[25] In cases of infant death, then, they were quick to condemn Black mothers.

In this instance, however, the physicians dismissed the accusations after they immediately recognized the distinctive visual signs of anencephaly. Nicoll and Arnold concluded that "no violence had been used to destroy the child, but that it was a monster of an interesting character."[26] It is striking to reflect on what it might mean for a woman to give birth to a "monster" within an institution already predicated on the forms of familiar, often sexual violence that the scholar Christina Sharpe calls "monstrous intimacies."[27] A decade before this birth, the Virginia Supreme Court had named the very condition of being born enslaved as legally "monstrous," though it limited this condemnation to the prospect of an enslaved child born to an emancipated mother: "A *free* mother cannot have children who are *slaves.* Such a birth would be monstrous both in the eye of reason and of law," the court declared.[28]

Any deeper connections between monstrous birth and enslavement, however, went unaddressed in Nicoll and Arnold's 1837 report. Though the broader clinical literature on monstrosity brimmed with discussion of prenatal maternal experience, Nicoll and Arnold did not offer any explicit details about the enslaved mother's conditions of life during pregnancy. They instead reported tersely that "the history of the mother affords no clue" as to causality, deeming her not salient to the field of inquiry—a notable departure from the comparatively extensive details of prenatal events, emotions, and internal sensations documented in Hildreth's report.[29] This omission may have reflected Nicoll and Arnold's disinterest in or inability to contemplate the experiences and complex interior world of an enslaved Black woman, perhaps influenced by a pervasive nineteenth-century discourse that cast racially marginalized bodies as "insensate" and unfeeling, lacking refined capacities to process and be affected by emotional and sensory impressions.[30] It also seems likely that the woman's position of extreme vulnerability throughout this encounter and her awareness of the explicit power these white physicians held over her life left her distinctly disinclined to share intimate information about her embodied, social, and affective worlds in the kind of granular detail that Hildreth's patient provided.

Later, Nicoll and Arnold worked with a colleague from New York to dissect the infant's body and present their findings to the Medical

Society of Georgia, one of the earliest professional medical societies in the United States. The two physicians published a case report in the *Southern Medical and Surgical Journal*, which was later reprinted in the *American Journal of the Medical Sciences* and the British medical journal the *Lancet*.[31] Beyond noting that the woman was cleared of the suspected infanticide, the physicians recorded no further details about her health, experience, or life following the delivery.

These two birthing stories are gleaned and interpretively reconstructed from a nineteenth-century medical archive authored primarily by white male practitioners. By imaginatively renarrating these reports to center the lives and experiences of the childbearing women, these vignettes as told here push against the decontextualization and abstraction from kinship that abetted the transformation of infant remains into standardized specimens of monstrosity. To become scientific specimens, newborn bodies were processed and stored in ways that obscured the varied social and relational worlds of their development and birth. Their prepared bodies were sealed in clear glass jars and cotton-lined cases, numbered as museum accessions, and made to stand in as generic referents of a monstrous "type," removing them both physically and conceptually from the sites of their familial origins.

For elite American physicians—a group composed overwhelmingly of white Protestant men in this period—the medical engagement with monstrosity underscored the rising authority of modern scientific medicine. In published rhetoric and portrayals, physicians presented themselves as the sole producers and authorizers of knowledge about bodies, reproduction, and human variation: men of science who calmly dispelled the vulgar ignorance of the laity, transforming a portent of "gravest fears," as the prominent physician and writer Oliver Wendell Holmes Sr. put it, into a specimen for an anatomy professor "to imprison in one of his immortalizing jars of alcohol."[32]

However, deeper attention to nineteenth-century case reports exposes a dynamic negotiation of knowledge making that was at once more collaborative and more contested than these self-fashioned images of singular scientific authority would suggest. By closely reading case reports to locate and expand on fragmentary details about childbearing women's experiences, this chapter situates the significance of diverse laywomen's social, affective, and embodied lives in historical processes of medical meaning making. It illuminates childbearing women's multifaceted involvement in medical knowledge production surrounding monstrosity—even while showing how the terms of their involvement were conditioned by hierarchies of gender, race, class, citizenship, and other social relations of difference. At the same time, the chapter offers insight into how predominantly white male practitioners increasingly sought to assert and consolidate authority over childbearing women's bodies over the course of the nineteenth century.

The chapter considers the roles and participation of a wide array of nineteenth-century women in the medical investigation of monstrosity, showing how they produced knowledge about the causes and meanings of anomalous births within gendered and racialized social imaginaries. This period's widely shared framework of "maternal impression" attributed anomalous births to mothers' experiences or emotions during pregnancy, establishing the relevance of women's subjective sensations, observations, and ideas to the medical study of monstrosity. By sharing their narratives of pregnancy, women participated not only in determining the proximate causes of anomalous birth but also in configuring and conveying the broader meanings of monstrous difference. Recurrent narrative themes and motifs variously situated the genesis of monstrosity in troubled contacts between humans and animals, in encounters with racial alterity, and in the upheavals of industrializing urban life in the mid-nineteenth-century United States. Distinctions of race, class, region, and familial status conditioned but did not foreclose this involvement in medical meaning making.

Yet even as some women used the theory of maternal impression to derive sense and meaning from an otherwise inexplicable experience, the framework could also be mobilized to deploy blame and assert medical authority over pregnant women's bodies and behavior. The chapter concludes by considering how late nineteenth-century trends, including the increasing ascription of anomalous birth to a mother's constitutional or hereditary pathology, further constrained childbearing women's participation in processes of medical knowledge production.

WOMEN'S KNOWLEDGE MAKING AND THE QUESTION OF CAUSALITY

Physicians such as Hildreth, Nicoll, and Arnold sought to establish their authority over the knowledge of monstrous birth at a time when physicians' authority over childbearing was neither self-evident nor secured. Physicians attended around a fifth of births in the United States at the start of the nineteenth century and around half of US births at the century's close, though the latter fraction remained significantly lower among many working-class, immigrant, Black, and Indigenous communities.[33] Few of these physician-attended births took place in hospitals and medical institutions, locations where physicians could expect to exercise a far more unilateral form of authority. Instead, for the nineteenth-century women who paid physicians to attend them in their homes, inviting an obstetric practitioner into the birthing room generally did not mean relinquishing control to him; a physician was usually one among a larger group of attendants, which often included a midwife, female relatives and female friends, and older women from the community. This female-dominated set of attendants and the birthing woman herself negotiated with the physician about interventions and interpretations rather than automatically deferring to his obstetric expertise.[34] While physicians took formal credit for the knowledge published in medical case histories of births, the embodied processes that produced this knowledge engaged these multiple kinds of actors.

To analyze these interactive processes of knowledge making, this chapter draws evidence from a review of several hundred case reports on the birth of "monsters," which appeared in national and local medical journals, medical museum catalogs, and medical society reports from at least thirty-five US states. These reports involved childbearing women from heterogeneous racial, ethnic, and socioeconomic backgrounds, including many private obstetric patients of physicians (usually white, Protestant, US-born, middle or upper class, and married) as well as childbearing Black, immigrant, working-class, and unmarried women. In age, the women ranged from their teens to their midforties.[35]

The negotiations of authority and knowledge making embedded in these case histories were shaped not just by hierarchies of gender but also by intersecting contexts of class, race, region, kinship configurations, and legal subjecthood. As the vignettes at the start of the chapter showed, such contexts could differentially shape the care a woman received, her relationship to the physician, and the way she was located more broadly in relation to the developing field of reproductive medicine. These contexts also conditioned the terms of women's participation in the formal medical narration and interpretation of monstrosity. In general, married, upper-class, Anglo-American patients—especially those with long-standing relationships to their attending physicians, like Hildreth's patient—were likeliest to be quoted at length in the case histories, and their knowledge claims about pregnancy and birth were likeliest to be explicitly treated as authoritative. By contrast, recorded contributions from women in more marginalized social positions, such as the enslaved woman in Georgia, were often comparatively minimal in scope. In this way, the attribution of epistemological authority, even in this already circumscribed capacity, was markedly racialized and classed as well as gendered.

However, a careful and attentive reading of the case histories illuminates how women from a variety of racial and class positions participated in medical knowledge making. For instance, reports frequently acknowledged diverse women's capacities of observational and quantitative knowledge making in matters such as assessment of gestational age, which was directly calculated by the pregnant woman, and the timing and qualia of sensations of movement in utero. This information contributed to a variety of medical knowledge-making projects, including debates over what monstrosity revealed about the function and development of the nervous system. Further, the interoceptive alterity of "monstrous" fetal movement functioned as one way for medical case reports to characterize and communicate the nature of monstrous difference.

Women provided granular observations of internally perceived fetal motions: One woman described "an intermittent, spasmodic and strange jerking movement, increased or prolonged by exercise or by jarring"; another "perceived most violent motion of the child" that felt as if it might rend her body from within.[36] In other cases, the fetal motions "were always feeble and peculiar"; one woman "felt feeble, and rather indistinct motions of the foetus, much lower in the uterus than usual, and she complained of great weight in the womb." Making clear the value attributed to such knowledge, one physician explicitly identified the "chief interest" of his report as consisting of the information it provided about "the difference of the kind of movement experienced" during a monstrous gestation.[37] This knowledge was necessarily produced and contributed by childbearing women, the only direct observers of their own internal sensations during pregnancy. Women also explicitly interpreted the observational knowledge they produced: One physician recorded that a woman was able to "foretell" the condition of her offspring based on the "unusual and anomalous symptoms" she experienced during pregnancy.[38]

A few physician-authored case histories also specifically credited female lay attendants or relatives as producers of authoritative knowledge. In an 1838 case involving the birth of twins, one born without any organs of the upper body, the elite Boston physician J. B. S. Jackson recorded the observations of a patient's mother, who "took charge" of her daughter's placenta after the delivery. The woman, he wrote, "observed that [the placenta] was small and divided into two portions; this last circumstance was noticed, as she herself once had twins, when, as she remembers, the after-birth formed one continuous mass." Noting that this woman "has frequently been with women during labour, and knows the appearance of a placenta," Jackson opined that her statement "certainly seems to deserve some credit," adding that her contributed knowledge, "if true," revealed that "the circulation of the blood must have been carried on by the vessels alone."[39] Drawing on her critical observational skills and experience, this laywoman produced the type of empirical knowledge—derived from and verified through direct observation—that elite American physicians such as Jackson claimed in this period as the foundation of scientific medicine.[40]

Childbearing women's participation in medical knowledge making notably extended into one of the foundational questions of scientific teratology: determining the cause of monstrosity. This question deeply concerned and motivated both physicians and laywomen, for both divergent and overlapping reasons. For physicians, understanding the cause of monstrosity was part of a larger project of asserting their scientific authority over the interpretation and management of human bodies. More concretely, the study and collection of teratological specimens could be a pathway for professional advancement and recognition: Presenting a teratological specimen offered an individual physician an opportunity for national or even international publication, and submitting specimens to prominent medical collections promised to "provide for the perpetuation of his name as that of a physician interested in the progress of the profession." Curators framed museum collections with robust holdings of monstrous specimens as points of pride for prominent medical schools or even for the "national prestige" of American medicine as a whole.[41]

The study of monstrosity held particular value within the growing subfield of obstetrics, where it helped establish the scientific legitimacy of obstetric education by linking it to the (largely Europe-based at this point) laboratory sciences of experimental embryology and teratology.[42] In the later nineteenth century, medical interest in monstrosity overlapped with rising ambitions toward the scientific management of pregnancy and motherhood.[43] The medical investigation of monstrosity was situated within an increasing assertion of reproduction as a proper area of interest and intervention for medical practitioners, aligned with emerging aspirations to establish the prenatal period as an object of medical supervision and regulation.[44]

Yet across the course of the nineteenth century, physicians remained acutely aware of a critical limitation when it came to their authority over monstrosity. Although they could confidently explain the genesis of monstrosity in an arrest or deviation of embryological development, they still could not explain what caused these deviations to occur and, relatedly, could offer no way to prevent them. The physician John Barry lamented in 1894 that "the etiology of monstrosities is as vague as ever, and medical pride bows in abject submission when confronted with the task of averting the misfortune, or even comforting the pangs of sorrow and distress incident upon a monstrous conception."[45]

Leading nineteenth-century physicians publicly sought to cultivate an image of aloof neutrality for the profession, contrasting their impartial scientific regard with the public's "emotional" reactions to monstrous births.[46] But individual case reports suggest a clear affective component to physicians' interest in resolving the question of monstrosity's cause: Physicians described feeling unsettled, fearful, horrified, repulsed, and "shocked, as well as astonished" by the material realities of monstrous birth, particularly by aspects that appeared to them "unnatural" or beyond explanation.[47] The elusive ability to explain the etiology of monstrosity (and, perhaps, to advise on its prevention) could appeal to physicians as a way to soothe not only their patients' emotions but also their own.

Though childbearing laywomen did not have the same opportunities as elite physicians to directly describe their interest in knowing more about monstrosity, many of them also appeared highly driven to understand the cause of their offspring's condition. A close and attentive reading of case histories yields a portrait of women as motivated and engaged participants in determining the origin of monstrosity: offering their own causal theories, expressing doubts and uncertainties, sharing and seeking knowledge that could help them interpret and make sense of an unexpected and often deeply troubling experience. For such women, the stakes of this search were singularly heightened. They intimately experienced the impact of monstrous birth on their own bodies and health, on their hopes and aspirations for a projected future, and on their role and relational standing in their respective social and familial worlds.

While a woman could draw on a variety of nineteenth-century religious, popular, and legal discourses to try to make sense of her monstrous birth, existing schematics of interpretation could sometimes be inadequate to fully reconcile her particular embodied experience, to fully satisfy her and her loved ones' desire to understand what had happened and why and what they were to make of it in the context of their own lives and relations. If so, an encounter with a medical practitioner who also aspired to know more about monstrosity could represent an opportunity to collaborate in a shared search for deeper context, meaning, and understanding—even as the premises, goals, and conclusions of that search did not always align among the participants.[48] The case histories reveal women's extensive involvement in attempts to determine the origins of monstrosity and show how physicians routinely acknowledged women's shared epistemological authority in this matter. Cases regularly detailed the "cause assigned by the mother."[49] Even in instances where the woman declined to provide a theory, case histories noted that her input had been solicited—inclusions that implicitly recognized the salience of women's information and ideas regarding questions of causality.

Recognizing this engaged, interpersonal dynamic complicates traditional narratives of this history, which portray lay and medical explanations of monstrosity as opposed forces and depict nineteenth-century medical experts sweeping in to replace women's folk beliefs in "maternal impression" with an improved scientific understanding of monstrosity's embryological origins.[50] On the evidence of hundreds of case histories published throughout the nineteenth century, though, "maternal impression" frequently served as a shared belief system for both physicians and childbearing women. Certainly, some physicians as well as some laywomen rejected the notion that a mother's mental and sensory experiences during pregnancy could shape the form of her developing offspring. But at midcentury the idea garnered support within even the most elite American medical circles, defended by leading Harvard physicians such as J. B. S. Jackson and David Humphreys Storer. In 1889, a Philadelphia physician described belief in maternal impressions as "almost universal with the laity" and "also shared to a large extent by the members of our own profession," while a Chicago physician in 1896 likewise identified a widespread belief in maternal impressions among American physicians.[51]

Indeed, many nineteenth-century physicians found the framework of maternal impression to be perfectly compatible with newer embryological explanations of monstrosity. Although scientific consensus now attributed monstrosity to arrests or deviations in embryological development, it remained to be determined what mechanism produced these arrests and deviations—and, here, experts entertained maternal impression as readily as any of the other major candidates (which included mechanical accidents, nutritional deficiencies, embryological disease, and hereditary pathology of the parental "germ"). Physicians seamlessly integrated theories of maternal influence within embryological frameworks of monstrous production, even proposing specific physiological mechanisms by which strong maternal emotions could materially disrupt development at critical points in the trajectory of gestation. One suggested that anencephaly could arise when a woman's experience of intense emotional shock early in pregnancy elicited a physiological impulse "to contract and gather" the uterine walls, inadvertently damaging crucial cells "at the superior pole of the developing embryo."[52]

Embraced by large numbers of nineteenth-century physicians and laypeople alike, the shared explanatory framework of maternal impression particularly facilitated the involvement of laywomen in the production of knowledge about monstrosity's etiology, establishing the relevance of mothers' subjective experiences, observations, and thoughts. Even physicians who doubted the reality of maternal impression often felt compelled to gather information about accidents and experiences that generated intense subjective sensation during the early stages of pregnancy. In some cases, physicians reported soliciting this information directly, urging their patients to recall any experiences that had elicited feelings of fear, shock, disgust, or grief.[53] In other cases, physicians recorded recollections that women offered unsolicited. Either way, the medical reporting of monstrous births became an occasion for gathering and recording information both about childbearing women's theories of monstrous production and about their subjective experiences and moments of deepest emotional significance during pregnancy.

Because childbearing women were best positioned to observe events and sensations during their pregnancies, they were recognized to have access to privileged forms of relevant knowledge. Some case reports indicated that a woman's knowledge of her offspring's condition preceded anyone else's, confirmed when she gazed for the first time on a "monstrous" infant whose exact condition she had known to expect before delivery. Following a birth in 1841, "after a few moments of recovery, the mother wished to know if it was a perfect child, for, said she, 'I did not expect it would be.'" Asked to elaborate, she explained, "'I thought there would be something the matter with its head, for I dressed the head of a calf last June, and when I took the axe to cut it open, I felt dreadfully, and thought I should faint or die for the next two or three hours.'"[54]

As in other matters, hierarchies of race, class, and social position shaped the way physicians solicited and recorded women's narratives of maternal impression; they influenced which women were more readily imagined as creditable reporters of subjective experience or were even imagined to be possessed of a complex subjective interiority at all. In a suggestive pair of cases, a South Carolina physician, Dr. A. A. Moore, published two reports of monstrous birth, one involving a woman described as "blonde" and the other involving a woman described as "colored." In the first case, Moore asked the patient to recount any memorable emotions or experiences during pregnancy; in the second, he did not.[55] Historians have argued that nineteenth-century physicians associated the phenomenon of maternal impression "almost exclusively" with white women, revealing "a racialized attempt to understand and explain disability among newborns."[56] Indeed, across nineteenth-century case literature, especially detailed descriptions of maternal-impression events usually involved white women—and often, more specifically, white upper-class Anglo-American women. Prevailing nineteenth-century medical discourse attributed to these women a heightened emotional and physiological sensitivity, positioning them as uniquely capacitated to receive and be affected by mental and sensory impressions.[57]

But, notably, an in-depth reading of the case literature shows that US physicians also solicited and recorded information on maternal impressions from racially and economically marginalized women, including numerous women of African descent.[58] In a few rare cases, nineteenth-century physicians even speculated on how conditions of marginality might systematically expose women to distressing experiences during pregnancy. For instance, a Wisconsin physician testified that the "nervous shock caused by her arrest and incarceration" could leave a woman in jail "liable to give birth to a monstrosity," while a New York physician cited a woman's reported "great privations" and "condition of poverty" during pregnancy as possibly relevant factors.[59] While maternal status differentially shaped some aspects of conversations about causality, narratives of maternal impression implicated the lives of women across a wide array of social and racial backgrounds.

WOMEN'S NARRATIVES AND THE MEANINGS OF MONSTROUS BIRTH

The narratives of pregnancy recorded in these case histories reflect women's participation not only in determining proximate causes of anomalous birth but also in configuring and conveying the broader meanings of monstrosity in nineteenth-century medical literature. In descriptions of their prenatal experiences, women often identified monstrosity as being presaged by a disruption of social, affective, and bodily boundaries. The themes and motifs that arose in these narratives tended to situate monsters within relational orders of kin and strangers, locating the origins of monstrosity in anxious contacts between humans and animals; encounters with racial Otherness, in particular white women's encounters with Blackness and Indigeneity; and physical dangers posed by the reformation of urban life in the mid-nineteenth-century United States. Some of these motifs bore continuities with classical, medieval, and early modern attributions of monstrosity—especially the association of monsters with transgressed human–animal boundaries—but they acquired new form and specificity in the context of nineteenth-century clinical encounters and the embodied interpersonal worlds of nineteenth-century American women.[60]

A motif running through many different women's narratives involved distressing encounters with animals during pregnancy. More than any other, these narratives of prenatal animal encounters cut across stratifications of race, class, and region. An enslaved Black woman in Tennessee was "much frightened by seeing for the first time, and very unexpectedly, an *elephant* belonging to a traveling menagerie" in 1850, while an upper-class Anglo-American patient of an elite Boston physician was similarly "much frightened" when she unexpectedly saw a "serpent" in 1849. Women reported fear and shock at the general sights and sounds of bellowing bulls, shrieking screech owls, and drowning hogs. One woman approached a "good sized dry log" on the Florida coast and was "in the act of seating herself" on it when she realized, with dawning terror, that the log was in fact an alligator.[61]

Several narratives described male relatives using animals to intentionally inflict distress. The husband of a white woman in New York "amused himself by walking around her" and dangling crabs in front of her, knowing "she was afraid of them," while the brother of a multiracial woman in Virginia "entered her room about midnight and threw a living opossum on the bed, frightening her much."[62] Some encounters involved multiple animal kinds. A Black woman in South Carolina was shocked by a sudden encounter with a buzzard devouring a pig and afterward felt "attacked with 'uneasy sensations'" in the pit of her stomach. A Methodist woman in Ohio tried to flee from agitated horses after being "badly frightened" at a camp meeting, only to be chased and jumped on by a large dog; another woman was "out with a friend gathering some whortle berries" when they came across a "huge rattle-snake, which first bit their dog and then made battle with them."[63]

A less ubiquitous but still recurring narrative in the case histories, more narrowly tied to a specific class and racial demographic, featured a married upper-class white woman's overly intimate attachment to a companion animal during pregnancy. In one case in 1840, a pregnant woman doted on a dog "which had been used to draw her breasts" after an earlier miscarriage. She sent for her private physician "in consequence of her anxiety" from the critiques of her friends, who believed her inordinate fondness for the animal would mark her developing child. A similar case in 1894 involved an affluent woman who was described as having "distinct predilection for lower animal tastes," being "much devoted during her pregnancy to the care of a dog and a pet rabbit, the latter of which was to be frequently seen nestled in her lap or poised on her shoulders." Her friends "repeatedly discouraged these attentions on her part, but to no purpose."[64] These narratives encoded general anxieties about the transgression of affective and bodily separations between humans and animals as well as more specific anxieties about excesses in the sentimental attachment to animals that was associated with nineteenth-century constructions of genteel, civilized white femininity.[65]

Taken together, the frequency with which animals appeared in these accounts suggests the ways in which monstrosity implicated anxieties over interspecies boundaries and, particularly, over the stability of the kinship boundary between humans and beasts—as in the case of the woman in 1840, whose friends disparaged her attachment to a dog she had suckled in place of a human child.[66] Recalling earlier classical and medieval notions of monsters as the promiscuous mingling of animal species, these associations of monstrosity took new shape in the contexts of nineteenth-century women's daily activities, relationships, and social imaginaries.

In another recurrent narrative, a monstrous birth was attributed to a woman's encounter with a figure of racial alterity during pregnancy. Typically, this involved a white Christian woman's encounter with a "deviant" racialized figure, inscribing racist tropes that conflated Blackness and Indigeneity with monstrosity. A birth attended by a

Pennsylvania physician in 1865 involved a married mother of five described as "of delicate organization" and "exceedingly nervous"—words typically associated with white, Protestant, middle- or upper-class femininity. Prior to delivery, she informed the physician "that her babe would be deformed," citing an incident that had occurred about nine weeks into her pregnancy: Her husband had left her home alone in the evening with their children, when "about dusk a large negro man, in soldiers' clothes, came to the door and asked for an axe; he was the worst featured and most disgusting human being she had ever beheld." The woman "was so alarmed as to faint; and lay upon the floor unconscious until her husband returned and lifted her to bed, where she remained much agitated and very feeble for several days."[67] In a similar narrative from an 1871 birth history, a "Christian lady" of "excitable, nervous temperament" reported to her physician that "a colored woman, with large protruding eyes and singular expression, suddenly approached her whilst in her ninth pregnancy, giving her a fright, to which cause she attributed this malformation of the foetus." A late nineteenth-century case history described a pregnant woman's trip to New York City to see "the Aztec children," referring to a popular circus or "freak show" exhibition in which individuals with microcephaly were presented as descendants of an ancient Central American race.[68] In all these cases, a narrative of maternal impression located the genesis of monstrosity in a white woman's encounter with racial alterity—part of a broader racialization of monstrosity that configured cultural meanings of monstrous difference in nineteenth-century medical literature.[69]

Finally, a number of narratives attributed monstrous births to women's experiences of physical dangers and maladies associated with industrialization and expanding urban populations in the mid- to late nineteenth-century United States. Some involved violent traumas related to new mechanized technologies of economic production and transportation: for instance, tending to an injured brother whose hand had been "torn off by machinery" or to an injured husband whose foot got "caught in the cogwheels" while "running a traction-engine on the public highway." In other instances, women witnessed a child run over by a streetcar, saw the disfigured face of a family member killed in a railroad accident, or suffered "fatigue and seasickness" while traveling "in cars and steamboat."[70] Other narratives implicated the emergence of new carceral systems in increasingly densely populated cities. During one pregnant woman's visit to her incarcerated brother, "a prisoner was brought in shackled, and she repeatedly spoke of the sight, and hoped her brother would not be treated in that manner"; throughout her pregnancy, she was haunted by dreams of "her brother in irons."[71] Here, women's narratives associated monstrosity with anxieties over the social, technological, and institutional upheavals of nineteenth-century industrial capitalism and the new risks to life introduced by mechanization and urbanization in this period.

MEDICAL AUTHORITY AND THE FACILITATION OF BLAME

While some women used the shared framework of maternal impression to voice and theorize their lived experiences within a medical literature that frequently sought to exclude them, this same framework could also be a source of distress for nineteenth-century mothers. Some women recalled how the entirety of their pregnancies had been subsumed by a sense of dread and foreboding after experiencing a fright early on and how they were tormented by the recurrent thought that their developing child had been harmed by the incident. One woman was "exceedingly troubled" at seeing a boy injure a hen with a stone, and "as her pregnancy advanced, [she] continually dwelt upon the subject, insisting that her child when born would be found to be deformed." Another, upon visiting an ailing friend and watching her suffer a hemorrhage, "was greatly shocked, so much so as to faint; and she subsequently thought frequently of the occurrence, fearing its effects upon the child she carried." A third woman was frightened by a snake during her pregnancy and "felt at once that the child would be 'marked'"; she "tried to forget it, but could not, and 'often' spoke of it to her friends in a nervous state."[72] In these instances, a shared belief in maternal impression clearly exacerbated the fear and anxiety that women experienced during pregnancy.

Popular medical advice manuals on childbearing and motherhood, written by credentialed practitioners for an assumed readership of white middle-class women in the mid- to late nineteenth century, also conveyed elaborate warnings about the dangers of maternal impression.[73]

In language that seemed likely to heighten feelings of anxiety, these manuals cautioned women about the perils of harming their developing offspring through their thoughts, behavior, and emotions during pregnancy. The physician author of one manual warned that "during pregnancy there is unusual susceptibility to mental impressions" liable to "operate on the fragile structure of the unborn being," and he enjoined pregnant women to remember that "the child, though unborn, lives within her; its life is a part of her own, and so frail, that any indiscretion on her part may destroy it."[74] Women sometimes heard similar advice from their own physicians. One physician wrote in to the *Medical and Surgical Reporter* in 1883 to decry colleagues who warned patients about the dangers of maternal impressions during pregnancy, lamenting that "I have had women to become frightened at a fish, and worry and fret because they were sure, from what they had been told by doctors, that the child would have scales."[75]

In addition to heightening fear and anxiety, the framework of maternal marking could also facilitate the assignation of blame—used to suggest that a mother was at fault for recklessly exposing herself to upsetting sights and situations while pregnant or used to exert control over pregnant women's behaviors in mandating they avoid such exposures. At a time when the medical oversight of pregnancy was not yet routine, the framework of maternal impression could be invoked to advance a rising medical interest in asserting authority over the prenatal period.[76]

This mobilization of medical authority involved not a direct assertion of physician control over gravid bodies but rather the inculcation of orderly norms at microsites of everyday living through self-administered changes of habit and practices of personal care. As part of their injunction for the reformation of daily habit, popular medical advice manuals still urged reliance on the oversight of an authoritative physician: As Elisabeth Robinson Scovil, superintendent of the Newport Hospital in Rhode Island, advised in *Preparation for Motherhood* in 1896, "The function of a medical man ought to be not so much to cure his patients of disorders as to keep them in order."[77]

To keep pregnant patients "in order," manuals freighted imperatives around maternal impression with an expansive moral weight, configuring women as responsible not only for the quality of their own offspring but also for society and humanity writ large. One explained that "the mother's influence upon her unborn child, and through it upon society, church, and state, is immeasurably great," while another averred that a pregnant woman's conduct during pregnancy mattered "not only for the sake of herself and her husband, but also for the sake of her forming child and for the welfare of the human race."[78] Authors explicitly moralized pregnant women's behavior through the invocation of Christian Providence and sin, warning that "Providence does not design monstrosities" or decrying the birth of "deformed" infants as resulting from "a sinful neglect of those special measures imperatively demanded in the ordering of the daily life . . . upon pregnancy." (A similar formulation also appeared in professional medical literature: One case report from the 1870s wrote of physicians' "moral and Christian duty" to instruct women on how to cultivate themselves during pregnancy for the benefit of their developing fetuses, "that they may improve the race and not retrograde it.")[79]

The potential to influence a developing fetus was extrapolated to specific directives for maternal conduct, environment, affect, perception, and thought. One manual advised that "during pregnancy, the minds of mothers should be watched, as well as their bodies, with the greatest care." Others stipulated that "all the surroundings and employments of the pregnant woman should be such as conduce to cheerfulness and equanimity"; she should "cultivate grace and beauty in herself at such a time" and "maintain serenity and calmness."[80] Conversely, a pregnant woman must guard against "violent and sudden emotion"; she should avoid "ungraceful positions and awkward attitudes" as well as "all causes of excitement." She should remove "disagreeable and unsightly objects" from her environment and refrain from "looking at, or thinking of ugly people, or those marked with disfiguring diseases."[81]

Similar prescriptions appeared in formal medical literature. In an 1853 case report, a physician suggested that women should be "cautious of needless exposure to unpleasant sights in the early months of pregnancy."[82] Another, in 1894, wrote that "it seems to be the concensus [*sic*] of opinion that one cannot go far wrong by assuming it to be his duty to discourage morbid reflection, worriment, or apprehension of defective progeny in the minds of nervous, impressionable, pregnant women." He added, "If the minds of our pregnant patients are schooled in the aversion of voluntary, catastrophal sightseeing . . . it is just possible that monstrous conceptions might be a less frequent misfortune."[83]

In these invocations, a discourse of maternal impression was mobilized to shape and assert an intimate form of control over the lives and habits of pregnant women in ways that seemed likely to direct blame and guilt at women who "failed" to avoid monstrous impressions during pregnancy. Friends as well as physicians could be the source of such shaming: One case reported that "Mrs. A–," after ignoring her friends' warnings that her excessively intimate attachments to companion animals would mark her developing child, was "constantly upbraided with her misfortune" after the birth of a child with anencephaly.[84]

Yet this does not mean that a belief in maternal impression had a singularly negative impact on pregnant women's lives and autonomy. For one, it seems that many women engaged the theory of maternal influence not as a way to assign blame to themselves but as a way to derive sense and meaning out of a distressing and seemingly inexplicable experience—and sometimes as a way to explicitly direct blame toward circumstances or other people's actions outside pregnant women's control. And the shared framework of maternal marking could provide a site where a woman might actively participate with her physician in the medical narration of her experience and the production of medical knowledge about her body and offspring, a site where she could contribute her concerns, ideas, and narratives of subjective experiences in a shared search to more deeply understand the causes, meanings, and contexts of monstrous childbirth. This was especially significant during a period of rising medical authority over the interpretation of bodies and reproduction and of a widening cleavage between medical and lay knowledge—a time when women were often excluded from becoming formally authorized producers of medical knowledge within the developing profession of obstetrics.

Further, though the theory of maternal impression could be mobilized to blame women for undesired birth outcomes, it could also be invoked to shield individual women from a more totalizing form of blame and stigma. In some case reports of monstrous birth, usually involving married white Anglo-American women, physicians took pains to distinguish an instance of maternal impression from a larger indictment of constitution or character: They invoked the theory of maternal impression to underscore that a monstrous birth had simply been caused by an isolated one-time incident and that its occurrence should not be taken as a broader reflection on the moral or social standing of the mother, who was emphasized to be "a highly respectable and intelligent lady of my neighborhood" or "the wife of one of our most respectable citizens."[85] Indeed, nineteenth-century sources often deployed the framework of maternal impression in a less overtly stigmatizing way than a theory that increasingly gained traction toward the end of the century, which posited a parent's constitutional or hereditary pathology as a potential cause of monstrous births.

STIGMA AND EPISTEMOLOGICAL EXCLUSION IN THE LATE NINETEENTH CENTURY

While a substantial number of late nineteenth-century case histories continued to invoke theories of maternal impression, reports also began more frequently to take note of mothers' and fathers' "constitutional" and "hereditary" conditions as possible causal factors, locating potential origins of monstrosity in a sustained pathology of the parental body or family line.[86] In an explicitly stigmatizing formulation, late nineteenth-century case reports often discussed these potential conditions as "taints," a word that appeared most frequently in cases concerning working-class or racially marginalized parents. One physician recorded that the mother, "a farmer's wife" in Michigan, had "a specific taint," in this case referring to a venereal disease. In a case involving a multiracial mother in Missouri, the physician assessed the presence of general "hereditary taint in the family."[87]

Late nineteenth-century authors cast "hereditary taints" as a form of generationally transmitted "degeneracy" that corrupted both parent and child.[88] In a period of rising cultural anxieties around venereal disease, the category of "hereditary taints" could also encompass syphilitic infections. Presented as a threat to the middle-class familial and social order, syphilis was discussed in stridently moralized terms: not just as an infection but also as a transmissible "taint" that contaminated a person's whole being and lineage. In the coming decade, physicians would make explicit the eugenic implications of this framing of venereal disease.[89]

A notation of the parents' venereal disease status became a frequent inclusion in late nineteenth-century reports of monstrous birth, with some physicians directly naming syphilis as the likely cause of the infant's condition.[90] Notably, case reports that assessed and recorded parents' syphilitic status (whether positive or negative) often involved patients of lower social or racial status. An 1886 report "ascribed the cause to syphilis" when discussing an infant born to a patient "at the dispensary," an institution that primarily served "the urban poor" in this period.[91] An 1888 report noted that the "the mother was unmarried" and that she "denied syphilis"; another, from 1899, noted that the mother, "a colored woman," had "no evidence of syphilis."[92] In an 1898 report involving an upper-class married woman in New York, the physician felt the need to defend the classed respectability of his patient, the married Mrs. M, by clarifying that her venereal infection was "believed to have been contracted from a water-closet seat used by a servant who was later found to be suffering from syphilis." Physicians proposed a variety of mechanisms to account for how a "syphilitic taint in the mother" might beget monstrosity.[93] Theresa Bannan, one of about seven thousand female physicians in the predominantly male American medical profession at this time, suggested in 1894 that both mothers and fathers with "syphilis, chronic alcoholism, and other constitutional affections" were liable to conceive monstrosities because of their faulty "ovum and spermatozoon"—showing how concepts of moral, constitutional, and hereditary pathology could merge in causal narratives of "defective" parental bodies.[94]

Unlike information related to maternal emotion and experience, which was communicated by the patient, knowledge about "constitutional taint" was to be gleaned by the physician through expert assessment of the patient's body.[95] In the case of venereal disease, a New York physician avowed in 1898 that it was "absolutely necessary" for physicians to learn "the signs by which we can determine the existence of syphilis," explaining, "It is proverbial that persons with syphilis or gonorrhea are liars. It is useless to question the father or mother in these cases for they will only mislead one."[96] The physician's trained discernment, then, not the patient's subjective input, was configured as the epistemological basis for such knowledge—thus shutting out childbearing women from what had formerly been, for some of them, spaces of interactive knowledge production.

The later nineteenth-century shift to harden and consolidate physicians' authority over their childbearing patients was reflected in other aspects of the case reports as well. Physicians in this period attended a larger proportion of deliveries, particularly among white middle-class women, and they assumed an increasingly interventionist role when present. Late nineteenth-century physicians established authoritative knowledge of monstrosity in part through their ability to recognize and clinically diagnose it before delivery, usually through the performance of increasingly common and extensive prebirth digital exams (and, in subsequent decades, through the advent of medical imaging technology). Through this avenue, physicians gained access to knowledge that they could then disclose to or conceal from the patient as they determined fit. The physician's rising authority in the birthing room was underscored by these kinds of shifts in the structure of access to knowledge, accentuating an ever-widening asymmetry of power and epistemological authority between physicians and patients in this period.[97]

Although these late nineteenth-century changes in obstetric practice further constrained women's involvement in medical meaning making, they never fully foreclosed that involvement. Despite physicians' increasingly adamant claims to unilateral epistemological authority, laywomen continued to shape the formation of medical knowledge on monstrous birth. Their experiences, insights, and ideas remained entangled in the interpersonal processes of producing knowledge about biological bodies and reproduction, even as ascendant institutions of medical science largely excluded laywomen from formal recognition.

In this way, attention to laywomen's often-obscured yet insistent presence in the case literature sheds light on medical meaning making as an ineluctably embodied, relational, and socially embedded historical practice. In the space of the clinical encounter surrounding birth, interactions between laywomen and practitioners configured and revised the category of biological monstrosity. Moving into the postpartum period, the next chapter continues to analyze social and embodied terrains of medical meaning making, exploring how affective practices configured the monstrosity of living newborns after delivery.

CHAPTER TWO

Monstrous Newborns

Emotions, Embodiment, and Sensory Relation

For the most part, Mrs. G found her fifth pregnancy easy and unremarkable. She could recall almost nothing out of the ordinary about it, with one marked exception: In the last few months, whenever she made a sudden exertion, she would feel in response an unexpectedly forceful motion inside her womb. Mrs. G considered this curious but not terribly perturbing; she appeared far less distressed by it, in any case, than another nineteenth-century woman in similar circumstances, who described the sensation as a "violent motion" that felt "'*as if it would break through her*.'" Mrs. G did remark, however, that the fetal movements seemed far stronger than any she had experienced during her previous pregnancies.[1]

At thirty-five years of age, Mrs. G was experienced in maternity. Her New York physician, Samuel Purple, described her as a "well developed English lady" with four children, "all of whom are perfect in physical organization." Her fifth labor, in 1850, was short and uncomplicated, lasting only thirty minutes from the start of pains to the finish. Upon delivery, attendants immediately noted her newborn's unusual condition. The entire upper portion of the child's skull was absent, exposing a vascularized "tumor" in the place where a brain would ordinarily be. Drawing on the scientific taxonomy of nineteenth-century teratology (the "scientific study of monstrosity"), Purple designated the child as a "pseudencephalous monstrosity," a condition of anomalous brain and skull development similar to anencephaly.[2]

To the surprise of those observing, the child was born living. The infant struggled to take any sustenance at first but eventually proved able to swallow sugared milk and water offered from a spoon. Encouraged, the physician Purple passed his own finger inside the newborn's mouth and found that the infant "commenced to suck with considerable force" on the proffered digit. The child then began nursing after being "applied to the breast" and coaxed to suckle. Ultimately Purple reported that the infant "took nourishment with as little difficulty as ordinary children at birth" and subsequently excreted waste "which appeared, in all respects, like the same discharges of the naturally formed child."[3]

Other aspects of this newborn's embodiment, however, diverged sharply from the expectations of the assembled attendants and relatives. The sounds and movements of the child drew particular notice. The infant exhaled freely, but on the inhale the breath became irregular, seeming to shudder and catch in their throat. They made "frequent and partially effected efforts to cry," as if trying to break into a more vigorous wail that would not come. After a few moments of these frustrated endeavors, their body would convulse in a series of rapid muscular flexions and extensions and then fall still again. Purple found he could elicit this same reaction by "pinching" or "pressing" parts of the infant's body and head. Though he noted that this treatment consistently caused the child to let out a "suppressed cry," this reaction did not lead Purple to alter his behavior in any way. Instead, positioning the infant above all as a source of abstractable scientific data, Purple repeated his actions enough times to be able to characterize the "invariable" response of the child, proclaiming that these results could shed light on the relationship between specific physiological functions and the gross anatomy of the human brain.[4]

The infant lived for two and a half days, and Purple felt confident that they would have lived even longer if not for a suspected "circumstance" over which he "had no control." While Purple conceded that his suspicions were "only a matter of presumption," his words strongly insinuated that the parents had acted to intentionally hasten the infant's death. He believed these suspicions were borne out by the parents' refusal to permit him to take and examine the infant's bodily remains, contrary to his strongest efforts to convince them otherwise. In contrast to the enslaved Black woman discussed in the previous chapter, the married, upper-class, Anglo-American Mrs. G was not subjected to any formal investigation or censure based on the suspicion of infanticide. Purple instead seemed to fault Mrs. G and her husband mainly for refusing him custody of the infants' remains, which he had hoped to present as a specimen to his colleagues.[5]

The philosopher Michel Foucault describes the monster as a figure that historically transgressed binaries, signifying the mixing of two ostensibly oppositional realms. One of these putative binaries is "life and death": "The fetus born with a morphology that means it will not be able to live but that nonetheless survives for some minutes or days is a monster."[6] Continuing to chart the trajectory of infants' transformation into specimens of monstrosity, this chapter moves into this fleeting time frame of paradoxical life: the birth and momentary survival of infants with inexorably life-ending conditions such as anencephaly. It explores how these newborn bodies were made into "monsters" in part through embodied encounters and interactions in the postpartum period. Although conditions such as anencephaly precluded sustained existence, some affected infants—lacking most structures of the brain but born with portions of the brainstem intact—lived for minutes, days, or, rarely, weeks following birth. During their short lives, these infants cried, moved their bodies, swallowed nourishing fluids, and voided waste. They interacted with family members, attendants, and physicians in intimately sensory and embodied ways: suckling on breasts and fingers, receiving care and touch, and evoking complex and powerful emotions.

FINDING AFFECT IN MEDICAL ARCHIVES

An emphasis on emotional interactions contrasts with the image that leading physicians attempted to cultivate for the profession in the nineteenth-century United States. Across this period, the ideal of the physician as a neutral, dispassionate, "ever unemotional" man of science increasingly came to animate the self-representation (if not the lived reality) of professional practice.[7] Accordingly, in remaking monstrosity as a scientific category, leading nineteenth-century American physicians portrayed themselves as stripping away the affective meanings of monstrous bodies, turning an emotionally charged portent of "gravest fears" into an emotion-neutral "specimen."[8]

But as this chapter will show, emotion was deeply implicated in the medical construction of monstrosity. Before being cataloged and exhibited in medical museums or lecture halls, infants were produced as monsters through affective interactions in the birthing room during and immediately following delivery. Practitioners configured medical cosmologies of the monstrous body not only in formal anatomical and physiological renderings but also at these natal and postpartum sites of emotional and sensory relation.

Historians writing about earlier periods have compellingly broadened understandings of the spheres in which bodies were historically constituted and made meaningful, showing, for instance, that early modern Europeans understood their bodies through discourses of kinship, religion, and relations of touch rather than primarily through "medical models and medical discourses."[9] Although also foregrounding the understanding of bodies as socially and relationally embedded, my analysis does not investigate relational and embodied interaction as a sphere apart from and in addition to medical discourse: Rather, it approaches affective practice as an integral component of nineteenth-century professional medicine and a core avenue of medical meaning making.

Affect—used here to refer to both the expression of and the capacity to evoke an emotion or feeling—is often an elusive object of historical study, particularly when working with a source base comprising primarily written nineteenth-century clinical texts. To access questions of affect, this chapter takes a creative interdisciplinary approach to its medical archive. I draw on frameworks from queer, feminist, and disability studies, which consider emotion not as an abstracted, static, self-contained property of an individual but rather as embodied, circulating, and relational. My analysis is influenced in particular by the scholar Sara Ahmed's concept of "affective economies," in which "emotions work to align some subjects with some others and against other others," playing a role in the demarcation of bodies, identities, and relationships.[10] The chapter also applies frameworks of narrative analysis to delve more deeply into the affective content of medical case reports.

Drawing on these insights, the chapter probes the affective configuration of monstrous bodies by examining how physicians, mothers, attendants, and relatives reacted to and interacted with liveborn "monstrous" infants, attending carefully to both explicit and implicit descriptions of emotional and sensory experience. What feelings did monstrous newborns evoke in those who encountered them? How were their bodies seen, heard, touched, and narrated? What sorts of actions and ethical imperatives did their presence occasion? In addition to containing semantic descriptors of the emotions that monstrous births evoked, case reports also reveal how postpartum interactions affectively configured monstrosity. The chapter explores enactments of emotions such as fear, disgust, tenderness, relief, and grief as expressed through visual, auditory, tactile, and other modes of embodied relation.

At these intimate interfaces of sensory encounter, physicians and family members positioned anomalous living infants in paradoxical relation to themselves and to the figure of the "nonmonstrous" human child. Their interactions configured monstrous newborns as particular kinds of subjects, locating them within—or outside of—networks of familial and racial kin as well as within broader moral and cultural imaginaries of the human. Affective practices positioned the monster as a paradoxical embodiment of both kinship and alienation, a being simultaneously recognizable and unrecognizable as a human child.

"FEARFULLY AND WONDERFULLY MADE": THE DRAMATURGY OF MONSTROUS BIRTH

Nineteenth-century physicians were eager to disclaim the emotions long associated with monstrous births, which in the early modern period had prominently included complexes of "horror, pleasure, and repugnance."[11] In 1855, the leading Philadelphia physician Charles Meigs explained that practitioners' knowledge of modern science rendered them immune to the unruly feelings that monstrous births tended to elicit in those "unacquainted with the doctrines of embryology." John Shaw Billings, another nationally notable physician, contrasted in 1888 the public's continued "emotional" interest in viewing monstrosities with the physician's impartial regard: "For scientific and professional purposes," he wrote, "the emotional element does not enter into it at all."[12]

Yet descriptions of emotions saturate the nineteenth-century medical case literature on monstrosities, heightened by the social and embodied contexts of encounter tied to the rising nineteenth-century practice of physician-attended childbirth in women's homes. Physicians might tout their ability to remain emotionless in reaction to the anatomized remains of a specimen in a medical museum, but they seemed less able to represent themselves as emotionless when narrating experiences in the birthing room. In case reports of individual monstrous births, physicians conveyed their own frankly emotional reactions to the birth of infants with conditions such as anencephaly. One felt "shocked, as well as astonished" by a newborn's appearance; another watched "with horror" as he realized an anencephalic infant was alive and breathing.[13]

Nineteenth-century physicians sometimes tried to differentiate their modern medical interest in monstrosity by downplaying any overt affect of "wonder," which they associated with reactions to monstrous births in earlier eras and in popular (rather than professional) cultures of display.[14] Nevertheless, words related to *wonder* still sometimes emerged in the professional case literature, often in response to witnessing liveborn infants with conditions presumed to preclude life—the paradox of inviable life that philosophers such as Foucault and Georges Canguilhem identify as characteristic of monstrosity.[15] In describing the brief life of an infant with anencephaly in 1860, the prominent US obstetrician Hugh Lenox Hodge wrote that "it is certainly wonderful that this child should have breathed for twenty-four hours."[16]

As the historians Lorraine Daston and Katharine Park observe in their canonical work on monstrous births in early modern Europe, the emotion of wonder was "itself protean, sliding on one side toward pleasure . . . and on the other side toward fear."[17] Following monstrous newborns' deaths, many nineteenth-century American physicians appeared to take an acquisitive pleasure in claiming their remains, describing the bodies they obtained as "gifts," "prizes," "trophies," "presents," and "treasures."[18] In the presence of living newborns in the birthing room, however, physicians' wonder seemed more proximate to fear. Attending a monstrous birth brought to mind for one practitioner the psalm of the Old Testament prophet David: "I am fearfully and wonderfully made."[19]

Indeed, of all the words describing emotions that appeared in the medical case reports, by far the most frequently invoked were those related to fear—a semantic cluster defined here to include anxiety, nervousness, apprehension, terror, alarm, dread, and horror. In a sample of several hundred nineteenth-century case histories of monstrous birth, words in the *fear* cluster appeared in roughly ten times as many reports as words from any single other cluster. Words from the second most frequently invoked semantic cluster, *disgust*, often appeared in conjunction with words related to fear.

While the taxonomic distinction between fear and disgust is central to Daston and Park's analysis of emotions associated with monsters in the early modern period, nineteenth-century clinical case literature frequently depicted the two as linked or even interchangeable in relation to lived experiences of monstrous birth. Critically, this evocation of emotion extended beyond just individual semantic descriptors. A creative analysis shows how medical case literature conjured a combined affect of fear and disgust that was produced and embodied at interfaces of sensory relation.

A common narrative across reports featured a climactic visual reveal that conveyed and constructed the horror of the infant's "monstrous" embodiment. This recurrent storyline can be understood as a "dramaturgic form" of the monstrous birth case history—a characteristic series of narrative elements that repeat across accounts. In the dramaturgy of the case report, the climactic visual reveal of monstrosity was presaged by ominous internal sensations during pregnancy, confounding tactile encounters during the predelivery digital exam, and/or harrowing sensory experiences during labor. These ominous signs and feelings functioned to build an escalating sense of tension, foreshadowing the emergence of the fearsome monstrous body through descriptions of the heightened distress that preceded its arrival.[20]

The narrative built this tension through accounts of both emotional and physical sensations. Women experienced prenatal moments "of great terror and excitement" or bouts of "strange and unaccountable feelings—such as she had not experienced in any of her previous pregnancies."

Reports described personality changes attendant on shifts in emotional disposition: One woman, usually "an exceedingly amiable person," became "peevish and irritable during her entire pregnancy"; another went through periods in which she became "highly excited," at times being "so unreasonable" that her friends had "fears she would become insane."[21]

Other accounts of prenatal distress foregrounded more localized bodily sensations, recording women's interoceptive (internal sensory) experiences. They described "uneasiness and pain in the abdomen" and "a 'burning sensation' in the stomach and bowels." Some gave dramatic and visually evocative reports of aggressive fetal motion. One woman "suffered greatly from the violent movements of the fetus which increased in force as gestation progressed and could be seen across the room as the abdomen was struck from within"; in another case, fetal movements were "extraordinarily violent and prolonged, enough to call the attention of the husband to it."[22] Breaking through from sheer force of their extremity into the realm of the visually observable, these private interoceptive experiences became a source of intersubjective sensory distress.

The premonitory signs of a fearful event to come might include both distress during pregnancy and uneasy tactile encounters during the digital examination immediately before delivery. In these cases, the physician reported feeling a confusing and "peculiar sensation" as their "exploring finger" or "examining finger" came into contact with an anencephalic fetal head, at times producing "unaccountable" fetal convulsions by inadvertently touching the open lesion.[23]

A final premonitory motif, marking the beginning of labor, involved descriptions of hydramnios—a condition characterized by an excess of amniotic fluid, which is frequently associated with anencephalic births. Read as a narrative element in the "drama" of the monstrous birth, physicians' descriptions of hydramnios—which could border on the operatic—heightened the premonition of a terrifying or "unnatural" reveal to come. Physicians reported that "rupturing the membranes" resulted in the release of an astonishing volume of water, described in one case as "the release of a miniature Niagara." One physician observed that "a deluge came down upon me that nearly floated me off the bed. It flooded the bed, from which we dipped up two and a half gallons, soaked the mattress, ran down upon the floor and through it and dripped into the apartment below." Another reported, "A gush of fluid came, as I had never seen before, saturating anything; shortly after, another gush, which ran off in streams from the bed, filling two large chamber vessels at the side of the bed; a third gush, and the carpet and several sheets, which had been placed over the carpet, were soaked." Yet another physician described "a flood which could not be stayed," continuing: "It gushed forth until the bed was soaked and the patient inundated. It filled the depression in the mattress where she lay and ran above her thighs. It went through the bed and floor and wet the ceiling of the room below. After the deluge enough water was dipped off the top of the mattress to fill an ordinary wooden bucket holding three gallons, and a conservative estimate of the fluid which escaped would make a total of seven gallons—fifty-six pounds."[24]

The intensifying sensory signs of something amiss set the stage for the "monstrous" reveal of the infant's body. When the moment of birth finally came, case histories underscored the drama of the newborn's visual reveal by emphasizing the reactions of others in the room or dwelling on the emotional evocations of the sight. One case report described how, "on the appearance of the child, a bystander uttered a sudden exclamation of surprise," while another report declared that "none could have looked at the monster and felt their usual calmness."[25] In some case histories, a language of delayed visual revelation added to the dramatic effect. A team of physicians wrote that "it was not until the child was fairly exposed to the light that it was discovered to be a monster." Another physician described how a newborn's initially hidden body was eventually revealed upon "throwing back the bed-clothing" to uncover the sight; explicitly summoning an affect of mixed horror and disgust, the physician wrote that "our surprise can better be imagined than told on beholding the horrible and repulsive looking monster."[26] After foreshadowing the birth with a plotline of escalating tension and ominous premonitions, case narratives presented the unveiling of the monster as a climax of embodied visual horror.

SENSORY DISTANCE AND SENTIMENTAL WHITE MOTHERHOOD

In addition to presaged moments of visual revelation, acts of visual concealment also functioned to establish the fearful monstrosity of newborns, setting up the emergent body of the anomalous offspring as a figure of anticipated dread. One physician, after hearing the mother describe the violent fetal movement and feeling something unusual during the digital predelivery examination, "prepared two ladies who were present for some unnatural production, and begged them to convey the child, as soon as it was born, into an adjoining room from the view of the mother."[27] This directive configured the monstrous body as an object of projected maternal fear: a sight that must be covered and removed from sensory perception, that the mother must be protected from for fear of the terrible distress it would elicit in her.

The imperative of visual concealment was a recurrent trope in mid-century case histories, typically involving mothers coded as middle- or upper-class white women whose "delicate" sensibilities needed to be shielded from the sight of their offspring. A Maine physician in 1841 reported that "when I discovered the defect in the child, I kept it covered." A New Hampshire physician relayed that same year that "as soon as she was delivered I wrapped the child in a cloth and placed it in an adjoining room" so that "its deformities were not known to its mother or her attendants." And a Midwestern physician in 1851 wrote that "a sheet was folded about the child, so that it was impossible for the mother to have seen it."[28] The tactic of visual concealment often did not turn out to be an effective move for pacifying anxieties: In the birth of an infant with anencephaly in 1842, the woman's "first enquiry was, is not something the matter with the head? Being answered negatively, she asked to see it, which, it was thought, prudent to refuse." The woman was not fooled: "She replied, despondingly, that she always knew something was the matter, and our refusal to let her see it confirmed her belief." Sometimes, the mother successfully insisted on being allowed the sight of her offspring. In one case of attempted concealment, the physician reluctantly revealed the infant to the mother after she repeatedly insisted that she was "anxious to see it."[29]

Sara Ahmed theorizes fear as an emotion that "works to differentiate," establishing "distance between bodies whose difference is read off the surface." She posits that "fear and anxiety create the very effect of 'that which I am not,' through the very affect of turning away from an object." For Ahmed, "fear does not involve the defense of borders that already exist; rather, fear makes borders, by establishing objects from which the subject, in fearing, can stand apart, objects that become 'the not' from which the subject" seeks distance.[30]

Read through Ahmed's framework, what could be called the "affect of fear" described in nineteenth-century case histories—the concealment of, separation from, and turning away from the monstrous newborn as an object of projected maternal fear—could work to differentiate the body of the monster as a particular kind of negated "other." In these case histories, monstrous newborn bodies produced an "affect of fear" in part through physicians' attempts to conceal them—explicitly framing the monstrous body as a sight that needed to be turned away from, to be distanced from sensory perception. This affective production also worked across fields beyond sight through the denial of physical contact as well as visual perception. In one case concerning a newborn with pseudencephaly who lived for several days, the physician relayed that "from a fear of alarming the mother, no attempt was made to see whether it would take the breast."[31] In preempting the intimate contact of breastfeeding, the physician likewise positioned the infant's body as an object of projected maternal alarm.

These attempts to distance infants from maternal sight and touch mainly appeared in case histories where the mother was white, married, and relatively well-to-do. Notably, they occurred during a period when delicacy, refinement, and sensitivity to sensory stimuli and emotion—a "heightened faculty of feeling"—were positioned as core racial and gendered attributes of middle- and upper-class white womanhood.[32] In this context, the act of sensory concealment worked to affectively construct the monstrosity of the newborn and simultaneously the delicate white femininity of the mother. Establishing distance between woman and infant, concealment configured the alterity of monstrosity through a literal and symbolic displacement from the impressible white maternal body.

The imperative to establish distance between monstrous infants and upper-class white mothers centrally implicated an affect of disgust as well as fear. Like the affect of fear, an affect of disgust was linked to the behavioral response of turning away, of averting eyes and body, of cutting off or desiring to cut off sensory and physical contact. Physicians communicated the repugnance of monstrous bodies by describing the "rude appearance," the "hideous whining noise," and the "unearthly shrieks" of living newborns with anencephaly.[33] Emphasizing the infants' aversive sensory qualities, physicians configured the monstrosity of newborn bodies at the interfaces of visual and auditory perception.

Such infants were positioned as particularly repugnant through narratives of mothers' direct refusals to provide intimate bodily care and nurturing. These refusals of care and nurturance assumed heightened affective significance against prevailing ideals of white, middle- and upper-class motherhood. In the early nineteenth century, burgeoning Anglo-American constructions of "sentimental motherhood" elaborated new imperatives to provide attentive, loving, and intimate care for young children.[34] Expressions of maternal love and caregiving played an important role in nineteenth-century doctrines of "true womanhood," which positioned women as nurturing, pious, and confined to the "private sphere" of home family life, foregrounding their gendered roles as wives and mothers. These aspirational ideals centered white, middle- and upper-class motherhood as the truest form of womanhood.[35] Even as discourses of true (white) womanhood valorized domesticity and sentimental maternal attachment, regimes of slavery and familial separation systematically severed and denied Black and Indigenous mothers' bonds of kinship to their children, while the necessities of working-class women's lives rendered confinement in a private home sphere patently unattainable.

Within prevailing nineteenth-century constructions of motherhood, breastfeeding represented a fundamental enactment of a deep maternal bond, an essential expression of women's vaunted "mother's love." For the racialized and class-coded category of "true" women, breastfeeding was supposed to constitute both a key demonstration of maternal virtue and a subjective experience of keen emotional pleasure.[36] In case literature, the alienation of the monstrous newborn could thus be potently articulated through a genteel white mother's emotional aversion to providing this form of intimate and nurturing care—revealing the infant's power to unsettle the bonds of true motherhood through monstrous affects of fear and disgust.

In a mid-nineteenth-century case report of a "pseudencephalic monster" born to a white, well-to-do patient in Maryland, the physician relayed that "the ready movements of the child's mouth attracting attention, the mother was besought to apply her offspring to the breast; but nothing could overcome her repugnance to nursing 'so hideous a monster.'"[37] In this narration, the tensions that animated the ontological category of "monstrosity" were shown in bold relief. On the one hand, the narrative communicated the child's legibility as natural human kin, depicting an infant seeking biological nourishment from the maternal body—an act that would function to affirm a relational bond, simultaneously physiological and emotional, between "mother" and "offspring." Yet through the woman's refusal of the enactment of this bond and her (physician-interpreted) affective orientation of "repugnance" rather than "mother's love," the newborn was rhetorically transformed from "offspring" to "monster." In Ahmed's terminology, "the affect of turning away" here creates "the effect of 'that which I am not'"—the displaced body of the monstrous other rather than the closely held body of the milk-bonded human child.[38]

This physical and symbolic rejection again established distance between the delicate sensibilities of the repulsed upper-class white mother and the "hideous" offspring, who, in eliciting this disgust, could not be recognized as an object of maternal love and care. In this way, the affect of repugnance and the bodily enactment of separation helped to construct the racialized alterity of monstrous infants born to middle- and upper-class white mothers. Disrupting the emotional and somatic imperatives of sentimental white motherhood, the monster was cast outside the imaginary of the Anglo-American familial sphere.

MODES AND BOUNDARIES OF TOUCH

While case reports frequently invoked descriptors such as *fear* and *repugnance*, some of the richest insight into the affective configuration of monstrosity can be gleaned from passages that never directly name emotions. This insight instead comes from attention to described or implied relations of touch and embodied interaction among physicians, family members, and infants. As a pervasive daily site of social practice, sensory processing, and meaning making, touch represents an important, if elusive, area of analysis. In an intellectual tradition where "sight is the icon of the rational," touch has often been denigrated as the "lowest" of the senses—described as cruder, baser, and less refined than the others.[39] Yet touch operates in complex, intricate, and powerful ways. The question of which bodies are touched, how, and by whom is intimately involved in locating and defining the relational position of individuals within broader networks of familial, social, and racial orders.[40]

Relations of touch with living newborns constituted a powerful site of affective practice in the configuration of monstrosity. Nineteenth-century case reports recorded or implied a variety of physical interactions among mothers, physicians, attendants, and liveborn infants following delivery. Mothers held newborns against their breasts to coax them to latch and nurse. Other forms of feeding documented in the case histories, such as inserting a milk-covered finger in the mouth of the infant for them to suckle on, likewise entailed intimate bodily contact between attendants and infants, as did practices of bathing, swaddling, and clothing. Tactile interaction also underwrote what I refer to as "experimental touch"—a form of contact in which physicians touched monstrous newborns to observe their reactions to a stimulus, with the intent to produce abstracted knowledge about human physiology.

The case reports that contain the most details about postpartum touch usually involved white, middle- and upper-class mothers. There were some practical reasons for this: These women were likelier than others in this era to give birth attended by medical practitioners in private family homes, and physicians might continue to visit their houses for days or weeks after the birth for follow-up care, offering them ample time to observe and interact with families and newborns. In addition to logistical factors, broader cultural discourses also contextualized the case literature's selective focus. As discussed, nineteenth-century ideals of motherhood foregrounded attention to middle- and upper-class white women, positioning the provision of nurturing maternal care to young children as essential to Anglo-American womanhood.

For all the emphasis on fear and disgust, case reports of monstrous birth also reflected practices of intimate infant caregiving, if often only implicitly. In one late nineteenth-century report of a newborn with anencephaly who lived for about two and a half days, several accompanying illustrations show the infant wearing a striped and patterned garment with a collar and buttons, resting their head on a small pillow trimmed with a ruffle. Though the case history did not directly describe these care practices, it can be inferred from the images that a family member or attendant took the time to dress the infant and gently place them on the cushioned bed.[41] Other case histories from this period included photographs of newborns with anencephaly on beds and in bassinets. The infants' bodies have clearly been carefully and scrupulously bathed, though the reports do not specify which adult performed this action. One physician referred directly to the "articles of clothing" placed on an infant with anencephaly, explaining that those who dressed the infant refrained from putting a "cap" on the newborn's head after doing so appeared to cause the child distress.[42] In implying or describing the way that infant bodies were cleaned, clothed, swaddled, and put down to rest, the case reports alluded to modes of touch closely associated with tenderness and nurturing.

While the previous section discussed reports of mothers refusing to breastfeed infants born with conditions such as anencephaly, the case literature also showed that not every woman experienced this aversion. An 1843 report noted that an attempt had been made to breastfeed a liveborn infant with anencephaly but stated that the infant "would not suck." An 1888 report of anencephaly described how "the child nursed a little, but had difficulty in swallowing," while an 1898 report recorded that "the baby nursed naturally."[43] Entailing an intimate form of embodied maternal contact and recognition, the act of breastfeeding firmly positioned the infant as a being who both elicited an imperative to be fed with and was capable of being nourished by a human mother's milk.

Case histories also recorded acts of giving nourishment other than breastfeeding. Adults prepared and administered mixtures of milk, water, sugar, or even wine to newborns using a variety of means. These narratives often portrayed infants being fed by attendants rather than family members, emphasizing the familial rejection of the infants even while acknowledging an obligation to provide nourishment to them. One physician recounted how a "nurse essayed successfully to feed the child with sugar and water administered with a spoon" when the mother could not bring herself to breastfeed; later, the physician personally spoon-fed the infant a "bland fluid" after relatives and attendants expressed continued aversion to the idea of going near the child. Physicians recalled how they "administered milk and water prepared for the purpose, a small quantity of which was swallowed with great difficulty"; reported giving "liquids from a sop"; and described an infant who "partook of milk and water from a spoon several times." In a case of particularly pronounced bodily contact, an infant "sucked the finger" of an attendant to ingest a prepared solution of milk.[44] The affective significations of these actions were complex. In reporting them, physicians positioned the infants not only as newborn children needing to be fed but also as sources of abstractable scientific knowledge that hinged on the infants' anatomical alterity. Physicians included descriptions of feeding in case reports not only to document care provided but also to provide data on whether physiological functions such as suckling and digestion could occur in the absence of major structures of the brain.

While it might be tempting to interpret these two objectives—to give care and to produce scientific knowledge—as mutually exclusive orientations, doing so would fail to recognize the affective ambiguity and complexity of practitioners' interactions with living infants in the postpartum period. Physicians' professed curiosity about infants' biological capacities could exist alongside and did not necessarily displace recognition of imperatives to perform traditional acts of infant caregiving such as cleaning, swaddling, and feeding.

However, in other instances, physicians' interest in infants as scientific data clearly did conflict with caregiving imperatives. Multiple case reports recorded a distinctive form of touch entirely unrelated to caregiving that powerfully configured the alienation of monstrous bodies. This bodily contact aimed to produce abstractable scientific knowledge—in the words of one physician, to "throw much light upon some of the most obscure points in physiology"—in the absence of intent to provide nourishment, comfort, or affection.[45] This mode of touch investigated rather than assumed the sentience of the newborns, who were suspected to be missing critical brain structures associated with consciousness and the processing of the senses.

The graphic descriptions of this form of touch recorded in case reports can be very challenging to read, especially when physicians recounted how they persisted in performing actions that elicited bodily responses strongly associated with pain and distress. In one report, the Ohio physician John Shaller explained that he provoked "violent convulsions" by "repeatedly" passing his finger into the open spinal groove of a newborn with anencephaly.[46] While other reports described how acts of attempted caregiving were discontinued after appearing to cause the newborn "much distress," in this case Shaller did not interpret the production of violent convulsions as an imperative to stop his actions.[47] In the 1850 birth introduced at the start of the chapter, involving a "pseudencephalus" infant born to the well-to-do Anglo-American mother Mrs. G, the physician Purple likewise described pinching and pressing on parts of the infant's body, observing the reactions to this touch as a way to examine what sort of movement and reactivity were possible in the absence of large portions of the brain. Purple noted that "pressure upon the tumor" at the back of the infant's skull "gave rise to convulsive action of the whole system." He wrote that, "To all appearance it possesses the full amount of sensibility—irritation by pricking produced movement of the limb touched, and if repeated several times a suppressed cry, followed by a partial convulsion, was the invariable result."[48] Like Shaller, Purple described performing these actions repeatedly in order to produce more robust scientific data.

Purple situated his actions as typical in the clinical investigation of a case of this kind. Indeed, he relayed several other cases in which colleagues interacted in similar ways with infants born with pseudencephaly. One described how upon touching the exposed tissue at the back of the head, "a general and violent convulsion was produced, as if it received the strongest electric shock," during which every part of the newborn's body went into full, rigid extension. In another case, a physician "blew upon [the newborn's head], and the most violent twitchings of the arms and legs took place for a few moments, and all was still again; on blowing upon it a second time; no such effect was produced." Purple praised his colleagues' actions for shedding "no small degree of light" on human physiology, offering evidence that certain physical responses could occur independently of the body's "large nervous centres."[49]

Here, when care and the production of scientific knowledge were in conflict, the positioning of such infants as a source of experimental knowledge—an epistemic object of medical science—seemed to supersede and displace their positioning as children, an affective category of human kin invoking primary claims to care and comfort. It is worth noting again that these positionings were not *inherently* in conflict: In some sense, any physician-administered treatment configures the body of the patient as an experimental source of knowledge, yet the very act of receiving medical treatment can hardly be said to preclude an affective recognition and affirmation of a patient's humanity. Instead, the alienating effect of the experimental touch described earlier was entailed in the relational nature rather than the scientific purpose of the action. It was repeated even in the absence of expected therapeutic benefit, despite producing physical reactions strongly associated with subjective bodily distress. The infant's "sensibility" and sentience—the ability to perceive and process stimuli, the existence of human consciousness and will—were objects of investigation in the physician's actions rather than their assumed predicate.

In a case report from 1862, the Baltimore physician Christopher Johnston recounted his interactions with a liveborn infant likewise classified as a "pseudencephalic monster." Johnston reported that the infant "moved its limbs, and grasped what it touched with the hands . . . but it appeared to be, and doubtless was, unconscious." Like Purple, Johnston was interested in evidences of "sensibility"—the capacity to perceive and respond to sensory stimuli. Describing the infant, Johnston wrote that "when undisturbed the little creature now made no effort to alter its position; it shrank, however, if flies crawled over its head, and started almost upright whenever the tumour, especially the posterior part of it, was touched." He noted, however, that "pressure exerted upon the same part was productive of very inconsiderable effects, although, at the moment of contact of the finger, sensibility seemed painfully heightened."[50]

While Johnston's account shared many similarities with Purple's, it also seemed to relay a more ambivalent affective orientation toward the newborn he described as a "little creature," perhaps as inspiring of pity if not fondness. Despite the earlier assertion that the infant "appeared to be, and doubtless was, unconscious," Johnston's comment that "sensibility seemed painfully heightened" positioned the child as a subject capable of either experiencing or evoking the sensation of pain—a being whose fitful reactions to touch could elicit a recognition and a seemingly intersubjective experience of pain in an empathic observer. In this respect, Johnston's account appeared to attribute to the infant some measure of relational subjective capacity.

Johnston reported that he himself fed the newborn after others refused to. The mother, he said, could not overcome her "repugnance" at the idea of breastfeeding the child, and the attendants were likewise "unwilling to satisfy the wants of so forbidding a creature." Johnston discovered that the newborn "could still practice suction upon a finger introduced into its mouth, and it swallowed a bland fluid which I administered in a spoon."[51] In showing the contrast between his own sometimes-tender interactions with the infant and those of the family members and attendants, whom he portrayed as vehemently refusing any bodily contact with the "hideous monster," Johnson appeared to offer a more ambivalent configuration of the child's affective subjecthood.

However, after his postmortem dissection of the newborn's brain and nerve structures—another mode of profoundly tactile relation that is explored in the next chapter—Johnston disclaimed his earlier affective ascriptions. He concluded that the newborn could not possibly have possessed any sensitiveness or subjectivity because their body lacked nearly all the vital structures of the brain and nervous system that allowed for consciousness and sensory perception.[52]

In the removed space of the dissecting room, Johnston felt confident in retrospectively characterizing the infant as a being without agency or sensation and therefore as a being who ought to elicit no feelings of pity, tenderness, or empathic pain. Yet, as Johnston's narration in the case report conveys, he felt considerably more uncertain about the infant's affective status when present with and touching the living child. These fraught and ambivalent interactions in the space of postpartum encounter underscored the affective ambiguity of the category of the "monster"—by definition a being whose intimate human relation and lineage could not be denied, even as their body was located outside "the range of variation of the species."[53]

COMPLEXITIES OF GRIEF AND AFFECTIVE ATTACHMENT

A final site of fraught affective production in the postpartum period involved family members' and practitioners' reactions to the deaths of liveborn infants with conditions such as anencephaly: the close of the brief window of "scarcely viable" life this chapter has traced.[54] The philosopher Judith Butler, in theorizing "bodies that matter," draws attention to the articulation of which bodies constitute "lives worth grieving," suggesting how the capacity or incapacity to evoke grief affectively positions a body as a particular kind of moral subject.[55] Critically tracing descriptions of grief and mourning (or lack thereof) can thus offer powerful insight into the affective configuration of monstrosity.

Words related to sorrow appeared infrequently in the clinical literature on monstrous birth in comparison to words denoting fear and similar emotions. However, the former were not entirely absent. One report described a mother as speaking "despondingly" about the condition of her stillborn child; in another, the physician referred in the abstract to "the pangs of sorrow and distress incident upon a monstrous conception."[56]

An 1872 report, in which the Chicago physician A. Woodward diagnosed his postpartum patient Mrs. H with "a case of melancholia," contains a singularly extensive description of feelings related to sadness (and many other commingled emotions) following the birth and death of a "monstrous" newborn. Two months after delivering a stillborn "monstrosity," Mrs. H descended into a deep depression. Woodward was summoned to treat Mrs. H's "anxiety on account of delayed menstruation, and fear lest she should have another" distressing experience of childbearing. Though this specific anxiety dissipated when her menstrual period began a few days later, she remained profoundly troubled. Woodward discovered that she had taken to sitting "unoccupied," moaning and weeping for hours on end; "nothing could be found to interest her," and her husband and living child now appeared repulsive to her. She struggled to sleep at night, and the only thing that seemed to hold her attention during the day was food: She began to eat constantly and insatiably in a futile attempt to mollify a suddenly boundless appetite.[57]

Months passed with no relief; indeed, her condition continued to worsen. Woodward described her "becoming more frenzied and violent in her behavior," which began to spill out of the confines of private family relation and into more public view. Whereas at first her bouts of visible mental distress were "paroxysmal and seemed to be under control in the presence of strangers," now they were "becoming more and more uncontrollable." Woodward read distress etched in every part of her body: "Her pulse was slow, the skin cool and clammy; the eye was wild and frightened, the face exceeding haggard; the tongue was heavily coated and the bowels constipated." Mrs. H felt her state to be unbearable; Woodward reported that she "beseeched me to do something to save her from herself. She made no threats, but it was evident she could endure in this frame of mind but little longer."[58]

Woodward interpreted Mrs. H's despondence as a reaction to her perceived failure in the role of wife to her husband. He wrote that "her mind seemed to dwell upon her own unworthiness and unfitness for being a wife; her constant moan and cry was—'Oh that I was dead! Oh that I was a girl again! Give me back my youth!'" Ultimately, the doctor felt confident he had figured out the root cause of Mrs. H's distress: an unendurable fear that, following the monstrous birth, she had lost her husband's love. On the brink of committing Mrs. H to an asylum, Woodward first consulted her husband. After asking the husband how much time he devoted to his wife's "company and pleasure," Woodward learned that Mrs. H's husband "hadn't visited with her for more than a year." To Woodward, this offered powerful support of his theory: Her husband's distant and unaffectionate behavior toward her was fueling Mrs. H's fear that she had failed at being his wife, causing her to spiral further and further into desolation.[59]

Woodward instructed Mrs. H's husband that "the cure remains with you. I can do no more." The physician beseeched the husband to "go home and court your wife over again; be as devoted and kind to her as you once was; try that prescription for one week and report." According to Woodward, the renewal of her husband's attention "worked a perfect cure. She is now as light-hearted and joyous as ever; and this was the whole cause—a doubt of his affection existing before her misfortune, and multiplied thereby beyond endurance."[60] In Woodward's account, the experience of monstrous birth had been emotionally upsetting for Mrs. H to the precise extent that she feared its impact on her husband's marital affection for her.

The narration of Mrs. H's emotions was of course heavily mediated through the physician's particular values, priorities, and interpretive frameworks, especially his understanding of the primacy of her gendered role as wife and the duties that role entailed. It is not clear if or how Mrs. H's narration of her own distress might have diverged from the doctor's account—though her quoted words about wanting to die, about wanting to be a girl again, and about wanting her youth back are intriguing not least in that the doctor's proffered interpretation of them does not seem to attend to all possible meanings.

Notably, this narrative did not frame Mrs. H's sadness as a reaction of mourning for the loss of her infant's life. The loss she mourned was, in her physician's interpretation, the loss of her husband's love or, in her own quoted words, the loss of her girlhood and youth. Her physician's interpretation of her grief configured monstrous birth as a perceived reflection of her "unworthiness" and "unfitness" for the gendered role of wife; her own quoted words seemed to configure it as something considerably more complex and poignant, potentially as an ordeal or experience of trauma that cut her off definitively from a younger and lighter-hearted stage of her life ("Oh that I was a girl again!"). In either rendering, the description of Mrs. H's grief did not seem to affectively position the lost child as a family member to be mourned but rather as a fearful disruptor of familial relations: a being whose affect of distance making and alienation was conferred onto the woman who gestated and birthed the monstrous body, cutting her off from her closest kinship ties—and from the happier and less freighted days of her youth.

In most other case reports that included words associated with grief, there was likewise ambiguity related to the source and object of the sadness. The content of many maternal-impression narratives—some of which described women witnessing the injuries or deaths of loved ones during pregnancy—broadly associated the phenomenon of monstrous birth with themes of tragedy, sorrow, and loss. Indeed, numerous physicians cited a woman's experience of grief during pregnancy as a possible cause of monstrous development.[61] Yet the case histories contain very little discussion of mothers' or other family members' grief after the delivery.

Several factors may contextualize the scarcity of references to grief as a reaction to infant death in the case reports. One possible factor relates broadly to historical contexts of nineteenth-century reproduction. This chapter earlier emphasized the idealized depictions of sentimental maternal love and attachment that proliferated in nineteenth-century cultural representation. But for women with large families and little means of safely and reliably limiting or spacing their pregnancies, the actual experience of repeated childbearing could be an ambivalent one; historians of childbirth show that pregnancy loss could evoke widely varied emotions for nineteenth-century women, including "comfort and relief" as well as grief and sorrow.[62] Further, nineteenth-century social scripts and conventions for noting and mourning infant death were forged in settings marked by elevated baseline infant-mortality rates. Because of the lack of standardized national data collection in this era, nineteenth-century infant-mortality rates in the United States are impossible to calculate with precision; however, it is certain that these rates were dramatically higher than they are today.[63] In contexts where infant loss was ubiquitous, it is possible that adults might develop ways to affectively distance themselves from offspring who did not survive early childhood as a way to cope with the frequency and awareness of probable loss.[64] Nineteenth-century sources routinely referred to both preterm and full-term stillborn infants as "foetuses," suggesting a historical understanding of neonates as remaining in a liminal, ambiguous state of fetal being rather than as already constituting fully realized persons.[65] One reason for the surprising scarcity of references to grief and mourning in the case histories, then, could be that present-day expectations and assumptions about the import of neonatal death do not adequately account for divergent historical contexts.

In the specific case of newborns with conditions such as anencephaly, the understanding that the infant's condition precluded survival past early infancy as well as observations of apparent infant suffering may have influenced both families' and attendants' reactions. Descriptions of living newborns with anencephaly often conveyed that these infants appeared to be in distress. Case reports described "cries more like sobs than the ordinary cries of a new-born infant" and reported that attempts at feeding "caused excessive strangling and convulsions." Many recounted infants continually "struggling and gasping" to breathe, which resulted from the absence of brain structures necessary to regulate respiration.[66] Perceptions of inviable life and/or infant suffering may contextualize descriptions of "the relief of the parents" upon the death of an infant with anencephaly some hours or days after birth.[67]

A number of case reports depicted parents as actively encouraging the death of newborns with such conditions. One Indiana physician wrote, "I informed the mother, as the head was being born, that a monstrosity was coming, whereupon she begged me to kill it," though the physician declined to do so. Other practitioners more obliquely recorded suspicions that parents had hoped for and acted to hasten the deaths of offspring, as in the case of Mrs. G in 1850.[68] Such narratives portrayed death as a desired outcome for parents rather than an outcome to be mourned.

At times, physicians highlighted and praised what they described as the medical profession's commitment to always abstaining from infanticide in cases of monstrous birth, contrasting this with female midwives' allegedly universal advocacy of the practice. In the latter nineteenth century, physicians connected these claims to their campaigns to end abortion nationwide, which they framed in part as an assertion of professional medical authority over the pervasive immoral conduct of women and midwives.[69] Conflating abortion and infanticide, some nineteenth-century physicians presented their opposition to infanticide as part of this same demonstration of medical morality over the supposed depravity of laywomen. Not all physicians, however, considered the morality of infanticide in cases of monstrous birth to be a resolved question. In 1883, a medical journal printed a letter of inquiry from a young physician who asked about the "legal, ethical, and moral rights and duties of the accoucheur" in regard to "acephalous monsters" born alive; he reported hearing from "an old practitioner" that "he always at once destroyed life" in these cases.[70]

These discussions make clear that the perceived moral status of monstrous newborns as "lives worth grieving" sometimes appeared to be in question, if not actively in doubt, from the perspective of some of the adults who interacted with them. Indeed, the scientific classification of monstrosity could itself perform the affective work of distancing a child from the position of recognized human subject, explicitly calling their human status into question by placing them outside of "the type of the species."[71] Under Saint-Hilaire's original taxonomy, the classification of teratological monstrosity aligned anomalous newborns with entities unlikely to be constituted as "grievable beings" under any circumstances, including dermoid cysts (large ovarian tumors filled with a motley assortment of tissue types). But even those unfamiliar with the intricacies of French teratological theory could easily understand the affective connotations of the term *monstrosity*: A mid-nineteenth-century textbook warned physicians that it would be "evidently both erroneous and unjust to call a child a monster" on the basis of only minor disfigurements, for "the very word conveys a horrible . . . impression."[72] As not just a professional but also a popular term used to refer to infants with conditions such as anencephaly in this period, the designation *monster* could frame the way that both physicians and laypeople perceived and understood such an infant's death—and perhaps tend to diminish reactions of grief and mourning.

However, another very plausible (and perhaps coexisting) explanation for the absence of recorded grief might be that many mothers and families *did* experience feelings of grief and loss but that physician-authored sources—which constitute the bulk of available historical documentation—are ill-suited for recovering evidence of these feelings. It is possible that physicians tended not to report emotions of grief and mourning in relation to monstrous birth even when such reactions did occur. Perhaps they failed to recognize the affect of grief in contexts where they presumed—or hoped—it would not exist. Whether physicians did so with conscious intent or not, they may have had ample motive to downplay and ignore expressions of parental grief in these cases. The positioning of anomalous infants as children to be mourned sat in tension with the professional imperative of obtaining, classifying, and producing these infants' bodies as teratological monstrosities. By denying the possibility that these newborns evoked parental grief, physicians could ease the way for the professional activities they wished to pursue.

Certain nineteenth-century institutions rendered the bodies of some infants already available to physicians. Within the system of chattel slavery, which configured an enslaved mother's body as property and violently denied the bonds of her kinship to her children, a physician needed no excuse to "obtain possession" of any "interesting specimen" he desired to seize for professional gain.[73] But when tending to middle- and upper-class white women, whose cultural identities as mothers were constructed around love and sentimental attachment to their children, physicians could make these infants "available" as specimens only by affectively displacing them as children to be mourned.

To physically transform a newborn body into an anatomical specimen of monstrosity, practitioners needed first to obtain from the family custody of the remains—a practice that tended to preclude any mourning rituals centered on the body of the deceased. Typically, the seamless narration of the nineteenth-century case history served to smooth over the negotiated vagaries and, in some instances, the violence of this process. However, every so often, an experience of friction—a family's refusal to part with the bodily remains of their infant—briefly illuminates the obscured social and affective dimensions of this process in the written historical record. A careful reading of these case histories supports the idea that some parents felt an affective attachment to their "monstrous" infants and a grief at their passing that went largely unappreciated and unacknowledged by the physician.

Descriptions of physicians' sometimes-thwarted attempts to "get the consent of the parents to take the child" suggests that the need to affirmatively secure consent constituted a recognized part of nineteenth-century practice (and not an anachronistic imposition of twenty-first-century expectations).[74] However, this imperative seems to have applied only to patients with certain kinds of social status. Out of a sample of twenty case reports that recorded successful parental refusal, most involved married, middle- or upper-class, US-born mothers, referred to as "ladies" and identified with racial descriptors such as "Anglo-Saxon" and "white, of good personal and family history."[75] There were a couple of notable exceptions, including a German immigrant woman in Chicago who did not speak English but who communicated along with her husband their refusal to allow the physician to "procure" their infant's remains and an unmarried teenaged mother named "Mary M.," who would not grant permission for a postmortem dissection of her infant.[76] But although exceptions like these existed, the overall pattern of evidence points to the aggregate gendered, racial, and class-based prerogatives that usually underwrote a family's ability to successfully refuse permission.

One such report, published in 1854 by the North Carolina physician N. C. Skinner, involved a married white patient named as Mrs. Ch. B. After ten hours of "alarmingly severe" pains, followed by a large dose of physician-administered chloroform, Mrs. B gave birth to a living infant described by Skinner as a "singular foetal malformation." Mrs. B attempted to breastfeed her child but noted the next day that the newborn had "not yet shown a disposition to nurse." When the infant died a few days later, Mrs. B and her husband refused Skinner's request to "procure the specimen for preservation" and further denied him permission to perform a postmortem examination of the body. Skinner attributed the refusal to "the very great (and natural) prejudices of the parents."[77] Although he did not elaborate further, it can be inferred that taking away the body would clash with parental imperatives regarding the respectful treatment and perhaps the burial and mourning of the infant's bodily remains.

Two late nineteenth-century case reports suggest further insight into affective dimensions of parental refusal. In one report, the physician wrote, "I was extremely anxious to obtain possession of the child in order to submit it for your inspection, but as this conflicted with the religious convictions of the parents I was unable to do so." In another report, this time involving conjoined twins (described by the physician as "a double monstrosity") who died shortly after delivery, the physician recounted, "I tried very hard to get the parents to give me the child, but I could not get it. They would not even let me have its picture taken, and they buried the child at one corner of the garden for fear I would have it taken up."[78] While the physician interpreted the act of burial primarily as an effort to thwart his own acquisitive desires, a burial can certainly also be interpreted as a classic ritual of mourning.

In these instances of recorded parental refusal, it seems quite possible that an understanding of these infants as constituting "lives worth grieving," as kin worth mourning, motivated the parents' actions. Further, the scarcity of references to obtaining permission in case reports involving more socially marginalized parents, in conjunction with broader nineteenth-century histories of documented racial violence and exploitation—including the widespread appropriation of Black and Indigenous remains—strongly suggests that many mothers were never given an opportunity to refuse. These mothers—enslaved, impoverished, or institutionalized women who were almost certainly never afforded the option to deny a white male physician's demand—were no less likely to have grieved the deaths of infants they were never given an opportunity to bury.

At these varied interfaces of postpartum encounter, then, affective practices positioned "monstrous" offspring in ambivalent ways. Visual and auditory encounters, practices of caregiving, modes and boundaries of physical touch, and reactions to infant death all served to locate and materialize the meanings of newborn bodies, configuring biological monstrosity as a category of simultaneous kinship and alienation.

These infants occupied an ambiguous and even paradoxical affective space: They elicited some but not all conventions of care, recognition, and emotional response associated with "typical" infant subjects in these contexts. Certain boundaries and modes of emotional and sensory relation—whether concealment from maternal sight, the denial of breastfeeding contact by a mother, or a physician's aggressive experimental touch—seemed to demote these infants' affective and relational status as human offspring, even as traditional rituals of infant caregiving and attachment appeared to affirm that status. If, as the theorist Margrit Shildrick writes, the monster is a being who is simultaneously "other" and "all too human"—that which is "not simply alien, but always arouses the contradictory response of denial *and* recognition, disgust *and* empathy, exclusion *and* identification"—then these practices constituted anomalous newborn bodies as truly monstrous.[79] In this way, the medical configuration of bodies as monstrous occurred in the birthing room as much as in the dissecting room, beginning well before practitioners started the physical process of transforming them into medical specimens of monstrosity.

CHAPTER THREE

Monstrous Specimens

Material Cultures of Collection and Display

Indexed as Accession 05820, the tiny cranium is more than one and a half centuries old.[1] Reflecting the passage of the years, much of the bone's variegated surface is now an ombre of deep yellowy oranges and browns, with patches of off-white that stipple the lower jaw and both sides of the nasal cavity. Two slender arches project above the orbital sockets, marking the highest point of the distinctly foreshortened cranium. The skull is affixed to a thin black rod that is oriented vertically and anchored in a small, rounded pedestal, prepared for a practice of professional visual display in a bygone era.[2]

These preserved cranial bones constitute the last bodily remains of a historical infant with anencephaly, born in 1859 to a woman in Dorchester, Massachusetts. The Dorchester of the late 1850s, in contrast to its present-day iteration as the largest and most diverse neighborhood in the city of Boston, was a "streetcar suburb," home to increasing numbers of wealthy white Protestants who flocked there from the city following the introduction of railroad lines and an electric tram service. Oliver Wendell Holmes Sr., in the years before embarking on his storied medical career, penned a well-known poem about the town's iconic "pudding-stone": distinctive rocky outcroppings that abounded in Dorchester and nearby Roxbury, their dark, multisize pebbles embedded in a matrix of stone like ossified lumps of fruit in a pudding.[3]

One of Holmes's colleagues, the physician Edward D. Miller, attended the woman in her labor. It was the twenty-four-year-old woman's first pregnancy. She had menstruated quite regularly before conceiving and could confidently date the start of gestation from her first missed period, which occurred soon after she married. About five months later, the woman felt the first indistinct fetal motions—the moment of "quickening" that marked the definitive confirmation of pregnancy in this era—and excitedly shared the news with her mother.[4]

The young woman gave birth in the fall. The labor was not an easy one; it lasted for twenty-four hours, and the infant's shoulders "came with some difficulty." The physician Miller described the stillborn child, who had a partial skull but "no trace of a brain," as an "acephalous foetus," which referred to a variant of anencephaly.[5] Just a few months after the delivery of her stillborn infant, the woman experienced another harrowing loss: the death of her beloved mother.

While the woman grappled with loss, the birth occasioned for her physician a professional gain. Miller obtained and presented the infant's body to members of the Boston Society for Medical Improvement (BSMI), an elite professional association that comprised leading Boston physicians such as Holmes. These practitioners eagerly prepared, exhibited, and cataloged the infant's remains in the Monstrosities Division of the society's sprawling anatomical specimen collections.

The Boston physicians began by performing a dissection, perhaps aided by student trainees at Harvard Medical School, where numerous society members taught as professors. The practice of dissection in this era constituted a central feature of American medical education, where its routinization helped desensitize practitioners to the intimate contact with bodily tissues and fluids that their professional activities often required.[6] In lectures, Holmes spoke rapturously of the "anthropotomic laboratory, known to common speech as the dissecting-room," which he described, with characteristic poetic flourish, as "that apartment of the temple of science where nature is seen in undress." According to Holmes, a sufficiently gifted educator could render the dissecting room "the sunniest of studios in spite of its mortuary spectacles."[7] Yet the men preparing the infant's remains may have been more struck by the studio's characteristic odor—a "putrid" and "exceedingly offensive" stench infamous for turning stomachs in the years before the advent of formalin (a fixative introduced in the late nineteenth century to prevent rapid tissue decay during dissection).[8] To protect themselves from cuts and the looming threat of deadly infection, practitioners were advised to wear sleeved aprons, smear their hands with lard or oil, and carefully cover sores with adhesive dressings.[9]

To perform the dissection, practitioners cut open the body and methodically separated the soft matter—flesh, muscle, nerves, connective tissue, viscera—from the hard matter of the bones. After exposing and clearing away an amorphous mass of tissue at the base of the Dorchester infant's skull, they isolated and prepared their cranium as a specimen of monstrosity.[10] Such preparations typically began with days of injecting, chilling, soaking, and draining the hard tissue, followed by months of immersing the treated skeletal tissue in a fastidiously maintained and retitrated solution of water mixed with a corrosive acid. After the bones were removed from the solution and dried, they could be suspended in oil of turpentine, varnished, reassembled, and mounted for display.[11]

Imbricated with these bluntly material dimensions of their labor, practitioners also claimed the dissecting room as a site for elucidating abstracted scientific knowledge. Seeking insight into the development of the nervous system, the Boston physicians carefully examined the abbreviated nerves that appeared to proceed from the "bulging spinal marrow" at the base of the Dorchester infant's skull. They excitedly noted the discovery of an intact pituitary gland—a structure that the French scientist Geoffroy Saint-Hilaire, in his seminal treatises on teratology (the "scientific study of monstrosity"), seemed to suggest did not develop in such cases.[12]

The resulting preparation was presented at one of the BSMI's regular meetings, which often entailed the exhibition of anatomical specimens to an audience of New England's most prominent physicians. Afterward, the preserved skull joined the BSMI's Anatomical Cabinet. In addition to skeletal "dry specimens" like this one, the cabinet's extensive nineteenth-century Monstrosities Division included drawings, paintings, plaster casts, wax models, and—perhaps most strikingly—abundant soft-tissue "wet specimens," which consisted mainly of infant bodies and organs sealed in containers of preservative fluid.[13]

When Holmes sought to convey the power of science to demystify monstrosity, he turned to this iconic image of a specimen contained in a jar of preservative fluid. "People used always to be terribly frightened by those irregular vital products which we now call 'interesting specimens' and carefully preserve in jars of alcohol," he wrote.[14] The entity of the anatomical *specimen*, a term derived from the Latin root *spectare*, "to look," linked the dominion of medical science to the capacity to see and make visible. Gazing at an anatomical specimen today can still proffer the sense of getting to see an objective biological reality, the clear-glass canisters allowing an ostensibly unmediated look at the preserved remains inside. With its emphasis on visual transparency, the preparation promises to lay bare the truth of the anatomized body before the viewer's penetrating eyes. The arrangement of the specimen jar works to isolate and expose the body of the monster—and to conceal the relational presence and embodied labor of the people who produced it.

In the present day, controversies over the display and stewardship of human remains abound. Museums publicly grapple with questions about how to exhibit remains without recapitulating an exploitative, objectifying, or dehumanizing gaze. Staff, scholars, and descendent communities attempt to reckon with the searing histories of bodily dispossession, scientific racism, and colonial violence that frequently underly the accessions of historical anatomical collections. Institutions face increasing pressure to attend to the ethical as well as the legal imperatives to know the provenance of the human remains in their custody—a mandate to consider the social and political contexts of the remains' acquisition and the lives of the people and communities from whom they derived.[15]

This mandate for context stands in stark contrast to the historical logic of teratological specimen creation. Producing bodies as specimens of monstrosity involved a process of pointed *de*contextualization that abstracted infants from their disparate familial origins—as well as from the social and power relations that rendered their remains available to professional physicians—and reconstituted them as generic referents of a universal biological type. Earlier chapters recontextualized such specimens in the circumstances of their birth and the worlds of the women who bore them. This chapter offers further contextualization, showing anatomical specimen preparations not as neutral and unmediated presentations of an objective biological reality but rather as contingent productions made within the particular physical, relational, institutional, and cultural worlds of nineteenth-century medical science. Just as social, narrative, and affective practices actively configured newborn bodies as monstrosities in the space of the birthing room, the concretely material practices of specimen preparation actively configured the monstrosity of their remains.

The chapter begins with a broad diachronic overview tracing the institutional collection of specimens of monstrosity in the nineteenth-century United States. It then delves into more vividly corporeal details of this history, revealing the messy material and sensory terrains on which physicians constructed and affirmed authority over monstrous bodies. The preparation and interpretation of such bodies entailed both embodied labor and the exercise of epistemological power. The chapter explores how practitioners dissected infant remains, transformed them into a wide variety of "wet" and "dry" specimen preparations, and rendered them legible to a "plurisensorial medical gaze" that encompassed both sight and touch in professional practices of pedagogy and display. It concludes by discussing how physicians engaged this multisensory authority over monstrous specimens to produce scientific knowledge more broadly about the nature of human bodies and deviance.

Producing and exhibiting specimens thus composed a multisensory process of making monsters visible on both physical and conceptual levels, reforging their remains as a text that could be read for "physiological truth" by the expert eyes of a largely white, male medical profession.[16] Through these activities, practitioners materialized the meanings of monstrosity as a condition of biological deviance and furthered their professional claims to authority over the anatomized human body.

SPECIMEN COLLECTION: A BROAD OVERVIEW

Across the nineteenth-century United States, medical institutions persistently created and amassed specimens of monstrosity for pedagogy and display. Practitioners presented these specimens at professional society meetings, exhibited them as accessions of medical museums, and used them to teach anatomy to students in medical schools.[17] As earlier chapters have shown, physicians obtained newborns' bodily remains through distinctive nineteenth-century practices and institutions that brought them into contact with diverse childbearing women, including rising obstetric attendance in private middle- and upper-class homes; new birthing locations such as lying-in hospitals and maternity wards, which primarily served poor patients in large cities; and medical participation in exploitative systems, such as racial slavery and imperialism, that exercised authority over marginalized women's reproduction.[18] For especially prominent institutional collections, the acquisition of infant remains might also implicate a spatially expansive network of exchange that crossed disparate regions of the nation and beyond.[19]

Monstrous specimens held many kinds of value for practitioners, who declared their general collection activities to be "forever devoted to the promotion of medical science."[20] A specimen might bolster an individual career or solidify relationships through a practice of professional gift giving. Leading physicians averred that large specimen collections could advance the status of institutions or even the international standing of American medicine.[21] Most abstractly but perhaps most enticingly, the production and display of monstrous specimens could expand professional authority by deepening medical knowledge of biological bodies.

In the first half of the nineteenth century, large US institutional collections with monstrous specimens were often located in Northeastern cities such as Boston, Philadelphia, and New York, reflecting the concentrated distribution of the nation's sparse professional apparatus in this period. Collections featuring monstrosities also existed in the antebellum South, where medical schools and professional societies amassed anatomical specimens in large part through the seizure of enslaved people's remains.[22] Likely the most elaborate collection of monstrous specimens in this era could be found in the Boston Society for Medical Improvement Anatomical Cabinet, later absorbed into Harvard Medical School's Warren Anatomical Museum.

Founded in 1828, the BSMI was an association of New England physicians, one of only a small number of professional medical associations that existed in the United States at this time. BSMI's membership comprised white Anglo-American men from New England's most elite social class, including physicians such as Holmes, Walter Channing, J. B. S. Jackson, Jacob Bigelow, John Collins Warren, and George Shattuck. Society members served as deans of Harvard's medical faculty, founded Boston hospitals, and launched the *Boston Journal of Medicine and Surgery* (precursor of the *New England Journal of Medicine*). BSMI members came together regularly "on a sort of medico-social basis" to discuss cases and exhibit anatomical specimens of particular interest in well-attended meetings that led to "the promotion of good feeling as well as of medical science."[23] If exhibited specimens were deemed to be of sufficient quality and interest, they would then be added to the Anatomical Cabinet and written up as case reports for medical journals, affording a prized "opportunity for speaking and publishing" for physicians in the early nineteenth century. BSMI's self-image traded in both the cultured gentility of upper-class New England society and the "ever unemotional" rigor of the idealized man of science, whose "steady, undeviating progress" was "unruffled by stirring events and men." The group declared a general dedication to advancing the cause of "scientific medicine," predicated on an expansion of its institutional and cultural authority, in American society more broadly.[24]

BSMI physicians' position as elite white men was formative, not incidental, to their professional activities and assertions of authority. Although many BSMI physicians opposed racial slavery, they were nevertheless invested in and to different degrees helped to perpetuate racial and ethnic hierarchy, in part through specimen-collection activities that produced, circulated, and legitimated concepts of innate biological difference between human populations. This was perhaps most overtly evidenced in the BSMI's National Skulls collection, which purported to document characteristic anatomical differences between racialized groups. But BSMI physicians also invoked imaginaries of human racial alterity to characterize specimens in their expansive Monstrosities Division—a collection that grew large enough to support the publication of its own separate indexing catalog in the 1840s.[25]

As the century progressed, the scope of US monstrous specimen collection extended far beyond elite groups in Northeastern cities such as Boston, reflecting more general trends in the proliferation of medical institutions. By the mid–nineteenth century, a variety of medical sects, each competing to assert itself in a pluralistic marketplace of practitioners, had established their own medical associations and credentialing schools. Practitioners of what their competitors termed *allopathic medicine*—the self-proclaimed "regular practitioners," who would go on to consolidate professional authority in the late nineteenth and early twentieth centuries—frequently engaged in the institutional display and collection of specimens of monstrosity, as did practitioners of homeopathic medicine and eclectic medicine.[26] This heterogenous group of midcentury physicians exhibited specimens of monstrosity to medical societies and medical museums in states across the Midwestern, Northeastern, and Southern regions of the United States.[27] By the 1870s and 1880s, exhibitions occurred at professional meetings spanning the coasts, from the San Francisco Medical Society in California to the Texas State Medical Association to the New York Obstetrical Society.[28]

In the later nineteenth century, the national scope of professional interest in monstrous specimens was affirmed by the National Museum of Health and Medicine, founded in 1862 as the Army Medical Museum. After the Civil War, the federally funded museum began to solicit specimens from "practitioners in civil life" across the United States, explicitly linking the development of the museum's collection to "the progress of the [medical] profession." Curator John Shaw Billings enjoined "every medical man in this country" to send at least one specimen, naming "monstrosities and malformations" as one of the institution's "special wants." Physicians from around the nation responded to the call.[29]

As late nineteenth-century conceptions of professional identity increasingly tied medical authority to ideals of scientific knowledge production, the American medical interest in monstrosity—which had long engaged transatlantic sciences of teratology, embryology, and anatomy—persisted.[30] In the 1890s, the University of Pennsylvania's Wistar and Horner Museum proudly claimed to have the premiere teratological collection in the nation. Positioning teratological collection as a key to "the development of scientific medicine in this country" and a potential point of national pride, the curator and obstetrics professor Barton Hirst wrote that "if members of the profession continue to contribute as generously as they have, we will soon have one of the finest collections in the world." Specimens entered the collection through a sprawling network of physicians that spanned the United States and beyond, reflecting transnational professional relationships as well as the expansion of the informal (and by 1898 formal) US imperial presence abroad.[31] By the end of the nineteenth century, substantial collections of anatomical specimens could also be found in medical museums associated with institutions such as Rush University Medical College in Chicago, Tulane University in New Orleans, and the Cincinnati Hospital.[32] In the Gulf Coast city of Galveston, the University of Texas Medical Department began to amass its sizable anatomical and pathological collections soon after its founding in 1891. The collections grew to include numerous specimens of monstrosity, such as an "anencephalic monster" born to a twenty-two-year-old woman afflicted by a "maternal infection" during pregnancy and a "monster with two fully developed heads" born to a forty-year-old woman.[33]

While practitioners engaged in monstrous-specimen collection varied in their class and regional backgrounds, the majority across this history consisted of white Protestant men, consistent with the demographic makeup of the systemically exclusionary medical profession. There were at least a few exceptions: Dr. Theresa Bannan, one of thousands of women practicing as credentialed physicians in the late nineteenth-century United States, presented a "case of monstrosity" to the Onondaga County Medical Society in 1894; Dr. Sara Welt-Kakels displayed a "twelve-weeks' fetus" with anencephaly before the New York Academy of Medicine in 1896.[34] Dr. Thaddeus Taylor "exhibited a foetal monstrosity, upon which quite a lengthy discussion of maternal impression was held" at a state chapter meeting of the National Medical Association, an organization of African American physicians founded in 1895 in response to pervasive institutionalized racism in the profession.[35] Overall, however, the professional collection and display of monstrous specimens remained a practice performed primarily by white men, whose claims to authoritatively displaying and interpreting the human body were grounded in part in claims to racial and gendered forms of social and political power.

SENSORY TERRAINS OF THE DISSECTING ROOM

The preceding overview provides important context regarding the institutional collection of specimens. But while this overview tells us much about where and by whom specimens were collected, it tells us rather little about the specimens themselves. Alone, it leaves unanswered critical questions about how medical specimens configured monstrous bodies and conferred epistemological authority. To engage these questions, the rest of the chapter turns to a more vivid and granular consideration of embodied practice, delving deeply into the material processes of medical monster making.

Previous chapters revealed how narrative and affective practices surrounding childbirth could configure the monstrosity of newborn bodies in birthing rooms and family homes, distancing infants from the status of human child, kin, and grievable moral subject. The practices of specimen preparation furthered this affective transformation of an infant's body into monstrous specimen but also added new, distinctly material dimensions to the transformation. Belying the presentation of the finished specimen as an unmediated depiction of the body's objective reality, these practices reveal the intricate physical, embodied, and sensory work that was required to turn bodily remains into an anatomical specimen.

This exploration takes us first into the multisensory terrains of the dissecting room, a space intimately connected to specimen making. Many types of specimens, including preparations of individual organs or skeletal tissue, required extensive dissection prior to preservation. The dissection of bodily remains represented a prominent and distinctive feature of general nineteenth-century medical education in the United States.[36] By the 1830s, dissection's role in medical training was pronounced enough to warrant the publication of multiple book-length instruction manuals, written by medical school professors at leading American universities.[37]

The activity of dissection constituted both an abstract epistemological practice—a way of knowing and interpreting the human body as pathoanatomical entity, reducible to its discrete constituent parts—and a concretely physical one. Manuals described a process of begetting specimens that demanded "long protracted labour and pains to finish"—a process where the practitioner's authority to cut open and prepare the bodies of others did not obviate his own vulnerabilities of embodiment. In a manual published in 1831, a section on "diseases occasioned by dissections" brought into sharp relief the bodily liabilities endemic to specimen preparation. The author warned of "derangement of the stomach" as well as "extensive and severe inflammation from slight wounds of the fingers." Ameliorating these concerns drew a physician's attention to both his embodied person and the environment in which he labored: Afflictions were to be prevented through means that involved a diet of "nutricious [*sic*] well seasoned food" and "attention to the air of the room both as respects temperature and cleanliness."[38]

While the aims of specimen preparation centered the visuality of the final product, the processes of dissection entailed, for practitioners, sensory experiences that both included and extended beyond the realm of sight. Dissecting rooms were infamous for their strong and unpleasant olfactory landscapes. Prior to dissection, remains were first treated with a hardening agent for preservation (favored compounds in the earlier nineteenth century included "white oxide of arsenic," "muriate of mercury," "nitrate of potash," and a simple solution of alcohol), but this did not entirely prevent tissue decay and its attendant odors. Mid-nineteenth-century manuals were straightforward on this point: "The air of rooms, where dead bodies are kept, as well as the walls and furniture, become exceedingly offensive," one stated. A caution about "putrid inhalations" made a similar point. Manuals instructed dissectors to keep a sponge on hand so that their dissecting table did not "become foul from blood or pieces of flesh standing on it" and offered technical advice on how to stave off rapid putrefaction of "the parts exposed" in the course of cutting a body open.[39]

Recommendations for mitigating the "diseases occasioned by dissection" likewise reflected an environment in which overwhelming odors were a prominent concern. These recommendations included keeping the dissecting room "freely ventilated"; sponging the cleared cavities of the body with "clean water" and sprinkling them "with chlorate of lime"; "never visiting nor remaining in the dissecting room with an empty stomach"; and taking "considerable exercise of the body in the open air" in between sessions.[40] To mask the odors in the dissecting room, some nineteenth-century medical students took to delegating one member of the dissecting team to continually smoke cigarettes or cigars while the others worked on the body.[41] By the turn of the twentieth century, technologies to prevent tissue decomposition had improved enough that the University of Texas Medical Department felt comfortable claiming (whether fully honestly or not) that its use of "thoroughly preserved" remains kept the dissecting room "free from offensive odors."[42]

In published case histories by physicians—unlike in practical guide manuals to dissection—the odors of dissection were rarely discussed. However, case reports that narrated the process of dissection often described or implied sensory experiences of touch, offering insights into explicitly tactile processes of dissection. In narrating dissections, physicians characterized the haptic qualities as well as the visual appearance of different structures they encountered. They described the "soft" texture of brain convolutions, the "rather spongy texture" of kidneys, and the "thickened, fleshy look and feel" of intestines. Reports variously described tissues of the body as "smooth and polished," "thickened and rough," "exceedingly thin and delicate," "coarse," "firm," "solid," and "gelatinous" in texture and consistency.[43]

In the case literature on monstrosity, narratives of dissection conjured and semantically configured a linked experience of touch and sight, portraying a process where physicians engaged with the tactility of the body to render it visible. In an 1881 report, the Ohio physician D. C. Lichliter described dissecting a stillborn infant with anencephaly, born to a woman who recounted experiencing two severe frights early in her pregnancy. Lichliter narrated the dissection in this way: "Upon making an incision through this membrane we exposed the spinal cord which was in appearance and reality flattened antero-posteriorly, but to all appearance possessed of its proper anatomical parts. . . . Carrying my incision upward to and through the much thicker membrane covering the cephalic tumor, we revealed to view the placental brain substance found in such monsters. Allowing my knife to pass deeply into the body of the tumor, several points of white brain substance were to be seen."[44]

In each sentence, the physician's tactile action served to render a part of the body visible. Something was "revealed to view" in consequence of "carrying my incision upward to and through the much thicker membrane"; something was able "to be seen" after "allowing my knife to pass deeply into the body of the tumor." The language specifically emphasized both the tactile elements of the lacerative process (the thickness of the incised membrane, the depth of the knife's passage into the body of the tumor), and the visuality of its consequence (allowing parts to be "revealed to view" and "to be seen"). The material processes of dissection thus engaged at the outset a variety of sensory modes in the medical transformation of remains into specimens of monstrosity.

MATERIAL CULTURES OF SPECIMEN PRODUCTION

The scope and nature of a dissection varied based on the type of specimen preparation practitioners wished to create. Phrases such as "preserved entire in spirit" could depict certain kinds of specimen making as a relatively uninvolved process that simply froze an intact body in time, conserving it just as it existed.[45] In reality, however, all methods of tissue preparation entailed numerous physical treatments and transformations. Preparation manuals and details from individual case reports suggest the granular details of the work that went into configuring bodily tissues as anatomical specimens. Each body, at minimum, needed to be injected, soaked, pretreated with a fixative and hardening agent, and "cleared of all unnecessary matter." Hollow parts and cavities were to be packed with "curled hair, wool, cotton, or the like" or, for smaller vessels, "exhibited by the introduction of bristles, quills, or bougies." These materials were to be left in for seven to ten days, until the tissue hardened around them, and then removed. Practitioners manipulated bodies in ways designed to visually emphasize particular parts or systems; for example, one later nineteenth-century case history described "injecting the vessels with a colored solution" to better visualize them.[46]

Perhaps the most iconic way of preparing a monstrous specimen involved preserving the body whole. Small "foetal" bodies (a word that nineteenth-century practitioners used to refer to full-term as well as preterm neonates) could easily fit intact in modest-size containers. In case reports, numerous physicians recorded hesitancy to make fuller dissections for fear of "destroying" or detracting from the holistic look of the specimen, thereby diluting its full visual impact when exhibited.[47] A Maryland physician in 1846 explained that he abstained from dissection in order to present "the specimen entire . . . as a present for the distinguished Professor of Obstetrics in the University of Pennsylvania." In an 1860 specimen exhibition before the BSMI, the presenting physician noted that the membrane covering the spine and cranial area "was not disturbed when making the dissection, as the *toute ensemble* of the monster would thereby have been injured before exhibiting to the Society."[48] These statements conveyed that monstrosity was best represented, in the words of the latter case, "toute ensemble"—that what was most essential about monstrosity might be lost or degraded if the monstrous body were broken down into constituent parts. Indeed, the medical definition of monstrosity, specifying an "extreme departure" from the "type" of the parental species that was "apparent on external view," explicitly predicated the diagnosis on holistic visual impression.[49]

Yet this directive to prepare the monstrous body as an undivided whole sometimes appeared to be in tension with an ascendant medical cosmology that increasingly conceptualized the human body as a series of separable organs, emphasizing dissection into discrete parts as key to understanding health and disease.[50] In the later decades of the nineteenth century, the practice of whole-body preparation sometimes came under criticism on exactly these grounds: An 1882 case history decried the "narrow-mindedness of museum curators who are satisfied with a general description of the exterior and are then content to suspend the specimens in jars," admonishing that "without a thorough dissection of the internal parts nothing, as to the causes producing deformity, can be determined." In 1888, the prominent physician John Shaw Billings, speaking on anatomical collection more generally, noted that "the kind of specimens most valued for illustrating anatomy in a museum is now very different from what was sought for in the first half of this century." He described increased demand for more elaborately deconstructed specimen preparations, including minute sections of thinly-sliced tissue mounted for microscopical examination.[51]

However, numerous late nineteenth-century case reports of monstrosity suggested that many physicians still felt an imperative, in the words of one 1882 report, to "preserve the specimen as nearly intact as possible." In 1889, at an exhibition before the New York Obstetrical Society, a physician explained that "no dissection was made, as it was desired to present the specimen with its original features." A Philadelphia physician in 1892 described how he "carefully sewed up" a dissected specimen so that the body appeared intact when added to a medical museum collection.[52] Despite a rising emphasis on studying the elaborately deconstructed interiors of bodies, these late nineteenth-century physicians continued to take pains in preservation to foreground the holistic exterior look that buttressed the classification of monstrosity, underscoring the quintessential visuality of the category.[53]

Beyond whole "foetal" bodies preserved intact, soft-tissue preparations took many other forms as well: individual organs or structures separated out in the course of dissection or infant bodies halved in the sagittal plane, positioned flush against the edge of the glass container to reveal the exposed organs inside.[54] Consistent with an emphasis on understanding the body through its breakdown into discrete constituent parts, these more deconstructed monstrous specimens might consist of isolated organs such as kidneys, renal capsules, bladder, spleen, lungs, heart, or eyes.[55] Before preservation, each individual organ was to be separated, injected, and arranged in a particular way, designed to achieve an organ-specific visual effect. For instance, manuals instructed that the stomach should be inverted "to show its vascular and villous coat."[56] As in all their specimen preparation activities, practitioners manipulated tissues in ways that configured and made visible the features they deemed most essential to conveying the "truth" of the body.

To finish creating a "wet specimen," whether whole or part, practitioners suspended soft-tissue remains within a glass canister, carefully selected for "the right size and figure" and filled with a clear preservative fluid. A commonly used method involved suspending the preparation by a thread, which was "brought over the rim of the glass, and fastened to another, round the neck." Another recommended method for positioning the remains involved the use of a glass float—but not, one manual warned, a cork float, as this was "apt to colour the spirits" and cloud the fluid's visual transparency.[57] As suggested by the reference to "spirits," earlier nineteenth-century specimen preparations used distilled alcohol as a preservative fluid, sometimes mixed with oils, alkalines, or acids. Later in the century, solutions of formaldehyde, including formalin (a 42 percent solution), came into use. A New York physician in 1894 praised the "marked hardening qualities" of the newly commercially available preservative, noting approvingly that "it is cheaper than alcohol, it causes little or no shrinkage, and bleaches the specimens but little."[58] Formalin turned out to be far more effective than alcohol for long-lasting preservation; some historical collections today still include remains prepared in formalin more than a century ago.

A second major mode of tissue preservation, which did not require permanent storage in preservative fluid, entailed preparing skeletal material as "dry specimens." This mode likewise implicated a lengthy and intricate material process. After "denuding the bony frame-work of skin and muscle," practitioners spent days injecting, chilling, soaking, and draining the remains, then months of submerging the preparation in a carefully maintained and retitrated solution of corrosive acid.[59] Once the bones had lain "in the liquor a sufficient length of time to complete the process of removing the earthy part" and "assume a beautiful transparency," they could be removed, allowed to air dry, and immersed in a glass jar filled with oil of turpentine. (Manuals cautioned that the resulting preparation "should be kept from the heat of the sun, which is very liable to burst vessels filled with oil of turpentine.") The delicate skeletal tissue "of a foetus or of a young child" was particularly well disposed to "demonstrate the vascularity of bone" after treatment with turpentine.[60] The bones could afterward be varnished for protection, although this often proved insufficient to keep away insects.

If sturdy enough, dry specimens might then be mounted and posed. For specimens of monstrosity, this sometimes involved arranging fetal and newborn skeletons in a straightened position and posing them vertically, as if standing fully upright, using an assortment of rods or small pillars for support.[61] Several nineteenth-century skeletal specimens of monstrosity, prepared from the remains of infants birthed by well-to-do Boston mothers, remain in the collection of the Warren Anatomical Museum today. In one, the tiny, varnished bones have been arranged in a vertical position and braced with a discreet support column against the far wooden edge of a little glass-front box. In another, the diminutive skeleton of an infant born months before term has likewise been posed and mounted to "stand" vertically; though an attempt was made to straighten the spine through bracing with a thin vertical support, the reconstructed torso curves to the side, hinting at the position of a fetus inside the mother's womb. In a third preparation, a set of tiny, separated cranial bones and cervical vertebrae are neatly arranged in a shallow wooden drum; the lid can be removed for access to the array of little pieces inside, upward of twenty in total.[62]

THE MULTISENSORIAL MEDICAL GAZE AND THE SPECTACLE OF SPECIMENS

In dissecting and preparing bodies, physicians rendered monsters visible in ways that underscored the rising (if often still aspirational) professional authority of medicine to see and know the truth of the human body. The significance of vision in modern medical discourse is perhaps most famously encapsulated in the philosopher Michel Foucault's concept of the "modern medical gaze."[63] Representing a distinctively new way of structuring knowledge and exercising power, the medical gaze produced the object-body of the patient as a source of hidden truth, a collection of localized signs to be expertly appraised and interpreted by the physician's penetrating perception.

While the idea of the medical gaze is understandably taken to foreground the sensory primacy of vision, in Foucault's original formulation it encompassed a far broader range of sensory fields "than is said by the word 'gaze' alone." The medical gaze instead constituted a "plurisensorial structure" that contained, cohered, and governed other modes of sensory perception, coalescing "into a sovereign unity that which belongs to a lower level of the eye, the ear, and the sense of touch." Through this "absolute, absolutely integrating" gaze, the expert practitioner could perceive, gauge, and bring to the surface the concealed meanings of the pathoanatomical body, projecting the data of life onto "the plane of absolute visibility."[64]

Foucault's schematic positions the emergence of medical modernity as a sharp and clearly demarcated epistemological break from the past, suggesting a radical discontinuity of eras that is difficult to perceive in the messy continuum of day-to-day embodied historical practice. Nevertheless, invoked as a broad analytic heuristic, the concept of the plurisensorial medical gaze helps contextualize and explain how nineteenth-century physicians engaged multiple senses to claim authority over monstrous bodies and render them visually legible through cultures of specimen making and display.

In practices of medical spectacle, monstrous specimens were subject to a plurisensorial gaze that both encompassed and exceeded the field of sight, integrating linked sensory modes of visual, tactile, and even olfactory revelation. The majority of nineteenth-century medical specimens were made to be both looked at and touched. Most were intended not to be permanently displayed behind glass in medical museums but as objects that could be viewed, taken out of their containers, and passed around by medical students and practitioners.[65] The visual and tactile qualities of the specimen enrolled it within larger pedagogical and epistemological projects of nineteenth-century medical science, including an increasing emphasis on "object-teaching" in medical training and education. These pedagogical activities foregrounded an entanglement of visual and haptic perception in which students were taught to "habitually think in terms of vision as interpreted by touch."[66] An 1884 case history described how a medical professor "laid open" the bodily remains of a preserved specimen before his medical students at Bellevue Hospital and led them through a partial dissection, enrolling the students not just in the visual apprehension but also in the tactile exploration of the monstrous body. The University of Texas Medical Department noted that its specimen collections, beginning in the 1890s, were "continually used in class-room demonstration"; school officials emphasized that "students and physicians have access to the shelves at all times" and that "many loose specimens are also constantly available for the purpose of study."[67]

This multisensory access to anatomized bodies played an important role in medical pedagogy, training, and professional formation and served in part to distinguish the privileged authority of the medical practitioner. Especially later in the century, a number of nineteenth-century medical schools and hospitals allowed the public in to look at specimens displayed in their museum collections, inviting laypeople to participate in the visual experience of anatomical exhibition.[68] But the more integrative and intimate multisensorial apprehension of specimens was reserved for practitioners and trainees in medical school classrooms, anatomical laboratories, and other nonpublic spaces of professional pedagogy and practice.

The history of multisensorial professional specimen exhibition occurred alongside this era's better-known history of popular display, including "freak shows" that exhibited unusual bodies as public spectacle.[69] Many medical practitioners disclaimed affiliation with such "sensationalist" commercial ventures, attempting to establish a bright line between the legitimate gaze of medical science and the tawdry or illicit gaze of the paying public. A late nineteenth-century medical journal editorial decried the "popular exhibitions" of "freaks and monstrosities," averring that "the exhibition of such monstrosities to miscellaneous audiences should not be permitted, while scientific men should be given the fullest opportunity of investigation."[70]

But while nineteenth-century practitioners drew distinctions between the purposes of popular versus medical exhibitions—the one for public entertainment and commercial profit, the other for professional pedagogy and scientific knowledge—in reality this division was far from impermeable. In practice, the medical study of monstrosity resonated and at times directly intersected with forms of popular commercial exhibition. In the later nineteenth century, medical museums such as the Mütter Museum in Philadelphia increasingly made their exhibits accessible to the public, conspicuously blurring the line between professional and popular interest. Meanwhile, some elite physicians and scientists performed private examinations on individual subjects of popular "freak show" exhibits, which they published as case reports in professional medical journals.[71] Physicians also readily gave comments for popular newspaper articles on the births and public exhibitions of particularly unusual "monstrosities" in the later nineteenth century, which were printed in publications such as the *New York Times*, the *Austin Daily Statesman*, the *Los Angeles Times*, and the *Washington Post*.[72] In contrast to the noted racial heterogeneity of patients in case reports published in medical journals, nearly all the parents and infants described in these popular newspaper reports were Black, suggesting how contexts of racial inequity affected who got exposed to the gaze of broader publics.

It is clear, then, that nineteenth-century medical professionals did engage with practices of popular and commercial exhibition. However, the connections between visual display and medical interest in monstrosity ran even deeper. Practices of exhibition scaffolded the medical engagement with monstrosity even—and especially—*within* formal medical institutions and professional activities. Even when medical specimens of monstrosity were never exhibited to a public, they were intended for the visual (and often extravisual) consumption of an audience, designed to be viewed and handled by practitioners and trainees in professional associations, universities, and teaching hospitals. As detailed earlier, physicians exhibited specimens to colleagues at the meetings of medical societies, displayed them to students in medical school lecture halls, and gathered them for the gaze of professional successors to come in the anatomical collections of medical museums.

In extolling the value of specimen preparations, practitioners described an explicitly visual exercise of authority that centered on the act of viewing. Leading physicians employed an operative metaphor of a penetrating medical gaze that could "render visible" what had "hitherto been obscure," lifting hidden truths of the body "out of the invisible and into the sight" of observers.[73] In claiming the authority to view monstrosity, nineteenth-century physicians sought to distinguish their gaze by emphasizing the importance of scientific training, knowledge, and skill. In rendering the body visible, specimen preparation more specifically rendered the body visually *legible*—as a text that could be read by those who had learned the language of anatomy.[74] Billings declared that a skillfully rendered specimen preparation, "whether seen at the post-mortem, or years afterward in a museum, is, to the scientific pathologist or the practical physician[,] . . . a sign or hieroglyph of the morbid process which has produced it." The professional interest in viewing a specimen, he wrote, lay in "the preceding phenomena which it connotes"—physiological truths of the body that the anatomical specimen revealed exclusively to eyes trained to read it.[75]

The visual and epistemological authority to see and interpret specimens was conferred not just on present-day practitioners but on the medical profession as a whole across a broadly projected futurity. Numerous physicians described their motivation to preserve and collect monstrous specimens for the benefit of professional successors' more enlightened (and more enlightening) gaze in the future as the scientific knowledge of medicine continued to expand. In an 1839 case report on monstrosity, a New England physician professed the hope that a specimen would be "of future use" to a more advanced successor who might one day "be able to clear up the doubts which envelope the present subject"—a subject that physicians could as yet only "'see through a glass darkly.'" In 1888, Billings continued to summon an imaginary of more clear-eyed successors to come when he explained that a well-made specimen preparation "is valuable, not only for what we can see in it, but also for what we overlook or misinterpret, and which our successor may see, and see rightly."[76] This discourse conceptualized the progress—and the foundational authority—of the medical profession as entailing an ever-increasing ability to see and produce knowledge about the human body.

In the case of monstrosity, the ability to see specimens was an act of doubled visual access: It made visible both the monster and the inside of the opaque maternal body. Extending an early modern medical discourse in which the uterus (and, through it, the associated figure of the female body) "came to stand for the body's hidden interior," nineteenth-century practitioners configured monstrous specimens as visualizations of internal secrets obdurately hidden from sight.[77] One physician declared that monstrous specimens offered insight into "a sphere so completely excluded from view that very little is yet clearly known"; two others wrote that "in monstrosities, we seem to catch forbidden sight of the secret work-room of Nature, and drag out into the light the evidences" of the "methods and means" of development.[78] Interpreted through the precepts of teratology, which understood monstrosity as an arrest or deviation in regular embryological development, a specimen of monstrosity represented a fetal body halted in developmental time and could thus reveal secrets of intrauterine development to those who knew the language of anatomy. Well before twentieth-century developments brought the prenatal period firmly into the plane of medical sight, specimens of teratological monstrosity helped nineteenth-century physicians establish a form of visual authority over the pregnant body, making visible the biological processes concealed within.[79]

SPECIMEN EPISTEMOLOGIES: MAKING THE MONSTROUS BODY BIOLOGICAL

The exercise of visual authority over monstrosity in this period was intimately linked to these broader assertions of biological knowledge. Whereas early nineteenth-century US physicians tended to foreground practice and experience as the basis of their professional identity, practitioners later in the century increasingly emphasized scientific expertise, linking the professional authority of medicine to the knowledge production of experimental science.[80] By the mid–nineteenth century, leading practitioners of obstetrics were already seeking to legitimize their clinical specialty by explicitly connecting it to fields of scientific study. In the introduction to his 1849 obstetrics textbook, Charles Meigs admonished those who would "call in question the claim of Obstetricy to be classed among the Sciences," insisting that the field "comprises the several sciences of Anatomy, Physiology, Pathology, in so far as they relate to the structure, the functions, and the diseases of the reproductive organs; it also includes the whole of Embryogeny."[81] At a time when physicians did not attend the majority of births in the United States and medical students rarely received hands-on obstetric training, practitioners could not claim authority over childbearing from an education built on direct clinical experience. Rhetorical claims of obstetric authority instead rested on the idea of expert knowledge—the promise of a rigorously scientific understanding of reproduction.[82]

Nineteenth-century practitioners' engagement with monstrous birth presented an opportunity to validate this claimed authority by linking the field to the burgeoning experimental sciences of embryology and teratology in Europe. Connecting American medical practice to the scientific work of prominent European scientists such as Étienne and Isidore Geoffroy Saint-Hilaire, Johann Friedrich Meckel, Étienne Serres, Camille Dareste, Willem Vrolik, and Karl Ernst von Baer, the professional interest in monstrosity bolstered obstetrics' aspirations to scientific status.[83] The production and collection of monstrous specimens allowed American physicians to engage with this field of scientific knowledge production in intimate and concrete ways, grounded in the material and sensory practices of dissecting, examining, and displaying bodies. In their reports of individual dissections, elite physicians emphatically noted whenever their discoveries of anatomical structures diverged from something Saint-Hilaire had suggested in his authoritative works on teratology. Others offered modifications of Saint-Hilaire's taxonomic scheme based on their own clinical observations and collections.[84] Later in the century, case reports on monstrosity cited scientific knowledge gleaned through "microscopical examinations and experiments" conducted by fellow US medical practitioners.[85]

The previous section discussed how physicians claimed the authority to see and read the truths that specimens made visible. By decoding infants' prepared remains, physicians could acquire and legitimate knowledge not just about the production of monstrosities but also broadly about anatomy, physiology, and embryology. In explaining the "scientific value" of monstrous specimens, physicians across the nineteenth century invoked ideals of knowledge production that emphasized the extrapolation of universalized scientific principles and laws.[86] In the 1830s, case reports from Ohio, Massachusetts, and Georgia used clinical cases of monstrous birth as an opportunity to discuss physiological laws and principles of development. In one, a physician expressed the hope that through the medical study of monstrosity, "the laws which govern in the development of these untoward specimens of humanity may come to be as well understood as any other physiological rule already established."[87] As ideals of scientific knowledge production became increasingly central to the broader professional identity of medicine later in the century, US physicians continued to emphasize this aspiration. By tracing "departures" and "deviations" from nature's "regular course," they averred, the medical study of monstrosity could reveal the "laws of life" that directed the development of "normal" human bodies.[88]

More particularly, the occurrence of anencephaly offered nineteenth-century practitioners a way to extrapolate general principles about the development, physiology, and anatomy of the nervous system. This knowledge production was tightly bound up in the material and visual practices of specimen dissection and examination. For instance, a Philadelphia physician in 1838 purported to provide evidence in support of the contention that the nerves and ganglia of the peripheral nervous system developed independently of the brain and spinal cord. Revealing the embodied, visual-tactile mode through which this information was acquired, he detailed his dissection of an anencephalic infant's remains, describing how the physical act of "tracing up these nerves" led to the discovery that they suddenly "terminated at the vertebrae and had no connexion with the spinal membranes." A report on anencephaly much later in the century, published in 1897, continued to use visual-tactile examination of specimen tissue to extrapolate knowledge about the developmental relationship between different structures of the nervous system, writing that "the development of the neuron of 1st order (spinal-peripheral) is shown, by this observation, to be in no way dependent upon that of the neuron of the 2nd order (cortico-spinal)."[89] In this later case, the physician generated knowledge through preparing the anencephalic infant's remains as a histologic specimen—a soft-tissue preparation designed to reveal tiny microscopical structures rather than the "gross" (large) anatomical structures visible without a microscope.

An extended consideration of another late nineteenth-century case report offers granular insight into the material and visual modes of this biomedical knowledge production. In 1888, the New York physician and medical professor Charles Dana described the birth of a full-term infant with anencephaly, born living to a woman who "was unmarried, but was healthy." The mother held and nursed her newborn at her breast; however, she found that the baby had difficulty swallowing, leading to bouts of breathing distress that caused the infant's face to turn a worrying blueish gray. The child, who lived for two and a half days, seemed to cry very little and then only in a "feeble" way.[90]

Dana took away the remains of the infant for dissection and microscopical examination. Like other forms of soft-tissue preparation, preparing a specimen to view under a microscope was an intricate and involved process requiring many treatments and manipulations. Dana noted that he first cut the brain stem into sections to submerge in "Muller's solution," a commercial fixative agent, and then in alcohol. Next, he stained the sections with dye to make visible their tissue-level structures under the microscope—a manipulation loosely akin to the way physicians used coloring agents to visualize gross anatomical structures such as the blood vessels in macroscopic specimens. For the stain, Dana used "Weigert's and ordinary haemotoxylon," which would color certain tissue structures a dark purple; carmine, a vibrant red pigment; and aniline blue. He next washed the stained specimens and placed them in a solution of hydrochloric acid.[91] An 1880s instructional guide on microscopy advised practitioners to dilute the hydrochloric acid with water "until it tastes about like sharp vinegar," suggesting yet another sensory field engaged by processes of specimen preparation.[92] (Perhaps Dana held off on tasting the solution until he had already diluted it a fair amount, given the intense corrosive properties of hydrochloric acid.)

After hardening, staining, and fixing the tissue sections, Dana embedded them in celloidin, a clear, semisolid substance that formed a sturdy transparent matrix. A recommended method involved wrapping a "strip of glazed paper" around a cylindrical cork, "fastened with a couple of pins," placing the tissue "in the box thus formed," and carefully pouring the celloidin over it. Following this, the tissue preparation was to be rehardened through immersion in a solution of alcohol for one to three days. Finally, cross-sections of tissue needed to be sliced with a special blade thinly enough to be mounted on glass slides and placed under the microscope for viewing.[93]

Reporting on his examination of the tissue under the microscope, Dana explained that "one of the chief interests in monsters lies in what they tell us post-mortem" about the microscopic structures of the nervous system. Based on a comparison of anencephalic spinal cord tissue with a comparable section of "normal" spinal cord tissue, Dana described what "must represent the mode of crossing of" a particular set of nerve fibers. Reflecting a strikingly granular level of visual observation, Dana explained that "in the anencephalic cord . . . these [fibers] crossed directly from one side to the other at a very acute angle. In the normal cord some fibres crossed in this way, but others ran along the edge of the fissure for a short distance and then cross at a more obtuse angle." In describing what he saw and how he interpreted the sight, Dana employed terminology unlikely to be understood by anyone without formal training in histology and the microscopic anatomy of the nervous system—noting, for example, that it "appears that the fibres of the raphe serve to connect the cranial nerve nuclei with the pyramids, and also with the lemniscus or corpus restiforme."[94]

The material and visual practices of preparing and viewing histologic specimens buttressed the ability of physicians such as Dana to configure the monstrous body as anatomical text—and to successfully read this text's increasingly esoteric language. Importantly, although histologic preparation represented an increasingly popular way of visualizing monstrous specimens, it existed alongside of rather than superseding ways of rendering monstrous bodies anatomically visible at a gross (macroscopic) level. As many other examples in this chapter have shown, late nineteenth-century practitioners also continued to produce, collect, and display organs and full bodies in clear jars of formalin. But these larger specimens were now joined in medical museum collections by slide-mounted microscopical specimens as well, and together the two types served as a visual assertion of monsters' legibility to medical science across multiple magnitudes of scale.[95]

In rendering and reading tissues and organs as anatomical text, practitioners gave material form to an epistemology of the human body—one in which knowledge of the body meant knowledge of anatomy and physiology.[96] The physical configuration of the specimen communicated that the important truths of the body were biological truths, that they lay in the secrets of physiology that might be read by an enlightened physician from the specimen's bared anatomical structures. This arrangement encoded the idea that the way to see the reality, the true reality, of a body was by viewing it inert and isolated from its social and environmental contexts, prepared in ways designed to emphasize particular anatomic systems, organs, and tissue structures. This might be accomplished through the manipulation and configuration of remains, the clearing out of "unnecessary matter," so deemed by practitioners, to produce gross anatomical specimens of organs and bodies "preserved entire."[97] Or it might be done through the elaborate hardening, staining, and sectioning of tissue that produced histologic specimens for examination under a microscope. In all cases, these profoundly mediated preparations were contingent, rather than inevitable, modes of presenting the reality of bodies. Other ways of knowing the body might involve, for instance, locating it within religious or kinship contexts, or they might require witnessing the dynamic flows and exchange of fluid within and between the living body and its environment.[98] By presenting specimen preparation as the way to reveal the singular truth of the body, medical practitioners of the nineteenth century conferred authority on those who could make visible and read the body as a pathoanatomical entity.

The ability to define and interpret the monstrous body—to lay bare and rightly see its biological truth—also bestowed on physicians an epistemological authority over the meanings of deviance and normality. By identifying what they considered the anatomical deviance of monstrosity, physicians located the state from which it departed. This shifted from descriptions of departure from a "perfect" state, which predominated in earlier nineteenth-century medical literature, to the descriptions of deviation from "normality" that came to typify later nineteenth-century accounts.[99] In quantifying the monster's anatomical and physiological deviation from the "perfect," "regular," or "normal" state, practitioners established an imaginary of deviance predicated on a particular biological understanding of the human body. This medical refiguration of monstrosity did not strip away the category's moral and cultural connotations but rather offered an intricate biological grounding for renewed moral and cultural valuations of the "monstrous." At the same time, it asserted the special authority of medical science to truly see and comprehend the nature of monstrosity.

In begetting and displaying specimens, then, practitioners located monstrosity within a larger project of making the human body visible and knowable to a largely white, male professional class. These practices established that the truth of monstrosity was to be gleaned through the collection and presentation of anatomized bodies isolated in transparent containers, understood in terms of anatomical and physiological information that could be seen and read as text off the exposed surfaces of the organs and tissues. The physical, multisensory processes of specimen creation asserted practitioners' authority not only over the infants they professed to "imprison" in jars of alcohol but also over broader conceptions of human bodies and deviance, rendering the "monstrous" legible as biological entity.[100] Far from passively revealing a fixed and preexisting corporeal truth, specimen production actively configured both the body and the meanings of the monster, highlighting material and visual practice as key modalities of medical monster making.

CHAPTER FOUR

Monstrous Images

Medical Illustration and Photography

The drawing accompanying Francis West's 1838 case report made a number of stark visual choices. Perhaps the most surprising one, for an image purporting to depict a stillborn infant, was the pose: The newborn is portrayed in a quadruped position, supporting their own weight on all fours, doleful gaze averted from the viewer. An especially muscular shoulder is textured with a shaggy coat of fur, while a thick band of hair starts by the prominent brow ridge and travels down the spine, forming a beastly mane from temple to tailbone. A broad flat ear projects from the side of the head, while the curving fingers and toes suggest nascent claws or talons. The eyes are large, round, and located close to the top of the head, a characteristic feature that underwrote historical descriptions of newborns with anencephaly as "frog-babies" or "owl-fetuses."[1]

West personally commissioned the illustration to represent an infant born to a woman he attended during a medically perilous birth in 1837. It was the twenty-eighty-year-old woman's first delivery, and it was an arduous one. Her difficulties started well before the birth, when she and her twenty-five-year-old husband were compelled to make a long and "forced journey" from Cincinnati. Exhausted, far from friends and family, and deep into her pregnancy, she sought lodging with her husband in a small Philadelphia hotel. She fell sick very soon after arriving and was in tenuous health when her labor unexpectedly began.[2]

For a woman in this period to give birth outside the home, unattended by any female friends or relatives, was an indication of dire circumstances. Both the woman and her husband were recent immigrants from England, with no family in Philadelphia. It is unclear what precipitated their expulsion from Cincinnati: Perhaps it was related to the woman's pregnancy or to the man she had wed around the same time—or, possibly, after—the pregnancy began. West had no existing relationship with the woman prior to her delivery; he met her for the first time after being summoned to the Philadelphia hotel to render emergency medical aid. When he arrived, shortly after the woman's water broke, she was in no state to answer questions about her situation. Upon delivery, West noted that the infant displayed the extreme arrests of cranial and brain development that characterized "derencephaly" (a "subspecies" of anencephaly) within the French scientist Isidore Geoffroy Saint-Hilaire's "classification of monsters."[3]

The woman fared poorly during labor. After the delivery of her stillborn infant, her fragmented placenta came away in pieces, accompanied by recurrent bouts of severe uterine bleeding. Her postpartum hemorrhage continued for several days, and West repeatedly feared for her life as he tried to treat her. Ultimately, however, she made a "perfect recovery" and was able to leave the city. She never saw her infant and was never informed by West about the "character" of the stillborn child.[4] While pointedly concealing the knowledge of the infant's congenital condition from the mother, West took the newborn's remains to produce as a specimen of monstrosity. He published a report of the case, accompanied by a full-page lithographic print of the commissioned drawing of the "anencephalous foetus" as a quadruped.

Illustrations such as this one frequently accompanied nineteenth-century US case histories of "monstrous" birth, offering visual representations of anomalous newborn bodies alongside written reports. Yet were these images to be laid out side by side, it would be difficult to guess that they all depicted the same referent. A sample of illustrations published in case reports spanning the 1830s to the 1890s seems to show many very different kinds of being. Several of the drawings clearly portray infant children. One leans over a pillow, eyes closed and little rosy lips seemingly pursed into a pout.[5] Another infant looks to be in a state of repose or gentle supplication: nestled on the ground, bending so far forward that their belly rests on the top of their thighs, face turned upward and mouth softly open, an exaggeratedly tiny infant hand held out in a little curled fist. The expression and somewhat cartoonlike style of the drawing give an impression of sweet, almost whimsical tranquility, juxtaposed with the large brainlike mass that sits exposed atop the child's upper back.[6]

Other images depict creatures that hardly seem human. Some, like West's, are clearly intended to appear beastlike. Several of this type similarly show a newborn on all fours, palms and soles in contact with the ground so that their weight is distributed evenly across hands and feet. One, crouched low on bent arms and legs, bears more than a passing resemblance to a big cat: massive jaw pulled menacingly agape as if midroar, slightly pointed ears jutting up and out, fingers hooked into the likeness of claws, a mane of shaggy fur ringing the head and shoulders.[7] The exaggerated bulk and volume of the facial features and body almost call to mind the proportions of a Botero cat sculpture. Others seem unlike any identifiable species: One, pictured in profile against a solid black background, appears to be a skeleton with the body of a miniature adult human, standing fully upright, tiny vertical spine topped by a narrow, lever-shaped skull.[8]

Though widely varied in their visual content, all these nineteenth-century images aimed to represent the same biological phenomenon: infants born with anencephaly or related conditions. These sorts of visual representations, which came to include medical photography as well as medical illustration in the later part of the century, constituted yet another modality through which medical practitioners configured and circulated newborn bodies as biological monstrosities. These disparate images positioned the monster in often contradictory relation to human and nonhuman orders of beings, locating and displacing infant offspring within projected ranks of familial, racial, and animal kinds.

This chapter closely analyzes a selection of the drawings and photographs that accompanied nineteenth-century medical reports of monstrous birth, tracing three major (and sometimes overlapping) genres of portrayal. The first of these involved images that visually distanced "monstrosities" from the position of a human child. Such images configured infant bodies as bestial and racialized "others," reflecting and mobilizing an entanglement of *species* and *race* in nineteenth-century imaginaries of difference and natural kinds. At the same time, a contrasting set of medical illustrations foregrounded signifiers of relational human status, portraying "monstrous" infants as babies who elicited care and comfort in contexts of familial home life. Finally, a group of later nineteenth-century images, which increasingly included photographs, began to incorporate visual conventions of scientific specimen and "physical type" portraiture used in fields such as zoology and physical anthropology. Such conventions presented an individual as a standardized representative of a separate species or ethnoracial kind, once again engaging linked notions of *species* and *race* to configure the alterity of the monster. Together, these varied genres of portrayal visualized monstrosity as a state of ambivalent kinship, situating monstrous bodies in the unresolved tensions between intimate familiarity and radical racialized difference.

A NOTE ON THE PRODUCTION AND REPRODUCTION OF IMAGES

Nineteenth-century medical practitioners used an array of techniques to produce images of monstrous newborns, including ink drawings, watercolor paintings, lithographs, woodcuts, copper engravings, etchings, daguerreotypes, and later forms of photography. The resulting images frequently accompanied published case reports and were sometimes preserved in institutional medical collections alongside tissue specimens for purposes of research, pedagogy, and display. Physicians explained that accompanying images served to clarify and at times stand in for the report's written descriptions of infants' appearances.[9]

Like other practices of medical monster making, the creation of images was often a collective endeavor. To create illustrations for their case reports, physician authors might enroll the labor of a variety of people, ranging from colleagues to medical students to commissioned artists and printers. In a few cases, professional illustrators were credited by name, usually in publications by elite physicians from densely populated cities. An account by the well-known Philadelphia physician Charles Meigs included "two lithograph illustrations from Daguerreotypes" by the prominent daguerreotypist Marcus Root, while the 1847 Boston Society for Medical Improvement collection catalog attributed an appended image to "Sharp, Peirce & Co.," a local lithography firm in Boston.[10] In addition to appearing in case reports, reproductions of these images also circulated more widely in a broader transatlantic network of knowledge production. One image commissioned by an elite New England physician ultimately appeared in a museum catalog, an obstetric textbook, and a seminal French treatise on teratology (the "scientific study of monstrosity").[11]

As can be gleaned from the descriptions at the start of this chapter, medical illustration did not provide a neutral, unmediated depiction of an infant body. Doctors and commissioned artists guided images in particular directions, both with and without acknowledged intent. The images' content was shaped not only by creators' individual idiosyncrasies but also by culturally established and perpetually renegotiated visual conventions for observing and representing the human body.[12] The analysis of such images, then, offers striking insights into how monstrous bodies were interpreted and configured within emerging discourses of medical science.

In the later nineteenth century, the rising prevalence of photography as a medical technology precipitated a major shift in practices of imaging monstrosity. By the 1860s, case reports began to mention photographs taken of anomalous infants; by the 1880s and 1890s, reproductions of these photographs commonly accompanied published reports.[13] At first glance, it might seem that photography as a medium would offer less latitude than illustration for medical practitioners to configure symbolic meanings of monstrosity. After all, practitioners explicitly lauded photography for its purported verisimilitude, its ability to "faithfully" and "objectively" depict reality free from the subjective mediation of illustrators.[14] This technology particularly appealed at a moment when the medical profession increasingly sought to claim an authority grounded in visual knowledge—that is, as explored in the previous chapter, the ability to see and read the body's biological truths.

Yet, as visual studies scholars have long contended, photographic images are also deeply culturally mediated, structured according to contingent visual rhetorics and conventions. In replacing artistic illustration with photography, practitioners did not eliminate artistic mediation. Instead, such mediation now occurred through choices that practitioners made in the process of photographic representation. These choices related to technical aspects of shooting, processing, and printing the image; selecting and posing the focal subject; and staging and composing the image within the pictorial frame.[15]

Although presented as neutral and unmediated likenesses of reality, the photographs accompanying later nineteenth-century case reports of monstrous birth drew on particular historical genres of aesthetic representation. These images enrolled emerging conventions of clinical photography, which arranged bodies in schematized ways that purported to reveal the truth of a patient's somatic affliction within ascendent medical cosmologies.[16] They also enrolled conventions of scientific specimen and ethnoracial portraiture, which positioned the focal subject of a photograph as a generic stand-in for a broader typological kind.[17] Both medical illustrations and medical photographs, then, constituted historical sites at which the monstrosity of newborn bodies was not passively reflected but actively and contingently made.

As chapter 3 revealed, the act of rendering newborn bodies visually legible and exhibiting them before an expert gaze played a key role in producing them as scientific specimens of monstrosity—the term *specimen*, as mentioned, comes from the Latin root *spectare*, "to look." A concern, then, is that reproducing and redisplaying these images could inadvertently recapitulate (rather than critically analyze) the historical practices that positioned bodies as monstrosities. At the same time, as chapter 2 argued, the visual *concealment* of infants with conditions such as anencephaly—the hiding away of them as a sight presumed to be too horrible and shocking for view—could also serve as a potent way to affectively construct their bodies as monstrous.

Informed by these considerations, I aim to avoid both voyeuristic overexposure and stigmatizing visual concealment in my presentation of historical images. I include only images that I directly describe and contextualize in the text, presenting them as a way to aid in understanding how specific visual aspects of a given image worked to constitute contingent historical meanings of monstrosity.[18] I have also opted to show only images that are very obviously mediated and stylized—images not likely to be mistaken, even if encountered out of context, as unmediated likenesses of the infants they purported to represent.

My choice to show only "obviously mediated and stylized" images may require a bit more explanation, especially because a premise of this chapter is that *all* images, including photographic ones, are mediated and stylized. Contrary to the representation of photography as a neutral medium that allows unmediated visual access to a purely objective reality, photographs, as just discussed, are ineluctably mediated cultural productions. Nevertheless, most of us are accustomed to viewing and interpreting a photographic image as a real and direct likeness of its referent in a way that is qualitatively different from the way we view and interpret line drawings or paintings. When viewed out of context and accepted at face value, clinical photographs of infants may tend to naturalize or reify the category of biological monstrosity: By presenting themselves as unmediated depictions of individuals and bodies as they truly appeared, photographs can render invisible the dense array of practices and interventions that went into configuring particular subjects as biological monstrosities. For the most part, then, I do not include reproductions of the photographs or photorealistic drawings that I discuss in this chapter. The sole exception is a photographic image that depicts an infant skeleton posed to stand perfectly upright in sharp profile against a featureless black background; this image is so heavily stylized and bears such obvious evidence of mediation that it is unlikely to be misinterpreted as a "true" depiction of an infant's natural bodily reality, even if viewed before reading the contextualizing analysis.

When photographic images of deceased bodies are viewed and interpreted as true and unmediated likenesses of the individuals they represent, they also raise issues related to the context-dependent ethics of displaying human remains. Physicians obtained newborn bodies from families and communities of varied racial, ethnic, religious, and class backgrounds, whose understandings of acceptable ways to view and treat dead bodies did not always align with those of the medical practitioners. Details in case reports indicate that at least some nineteenth-century parents explicitly refused to allow physicians to photograph the bodies of their "monstrous" infants (see chapter 2).[19] In cases where photographs were produced, it is often not clear whether and how this practice may have conflicted with the practices and beliefs of that infant's kin and communities. Given what we know about the asymmetries of power that structured physicians' encounters with different childbearing women and families as well as about the histories of exploitation and racial violence associated with the collection and exhibition of human remains in the nineteenth-century United States more generally, extra caution seems warranted in the handling of these historical sources.[20]

VISUALIZING ALTERITY: IMAGES OF NONHUMAN KINDS

To examine how practitioners configured monstrosity in visual representation, we first return to the image commissioned by the Philadelphia physician Francis West to accompany a case report of anencephaly in 1838. As shown in figure 4.1, this drawing pictured a shaggy, maned, and muscular creature posed on all fours, palms and soles flat on the ground. West explicitly intended this posture to communicate to the viewer the newborn's bestial status. He chose the quadruped position to evoke not a crawling human child but rather the "horizontal posture" of "the lower order of animals"—the beasts who walked their whole lives on four legs.

West visualized the downy hair on the newborn's body as the mane and fur of a beast, depicting "an abundant growth of very dark hair" that extended from the top of the head and down the length of the spine as well as thick shaggy hair on the arms and thighs. The infant's pose in the illustration aimed to foreground the significance of the child's "peculiar configuration and structure," which West claimed "would not by any possibility have permitted [the infant] to assume the erect position, supposing it capable of maintaining an independent existence." West here referred not just to the absence of brain and skull, but rather to what he considered the "peculiar deformity" of the newborn's entire physical being. He presented numerous aspects of the infant's external anatomy as proof that the child would have been naturally suited to move in the manner of a four-legged animal, emphasizing the "extraordinarily developed" deltoids, the "very long and muscular legs," and the "perpendicular" attachment of the limbs to the torso. He described how the infant's "very loose" joints easily admitted extreme flexion of the ankle, enabling the child to keep their feet fully planted on the ground while standing on all fours.[21]

To explain these "remarkable" physical features, West invoked the "scale of being," a concept that scaffolded long-standing imaginaries of

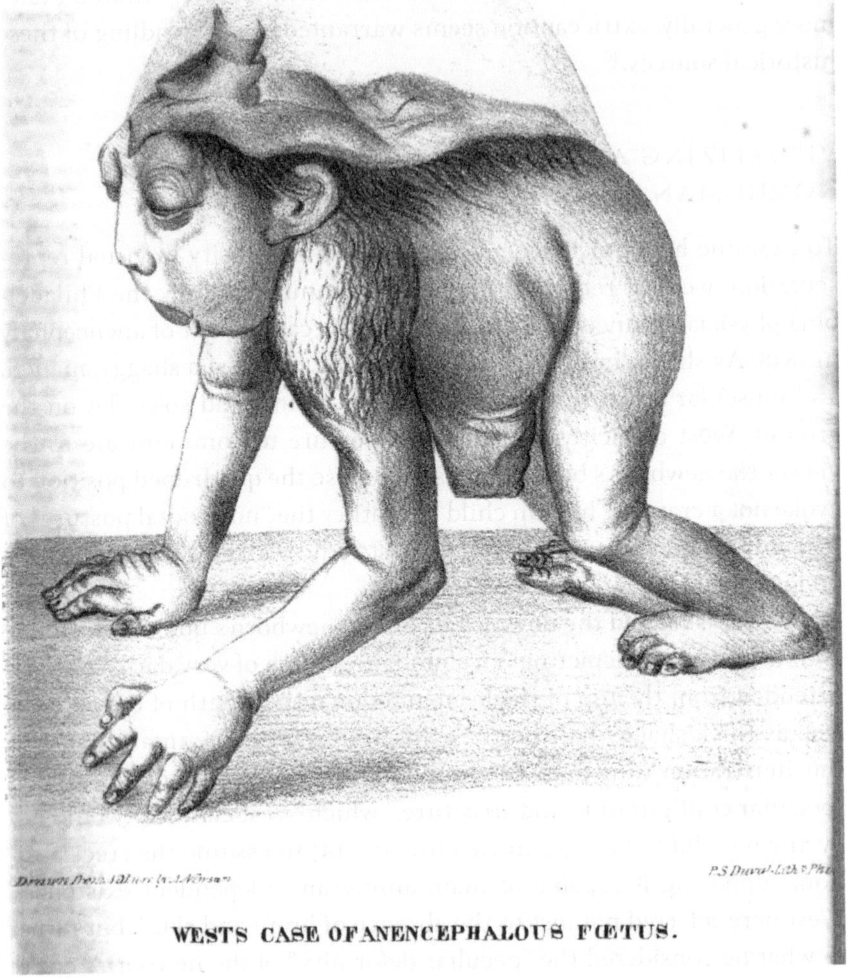

FIGURE 4.1 Drawing of infant with anencephaly as a quadruped, printed in Francis West, "An Account of an Anencephalous Foetus," *Medical Examiner* 1, no. 4 (1838): 60–61.
Source: Courtesy of Stanford Medical History Center.

a ranked continuum of species. He wrote that "by some very essential and radical vice of formation, this human foetus has been so materially degraded in the scale of being, as very closely to approximate, the lower order of animals." West's interpretation located the infant in a formally inferior position within a hierarchy of natural kinds. Even as the physician discussed anencephaly as a medical pathology of the human body, he simultaneously positioned the "'Anencephalus'" as a different species of being.[22]

West's representation of the infant as "materially degraded in the scale of being" situated monstrosity within a broad tradition of what the scholar Zakiyyah Iman Jackson calls "the racialization of the human/animal distinction," which mobilizes proximity to "lower animal orders" as a way to communicate debased or subhuman status. Describing how racialized Western imaginaries of a human/animal hierarchy construct Blackness as a state of degraded and bestial being, Jackson explains *race* and *species* as *"mutually reinforcing terms"*: "To put it plainly, the discourse of race is a discourse of speciation," she writes.[23] In images like West's, then, the portrayal of a "degraded" infant as a bestial species linked the category of monstrosity to discourses of human racial alterity.

Other illustrations used a similar visual iconography to likewise show monstrous infants as particularly bestial, employing signifiers such as quadruped posture and beastlike hairiness to depict them as distanced from human status within the order of animal kinds. In an 1862 report, the Maine physician D. S. Conant offered two illustrations of infant bodies posed on all fours, captioned "Anencephalous Monsters." As shown in figure 4.2, one sketch portrayed a creature with a horselike mane and four long, recognizably human limbs walking on fisted hands and toes, while the other depicted a skeletal specimen that Conant had prepared for display in his personal collection. The second drawing showed the skeleton posed on all fours, hands articulated at right angles from the wrist joints and carefully elevated on blocks to maintain a perfectly horizontal spine with arms and legs in full extension. The temporal bones of the face were drawn winged to the side, giving the impression of large and pointy ears.[24]

Another illustration in this genre, shown in figure 4.3, appeared in the Georgia physician P. H. Thompson's 1885 case report of anencephaly. The infant in this case was born to Thompson's private patient, a twenty-year-old woman in "excellent health, and a model of physical development." Thompson wrote that the infant's unusual facial features "gave to it the appearance of a cat's head," and the accompanying illustration depicted the infant with distinctly feline features.[25] The infant

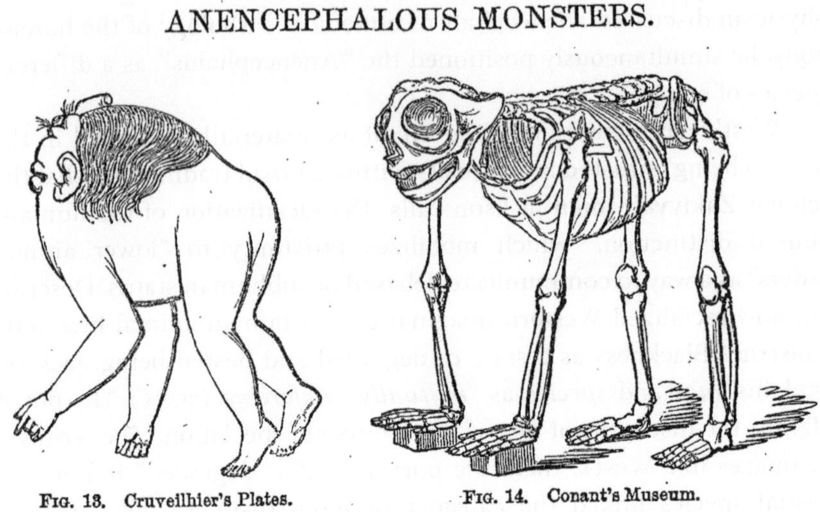

FIGURE 4.2 Drawing of infant and infant skeleton with anencephaly as quadrupeds, printed in D. S. Conant, "The Science, Causes, and Anatomical Peculiarities of Human Monstrosities," *Transactions of the New York Academy of Medicine* 2 (1862): 274. *Source*: Courtesy of Stanford Medical History Center.

was shown crouched low to the ground, resting on their forearms with feet folded under, so that their weight was supported on the balls of the feet rather than on the knees. The ears were slightly pointed and projected to the side, and the fingers were curled into hooks resembling claws. The mouth was drawn wide open, calling to mind a big cat in midroar, while the shading of the picture suggested a mane of fur around the face and back.

In addition to explicit portrayals of monstrous infants as akin to quadruped beasts of the "lower animal orders," illustrations could also communicate the species alterity of monstrosity through choices that visually distanced them from the life-cycle stage and accompanying kinship position of a human baby. One example of this involved posed infant skeletons standing fully upright in the biped stance of an older human being, as shown in figure 4.4. This remarkable late nineteenth-century image of a "dry specimen" in the University of Pennsylvania's anatomical collections, labeled "Skeleton of Anencephalus," pictured an upright fetal skeleton in profile against an austere black background.[26]

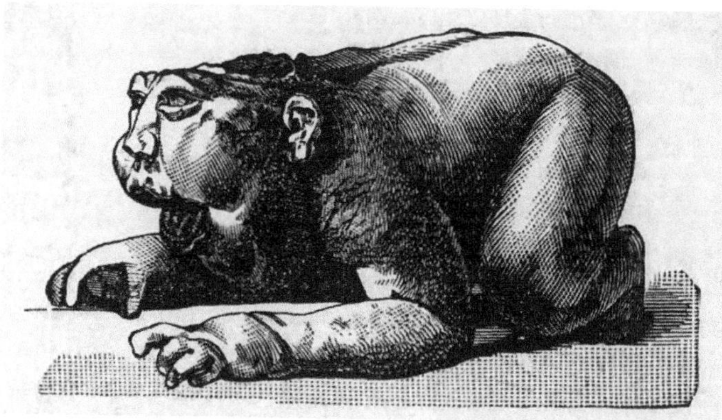

FIGURE 4.3 Drawing of infant with anencephaly as catlike, printed in P. H. Thompson, "Three Monstrosities," *Atlanta Medical and Surgical Journal* 2, no. 10 (1885): 593. *Source*: Courtesy of US National Library of Medicine, Bethesda, MD.

No pedestal or mounting apparatus was made visible in the plate, giving the illusion of a free-standing body. In contrast to the curled-up posture of the classic "fetal position," the diminutive skeleton's spine was straightened to full verticality, the hips and knee joints completely extended, so that the body-line was wholly upright. Only the ankle joints were bent at a ninety-degree angle so that the specimen stood in the likeness of an adult biped. The specimen's distinctive cranial shape seemed to further the illusion of a miniature adult hominid: Because of the skull's diminished size, the figure's head-to-body proportions more closely matched the proportions associated with human adults than with human infants, whose heads are characteristically very large in comparison to their bodies.

The visual iconography of an upright hominid skeleton with an unusually shaped and flattened skull, pictured in stark side profile, held pronounced racial meaning in nineteenth-century contexts. Medical and scientific discourse in this period cast skull profile and head shape as primary indexes of human racial classification. Prominent US physicians played a central role in producing concepts of race within burgeoning mid-nineteenth-century studies of physical anthropology and anthropometry, which quantified and compared "the conformation of racial crania" as a way to visualize and designate purported anatomical

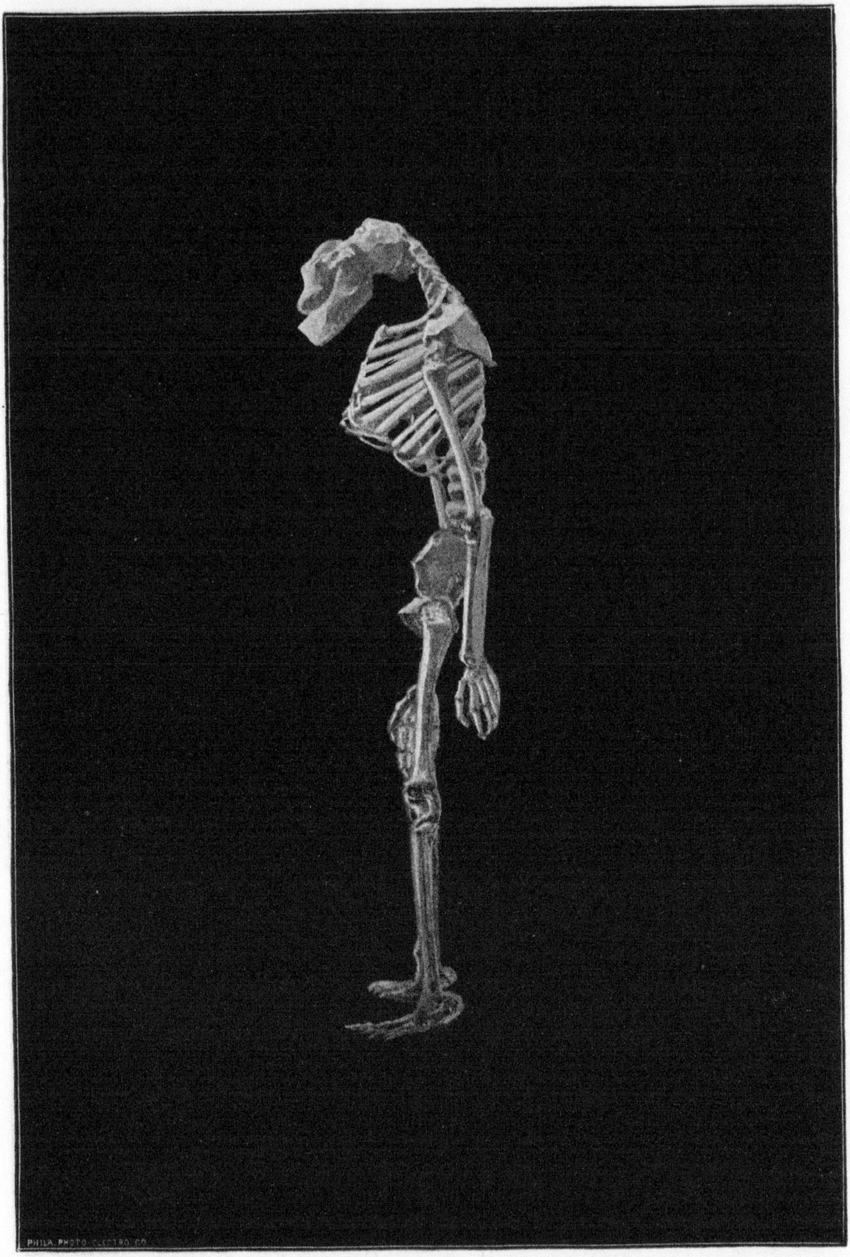

FIGURE 4.4 Photograph of infant skeleton with anencephaly posed standing upright, printed in Barton Cooke Hirst and George Piersol, *Human Monstrosities*, 4 vols. (Lea Brothers, 1891–1893), 2: plate XIX. *Source*: Courtesy of the Truman G. Blocker Jr. History of Medicine Collections, Moody Medical Library, University of Texas Medical Branch at Galveston.

differences among disparate races of humans.[27] In many cases, the same prominent US physicians who curated institutional collections of monstrous specimens also collected "racial crania" or "national skulls."[28]

Directly connecting the science of racial craniometry to medical interest in anomalies of development, the influential physician Abraham Jacobi wrote in 1859 that an existing anthropometric terminology for "discriminating the varieties of races by their skulls" could be deployed to classify anomalous cranial development in individuals. In nineteenth-century taxonomies, the "anencephalus" might join racial designations such as "dolicocephalus" and "brachycephalus" in indicating a taxonomic type defined by skull morphology.[29] Late in the century, physical anthropologists likened the skulls of a prehistoric hominid species to the skulls of the "lowest savage races" and to the skulls of individuals with arrested cranial development in the "civilized races."[30] This formulation related congenital anomalies both to present-day nonwhite populations and to an ancient hominid population (now known as *Homo erectus*) through a racialized imaginary of cranial alterity. Entangled in this dense late nineteenth-century discourse surrounding the racial evolution of skull type, the portrayal of the skeletal body in figure 4.4—posed as an adult of a hominid species but visually distinguished by a unique cranial shape pictured in sharply outlined profile—powerfully coded the "Skeleton of Anencephalus" as a specimen of racial and species alterity rather than as an infant human child.

Collectively, the images discussed in this section served to distance the subjects portrayed from the relational status of the human either by emphasizing their likeness to "lower" beasts or by displacing their signifiers of the life-cycle-specific position of human infancy. By representing these infants as anatomically and biomechanically outside the norms of the human species, practitioners visually configured monstrosity as, in the words of one nineteenth-century physician, "unfitted for the course of life proper to its species."[31]

Notably, images that associated infants with species alterity did not map in a predictable way onto the mother's racial and social status. In some reports that visualized infants as bestially degraded, the infants' mothers also occupied markedly subordinated social positions. For example, one antebellum case report emphasized in illustration and text the "abundance of hair" covering the body of an infant born to an enslaved woman, who gave birth within a violent system of racial and reproductive exploitation.[32] In the 1838 illustration commissioned by West, as seen in figure 4.1, the infant's mother was an immigrant woman whose indigence was revealed in the circumstance of her giving birth far away from family and friends in a strange hotel.

Yet in many other cases, physicians particularly emphasized the biological alterity of a "monstrous" infant in ways that could not be explained with reference to the racial and social alterity of a marginalized mother. In Thompson's illustration of an infant posed as a feline beast, the mother was a private upper-class white patient, whose more privileged status did not impede the physician from depicting and interpreting her offspring as particularly animalistic.[33] Indeed, as discussed in chapter 2, some reports seemed to particularly emphasize the contrast between a mother's well-developed white gentility and her monstrous infant's implicitly or explicitly racialized degradation. As a figure of bestial alterity born even to the most "respectable and well-to-do" of human mothers, the monster emphasized the proximity of that alterity to the imagined sanctum of the white Anglo-American family.[34]

FAMILIAR SIGHTS: IMAGES OF KIN

In contrast to these images of alterity, other case report illustrations appeared to emphasize characteristics that positioned the infants as human kin. These images signified the newborn as occupying the stage of life appropriate to human young rather than as a degraded or incommensurate species. In this way, such illustrations served to communicate a monstrous newborn's affective humanity—a recognized social or moral status of human child and family, with the capacity to evoke the associated emotional reactions.

Sometimes these affective signifiers were subtle. Consider the woodcut that accompanied an Ohio physician's case report of an infant born in 1853 to a "healthy, well-formed" married mother of "good constitution."[35] In this image, shown in figure 4.5, several small details emphasized the offspring's position as a baby child. In contrast to the illustrations shown in figures 4.1–4.4, the child here was depicted leaned over, the weight of their torso resting against the tops of their thighs, rather than supporting their own weight against gravity in a way that a

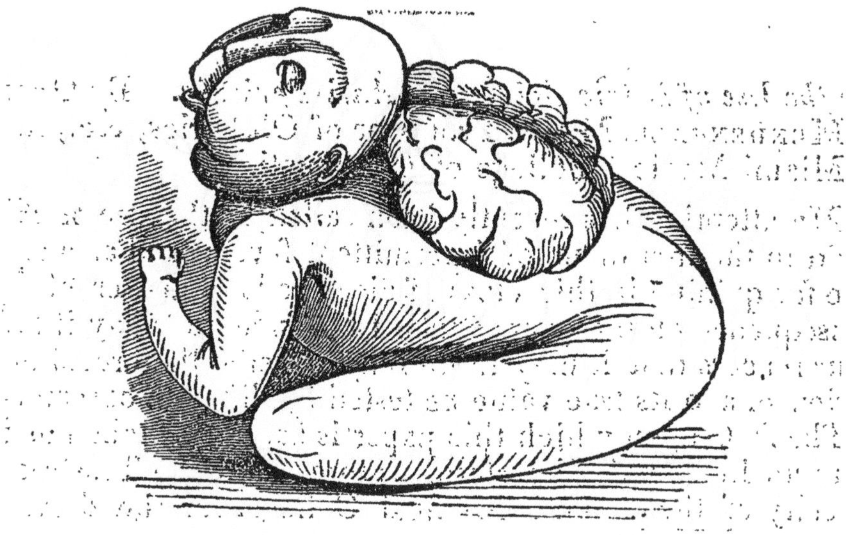

FIGURE 4.5 Drawing of infant with exencephaly in repose, printed in Julius Taylor, "Case of Monstrosity," *Western Lancet* 15, no. 7 (1854): 470. *Source*: Courtesy of Stanford Medical History Center.

newborn human would be physically incapable of doing. The exceptionally large head-to-hand proportion underscored, through exaggeration, the head-to-body proportions of a baby human rather than those of an adult.

In a drawing that accompanied an 1890 case report of anencephaly from Tennessee, as shown in figure 4.6, these signifiers of human childhood were even more pronounced.[36] Aspects of the illustration firmly located the infant within the comfort of domestic familial life and the conventional imperatives of care elicited by a newborn child. The drawing depicted the infant wearing a patterned and striped garment with a collar and buttons. Resting their head on a ruffle-trimmed pillow, the child appeared to be in a state of repose. The infant's closed eyes and position on the pillow seemed to suggest the tranquil sleep of a baby; the trimmings and intricacy of the garments and bedding implied a level of care, affection, and familial recognition. Compared to the maned, quadruped-posed creatures represented in other case reports of anencephaly, this illustration seemed far likelier to inspire tender feelings and affective recognition of a human child.

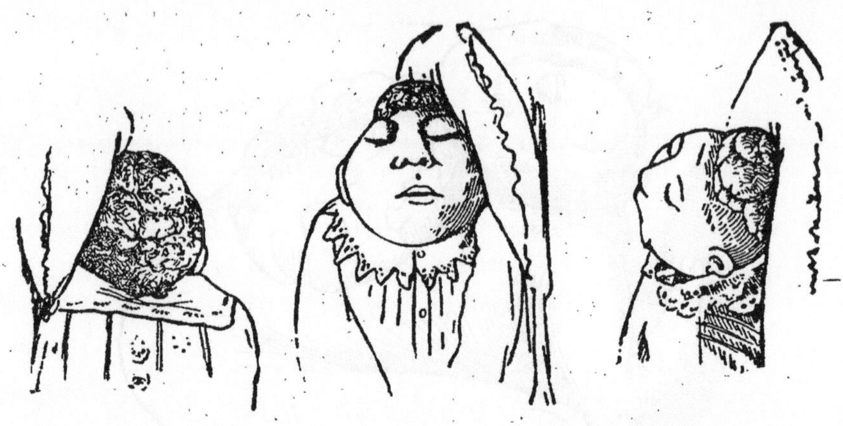

FIGURE 4.6 Drawing of infant with anencephaly wearing patterned garment and resting head on pillow, printed in J. Edwards, "Case of Acephalous Monster," *Nashville Journal of Medicine and Surgery* 45, no. 6 (1890): 228. *Source*: Courtesy of Stanford Medical History Center.

If the designation *monster* served to indicate a serious departure from a familiar "human shape," then the clothing and posing in this drawing served to reestablish a measure of that familiar human phenotype. Against the condition of alienated kinship that inhered in the formal definition of "monstrosity"—a being born of human parents but not immediately recognizable as the type of the human kind—this drawing offered the visual trappings of a cared-for child.

Photographs, too, could be composed in a way that contextualized infants as human children, showing elements that foregrounded the infant's social and biological connections to human family. One late nineteenth-century case report contained a photograph of an infant, born to a mother described as "a colored woman, 25 years old and apparently healthy," lying in a bassinet-like structure atop a thick, fringed blanket. This infant lived for one hour and ten minutes and received "artificial respiration" to aid with breathing for that time.[37] An 1896 case report published in the *American Journal of Obstetrics* included photographs of a newborn with anencephaly, born to thirty-year-old "Rosa M.," a patient in the "polyclinical service" of the senior class at Rush Medical College in Chicago. Her child, born after a "tedious labor of sixty hours," lived for only fifteen minutes after birth. The photographs show an infant posed on a bed or cot of some kind, resting against the raised headboard in an approximation of a seated position. The child's clean body suggests they had been carefully bathed after birth. The attached placenta, which is roughly the same size as the newborn, sits next to the child on the bed, taking up a roughly equal amount of space in the frame.[38]

These photographs stand out because most medical photographs of monstrous births did not show infants with contextual trappings of domestic life, such as beds, blankets, and bassinets. This was in part because many infants were not photographed until they had been taken away to other settings to be prepared as anatomical specimens. It was also the case that at least some parents actively refused physicians permission to photograph infant bodies in their homes. As discussed, evidence suggests that the mothers afforded this right of refusal were likely to be white, married, and well-to-do private patients of the physician in question, in contrast to a patient at a polyclinical service that served to give medical students experience in obstetric practice. While Rosa M.'s infant was likely photographed on a bed in a clinic or dispensary rather than a family home, the inclusion of bed and attached placenta offered visual signifiers of the infant's simultaneous social and biological connections to an implicit world of human family.

While the photographs in these two late nineteenth-century reports did suggest contexts of domestic life and the life-course stage of human infancy through their inclusion of beds and bassinets, in other ways they deployed elements of a new visual rhetoric predicated on decontextualization. Both case reports included a stylized series of photographs shot from a set of standardized angles—a genre of "type photography" discussed in the next section.

RACIAL RHETORIC OF SPECIMEN PORTRAITURE

The types of images surveyed thus far—those that portrayed infants as bestial; those that portrayed them as displaced from the life stage of a human baby; those that portrayed them as infants in contexts of kinship and familial care—accompanied cases throughout the nineteenth century. Illustrations of each type could be found accompanying case reports published at different points in the century, a phenomenon marked less by diachronic change than by continuity across this period.

Another distinctive visual convention, however, began to appear with great frequency in case histories in the 1880s and 1890s. This convention entailed a subject pictured from a prescribed series of angles labeled "front," "side," and/or "rear" views, centered and posed against a featureless background. Stripping away individuality, context, and idiosyncrasy, the visual language of standardized "type" portraiture—also used in fields such as botany, zoology, and physical anthropology—presented an individual subject as a representative of a broader typological category.[39] In teratological image making that partook of these conventions, an individual infant body was made to stand in as the generic referent of a distinct monstrous type.

This is conspicuously evident in the late nineteenth-century medical reference work *Human Monstrosities*, a four-volume series authored by the University of Pennsylvania physicians Barton Cooke Hirst and George Piersol in the 1890s. Hirst, professor and chair of the Obstetrics Department at the Medical School, had previously published a widely used textbook on obstetrics; Piersol, professor of embryology and anatomy at the Medical School, had written textbooks on anatomy and histology. With *Human Monstrosities*, the professors intended to provide an American work comparable to the seminal teratological treatises of Geoffroy Saint-Hilaire.[40]

Hirst and Piersol illustrated the four volumes with plates that showcased preserved fetal and infant remains from the University of Pennsylvania's medical anatomical collections. Each specimen was selected as a representative example of a different "species" of monstrosity described in the volume, evoking the taxonomic concept of the "holotype" or "type specimen"—an individual organism used to designate or model a broader organismal kind.[41] Making explicit these evocations of botanical and zoological study, one nineteenth-century physician explained that "orders, genera, and species" of monstrosities could be "represented by a typical form, that may be regarded as the center of a natural group." Thus, in *Human Monstrosities* the pictured remains of one infant, born without most structures of the brain, became a representative type of the species "Anencephalus"; the pictured remains of an infant whose brain developed outside their cranium became a representative type of the species "Exencephalus."[42]

The preserved specimens were pictured from precisely angled front, side, and rear views, harshly lit against a uniform black background so that the contours of the anatomical body appeared sharply outlined. Each subject was centered in the close-cropped pictorial frame, their body oriented as close to vertically as possible. Presented against a featureless black expanse, all background elements and support structures omitted from sight, the formalin-preserved bodies were made to look as if free-floating outside of their containers of fluid; a preserved skeleton was made to look as if freestanding, as seen in figure 4.4.[43] In these images, decontextualized individual bodies became representatives of an abstracted species type, located within a taxonomy of separate monstrous kinds.

The visual rhetoric of "type" portraiture appeared with increasing frequency in individual late nineteenth-century case reports of monstrous birth, even when accompanied by drawings rather than photographs. Multiple reports of monstrous birth from the 1880s included sketches of infants posed in this visual style. These illustrations depicted the infant body configured in standardized vertical orientation against a blank background, arranged to emphasize gross anatomical structures, and presented in a series of figures labeled "front view," "side view," and/or "rear view."[44] Drawn from observations of the remains of deceased infants, they were often quite graphic in their portrayal of exposed viscera and soft-tissue decay, presenting themselves as faithful and objective representations of bodily reality even as they deployed stylized aesthetic conventions of type portraiture. (Owing to considerations discussed at the beginning of this chapter, I have opted not to include visual reproductions of these images here.)

Photographs accompanying late nineteenth-century case reports incorporated similar visual conventions. Even in the case of photographs taken soon after birth, before removal and preparation of the body as an anatomical specimen, these conventions presented individual infants in their family homes as decontextualized scientific specimens. These images showed recently deceased infants photographed close-up; centered in the frame; and once again pictured from the front, side, and back, with background context omitted or minimized. In some case reports, infants were photographed against a black background, even more closely approximating the curated photography of museum collection specimens published in *Human Monstrosities*.[45] Absent the contextual trappings of family life and domestic comfort, these newborns were visually coded as standardized, atomized, and abstractable specimens of science. While practitioners lauded the medium of photography for its ability to represent the unadorned truth of the body "just as it was," free from an artist's subjective mediation and interference, the photographic images they produced continued to be structured by stylized and contingent visual rhetorics.[46]

Notably, this visual rhetoric aligned monstrous infants with a burgeoning anthropological genre of ethnoracial portraiture. In the second part of the nineteenth century, Anglo-American anthropologists attempted to standardize the use of photography as a way to produce data about human racial types. They sought to codify visual conventions that included photographing subjects isolated and centered in the pictorial frame in "established anthropometric poses," pictured both from the front and in profile. Indeed, serial images of isolated subjects shown from front and side views became a "hallmark of anthropometric photography" in the late nineteenth century.[47] Within ethnographic and colonialist photography that adopted these conventions, individual subjects from regions outside Europe were presented as fungible referents of an ethnoracial "type," used to buttress white-supremacist taxonomies of human racial classification.[48]

The visual coding of monstrous bodies through the aesthetic conventions of specimen and ethnographic "type" portraiture underscores the way these images produced a racialized imaginary of monstrosity—an understanding of the monstrous body as representing a distinct and separate type of being. Recall that nineteenth-century Anglo-American practitioners used the term *race* both to designate an entire animal species and to designate divisions within that species, broadly defined with reference to geography, ancestry, and/or phenotype. The word could describe populations that were both far broader and far narrower than those delineated by contemporary racial categories. Medical journals from this period used *race* to designate a distinct animal species, referring to the full "human race" or to the "race" of snakes.[49] The reports also named a dizzying assortment of intrahuman "races": They included the "race" of "ancient Romans," the "Anglo-Saxon race," the race of "Indo-Europeans," the "colored races," the "indigenous races" of the Americas, the "white race" (singular) and the "white races" (plural), the "black race" (singular) and the "black races" (plural), and "races such as the Egyptians and the Chinese," as well as designations of "civilized races," "primitive races," and "the lowest savage races."[50]

These sources used *race* in seemingly contradictory and inconsistent ways: the singular human race, the many human races. However, the multiple nineteenth-century significations of race did not constitute distinct and unrelated concepts but were instead inextricably entwined. Whether used to delimit the entire human species or a particular population within it, the term *race* in all these contexts denoted a typological category of being, located within an implicitly or explicitly graded hierarchy of human/animal kinds. While the demarcation of boundaries between "races" differed wildly across examples, on another level the broader logic of typological demarcation unified them all.

This historical formulation underscores Zakiyyah Iman Jackson's interpretive contention, discussed earlier in the chapter, that race fundamentally constitutes "a discourse of speciation."[51] It was in this context that the linked aesthetic conventions of specimen and physical type portraiture helped to produce the compounded racialized alterity of the monster as a race of being set apart from both the white Anglo-American family and the broader human species.

Across these wide-ranging visual representations, medical practices of illustration and photography charged monstrous bodies with sometimes contradictory valences and meanings. As in other arenas, the configuration of monstrosity in medical images foregrounded the tensions and paradoxes of the category. On the one hand, a recurring theme involved the positioning of a monstrous newborn as a separate type of being, distanced in some way from the ontological status of a human child. In some of the examples discussed, this was accomplished by depicting monstrous specimens in positions that a newborn human subject could not attain or by removing contextual signifiers of existence within familial life. Recall the drawings of infants posed on all fours to highlight similarity to "the lower orders of animals"; the "skeleton of anencephalus" posed standing fully upright, as if in the likeness of a miniature adult biped; and the infant body photographed in profile and framed against a featureless black background in the stylized tropes of specimen or ethnographic portraiture. Both the drawing as quadruped and the posing as biped served, in different ways, to aesthetically position the monster as exemplar of a separate and unfamiliar species, dissociated from relational contexts of human sociality and the life stage of the human child. The conventions of scientific specimen and physical type portraiture further constructed monstrous bodies as a separate classificatory kind, hinting at the deep links between the study of monstrosity and taxonomic logics of race and human difference.

These portrayals visualized the deviant body as a species apart, as holotype of an othered being: alienated from the anatomy, familial context, life course, and the racial/species descent of a human infant. Yet other medical images of monstrosity—case report illustrations of newborns resting on pillows and in bassinets, clothed in trimmed garments, proportioned to emphasize the visual signifiers of biological human infancy—situated such newborns within familial and familiar contexts, locating them as infant human offspring within domestic settings of birth and encounter. Visualizing anomalous offspring as both foreign species and domestic kin, the images of monstrosity in medical science elaborated tensions and contradictions that had long structured the category of monstrosity: the tense and resonant commingling of alterity and familiarity, stranger and relation, other and self—paradoxical conditions of alienated kinship and bestial humanity, beings both too unlike and too like for comfort. Far from quelling the cultural and symbolic resonances that animated the category of monstrosity, this modality of medical practice once again refigured and circulated them in new ways. Further, these visual productions revealed entanglements of medical monster making with multivalent discourses of race, suggesting how nineteenth-century logics of racial classification intimately interfaced with new teratological conceptions.

CHAPTER FIVE

Monstrous Logics

Concepts of Race, Sex, and Disability

1868: "ORDERS, GENERA, AND SPECIES"

The woman, named as Amelia H., gave birth in 1868. She was attended in a difficult labor by an Anglo-American physician who worked for the Panama Railroad Company, the US corporation that "effectively ruled" the port city they called Aspinwall.[1] The company had overseen construction of the Panama Railroad in the 1850s, a project of "informal U.S. empire" that occurred before the formal expansion of US empire overseas at the close of the nineteenth century. Like much of the migrant labor force recruited by the Panama Railroad Company, Amelia H. was from Jamaica.[2] She was twenty years old and of mixed African and European ancestry. Early in her pregnancy she had attended an acrobatic performance, perhaps as part of a traveling show that came to entertain those passing through the bustling Atlantic terminus of the railway line.

Amelia went into labor about a month before expected, early on a September morning. After sixteen hours of pains, a single infant arm was presenting, but despite the "forcible and frequent" contractions no further progress seemed to be made. George Badger, a US physician employed by the Panama Railroad Company, was at this point called in to assist. Ultimately, with the aid of chloroform administered to relax her muscles, Amelia delivered stillborn twins: as recounted in the published case report, "*two girls united by the tops of the heads.*"[3] When the young mother saw her conjoined infants, she recalled the intertwined bodies of the acrobats she had seen months before.

Accounts of this birth appeared in at least two US medical journals. In one, a New York physician classified the infants as a species of "compound monster" belonging to "*Genus I.*—CEPHALOPAGUS," which fell under "ORDER II—*Terata anadidyma*" in an elaborated taxonomic system created by a fellow US physician. Using the same taxonomic categories deployed to classify plant and animal kinds, the physician identified several other instances of this same "species" and "genus of monster" in transatlantic clinical literature. Notably, the childbearing women involved in the cited case histories came from countries in Western Europe, Eastern Europe, and South Asia.[4]

Nineteenth-century classification schemes often sought to draw pronounced divisions between human racial groups. Indeed, the derogatory term the physicians used to identify Amelia H.'s mixed racial ancestry—*mulatto*—implied that a child of an African-descended and a European-descended parent constituted, like a mule, the offspring of two unlike species. According to the precepts of *polygenesis*, a mid-nineteenth-century theory taught widely in both Northern and Southern US medical schools, different continental populations of humans represented distinct and separately created species.[5] Yet in this case history, women of African, European, and Asian descent birthed infants classified as the same "species" of monstrosity, belonging to Class I, Order II, Genus I of the "compound monsters."[6] Within the prevailing taxonomies of mid-nineteenth-century US medical science, these mothers might not belong to the same species as one another—but, remarkably, they could bear monstrous infants who did.

1885: "MUCH LIKE THE AZTEC CHILDREN"

Early in her pregnancy, in 1885 or 1886, the unnamed Anglo-American woman attended a traveling circus exhibition with her husband. The pair were drawn, perhaps, by the chance to see the "extraordinary living curiosities" featured in Barnum's American Museum, advertised as "the wonder of America" in a breathless broadside. Promotional materials for the exhibition promised "family amusement" of the most "instructive and moral character."[7] There, as her husband later reported to their physician, the woman had viewed the "Aztec children."[8]

The "Aztec children" referred to a long-running exhibit that featured a brother and sister called Máximo and Bartola. The siblings, both of whom had congenital microcephaly, were advertised to audiences in the United States and Britain as the lone survivors of an ancient Central American race. Popular late nineteenth-century circus exhibits such as the "Aztec children" drew on a white-supremacist discourse of civilization that positioned individuals with variant anatomical forms as representatives of primitive nonwhite races marked for extinction or as "missing links" between beasts and "civilized" Anglo-American societies.[9] The conflation of racial difference and congenital anatomical difference permeated both popular culture and medical discourse in this era. Indeed, some nineteenth-century medical literature used the phrase "Aztec type" to refer to congenital microcephaly.[10]

There is no indication that the woman herself felt particularly affected by her trip to the circus. She did not describe having any difficulties with the pregnancy until toward the very end, when she felt afflicted by "a peculiar train of symptoms." She continued to feel active fetal motion, but her belly swelled so suddenly and so dramatically that she now appeared as if she were carrying twins. The source of this mysterious swelling was revealed during labor with the release of a "deluge" of amniotic fluid. Her physician reported filling "a twelve quart pail full to the brim," which he dipped with a basin from the bed. He described the infant's emergence with an affect of particular repugnance, writing that, "with another pain, this *thing* was born." The stillborn child had no upper skull, exposing a "rudimentary brain no larger than a hickory nut."[11]

The woman's husband immediately felt sure that the infant's condition had been caused by their excursion to the Barnum exhibit months earlier. While not prepared to confirm or deny, the physician averred that "the shape of the lower head was very much like the Aztec children, sloping downwards and backwards."[12] Yoking together imaginaries of monstrosity and Indigeneity, the infant in this telling came to embody the figure of racial alterity encountered by the white mother during her pregnancy.

1888: "THE LOWEST IN THE HUMAN RACE"

Upon touching what felt like a crowning head, the midwife felt sure that a second infant was coming. Just fifteen minutes earlier, she had delivered the sixth child of her patient, a thirty-three-year-old woman. Now, the women prepared for the birth of the "perfectly formed" newborn's unexpected twin.[13]

The midwife was not certain what to make of what happened next. Nor was the physician—a noted New York gynecologist and, later, avowed eugenicist—who arrived afterward to examine what he described as a "monster without a trunk." The "head-like mass" measured under four inches in diameter; it was covered in short thin hairs and large pores but contained no other clearly recognizable structures. The physician discerned indeterminate protuberances that resembled "rudimentary" facial features and extremities as well as "the outlines of cartilaginous plates" that might represent precursors to the bones of the skull. There was also a "tail-shaped" structure, which he associated with a primitive ancestral form that human embryos typically passed through on their path to completed development.[14] The physician described the infant as neither male nor female.

Exhibiting the preserved remains to colleagues, he proclaimed that the "globular monster" represented "the lowest degree of organization known in mammalia and the human race." Finding no precedents in case literature, he declared that "it is the first time that a specimen of so low a degree of organization has been found in a woman." The doctor marveled at the contrast between the "perfectly formed child" and the amorphous twin.[15] He presented the ovoid body as a grim manifestation of the potential for racial degradation of the individual—a regression from the advanced physical organization of the species type to the most rudimentary of biological forms—that haunted the highest orders of human reproduction.

These vignettes reflect three of the varied racial logics that animated the nineteenth-century medical engagement with monstrosity. White American practitioners constituted biological monstrosity simultaneously as a race or species apart from humanity, as an analogue of racially marginalized populations (especially Indigenous American and Black populations), and as an embodiment of human racial degeneration.

As the preceding chapters have shown, medical meaning making around monstrosity was not confined to abstract intellectual theorizing by credentialed practitioners. It instead comprised an interactive, multisited, multimodal process that engaged a variety of people and practices. But although theorizing by medical professionals was not the *sole* avenue through which meaning making occurred, it nevertheless constitutes a critical part of this history. As historians such as Deirdre Cooper Owens and Rana Hogarth argue, physicians' knowledge making played a critical role in producing and circulating historical concepts of racial difference.[16] Drawing especially on Owens's insight that "medical journals were critical sites where 'race was daily given shape'" in the nineteenth-century United States, this chapter analyzes how practitioners conceptualized and configured intimately entwined categories of race, sex, and disability through their treatment and theorization of monstrosity in the medical press.[17]

For nineteenth-century practitioners, the term *race* referred both to a broad designation of the human species (the singular "human race") and to taxonomic divisions between human populations, usually defined with reference to geographic origin, ancestry, and/or phenotype. In this capacity, race served as an unstable yet central lens for constituting, assigning, and ascribing meaning to human variance. As a political category, race served to naturalize arrangements of power by appealing to the "givenness" of the physical order, anchoring social and economic hierarchy in the putative solidity of natural biological distinctions.[18]

Rife with ambiguities and contradiction, many different concepts of human racial difference existed in the nineteenth-century United States. A common early nineteenth-century discourse attributed racial variation to contingencies of climate and place, casting racial traits as environmentally malleable. At the same time, the institution of slavery defined race—and, more particularly, Blackness—as a permanent hereditary trait transmitted through the body of the mother. At midcentury, proponents of the theories of polygenesis and monogenesis clashed over whether different human races constituted separately created species or not. Later in the century, assorted notions of immutable biological difference, rooted in claims about racial anatomy and evolutionary descent, proliferated. Though experts and practitioners expended a tremendous amount of energy in their attempts to reliably define racial difference, their object proved elusive as the boundaries between coexisting and often contradictory schematics of race shifted, merged, fragmented, and blurred across the course of the century.[19]

Despite its unstable multiplicity, race remained a central category in the social, political, and economic life of the United States. Indeed, some scholars argue that the "protean character" and "mercurial nature" of race has directly enabled its historical "persistence" and "abiding power." The sustained processes of forming and maintaining contested distinctions of race ramified through nineteenth-century US histories of slavery and segregation, immigration, settler colonialism and Indigenous displacement, and the expansion of empire overseas.[20] The historical concept of "race" also encompassed and signified a broad range of other social and power relations, including constructions of gender, sexuality, class, citizenship, and nation. Recognizing what the historian Evelyn Brooks Higginbotham describes as the formative "role of race as a metalanguage" in US history, this chapter's analysis understands race as mutually constituted with other discourses of social difference and relation, particularly foregrounding the multivalent intersections of race with sex/gender and disability.[21]

Nineteenth-century medical case literature frequently referred to categories of "sex," which practitioners used to signify the division of both biological bodies and social roles into a gendered binary of male and female, defined with reference to imputed reproductive function. Like schematics of race, schematics of sex/gender in the nineteenth-century United States were messy, contested, and multivalent. Newer understandings of sex difference as a categorical biological binary coexisted with much older understandings of female and intersex bodies as less perfectly developed versions of male bodies.[22] In their nineteenth-century iterations, these categories of sex difference implicated and intersected categories of race in sundry ways. The notion of a sharply defined sex binary—made manifest through clear gendered distinctions between males and females in civilized societies—underwrote imaginaries of Anglo-American racial progress. Aspirational categories of "true" womanhood and manhood both defined and hinged on ideals of middle- and upper-class whiteness.[23]

Unlike the terms *race* and *sex*, the word *disability* almost never appears in the nineteenth-century medical literature on monstrosity. Late nineteenth-century sources occasionally referred to "disability" to denote acquired incapacity for labor (especially military service) but did not use the term to describe conditions of congenital anatomical variation.[24] However, informed by scholarship in disability studies, this chapter uses *disability* as an analytic concept to refer to the shifting social, cultural, and political discourses that constitute "othered" embodiment.[25] The chapter analyzes medical monstrosity as a particular cultural construction of disability—a contingent way of ordering and signifying variations of physical form. Understood in this sense, the category of biological monstrosity powerfully illuminates how nineteenth-century practitioners constituted and linked concepts of race, sex, and disability in emerging biomedical discourse.

The formal classification system of nineteenth-century teratology (the "scientific study of monstrosity") positioned monstrosity as a "race apart," seeming to set it in a separate taxonomic universe from the rest of humankind. Monstrous offspring received their own species and subspecies designations, distinct from and independent of their parents' racial categorization, and their medically identified sex frequently fell outside a male/female binary. Yet even as teratological taxonomy could ostensibly supersede classifications of human race and sex, teratological frameworks drew on and amplified particular nineteenth-century logics of racial and gender hierarchy. Practitioners conflated significations of racial, sexual, and anatomical variation within a common scientific framework of development that aligned "lower" races, nonmale bodies, and monstrosities as inferior versions of humanity arrested in a primitive stage of formation—monstrous-racial Others dislocated in organismal and evolutionary time. Framed as an extremity of racial degeneration, biological monstrosity became a warning about the fragility of racial inheritance and the liabilities of women's reproductive bodies during a period of rising cultural anxieties around Anglo-American decline.

Significantly, this deepening entanglement of monstrosity with cultural discourses of difference did not occur *despite* monstrosity's scientific framing but rather (in part) directly *through* that framing. Through the scientific framework of teratological development, monstrosity gained specificity as a way to articulate the nature of racial order: as hierarchical, temporalized, biologically embodied, and vulnerable to the perils of women's reproduction. Linking together racial and reproductive deviance in the figure of "defective" biological embodiment, medical monstrosity forged an imaginary of disability that was intimately connected to later eugenic logics of racialized reproductive control.

The chapter proceeds by exploring how three contrasting yet interwoven logics of human difference both structured and emerged from medical theorizations of monstrosity. These logics comprised the classification of monstrosity as an ontologically separate kind of being, existing outside of human racial and sexual taxonomies; the conflation of monstrosity with "inferior" human races and sexes within a unifying framework of hierarchical biological development; and the interpretation of monstrosity as racial degeneracy, materializing the feared fragility of white Anglo-American reproduction and descent. The paradoxes of teratological monstrosity, as an embodiment of difference that was simultaneously categorical and relational, offered practitioners a way to accommodate and reconcile contradictions in changing concepts of racial-reproductive order. Analyzed together, these multiple logics foreground the significance of biological monstrosity as a figure that could both expose and shore up the tensions, ambiguities, and instabilities in ever-shifting social imaginaries of difference.

A TAXONOMY OF SEPARATE KINDS: MONSTROSITY AS A RACE APART

The classification system of nineteenth-century teratology ostensibly positioned monstrosity as a race or species apart, seeming to set it in a separate taxonomic universe from the rest of humankind. Nineteenth-century practitioners categorized monstrosities through the "usually adopted" taxonomy of Isidore Geoffroy Saint-Hilaire, the French scientist whose "classical and authoritative work on Teratology" was, according to one US physician, "more frequently referred to in this country than any other authority."[26] Saint-Hilaire's system deployed the nomenclature of the eighteenth-century naturalist Carl Linnaeus—still widely used today to name biological organisms—to designate varieties of monstrous kinds. It assigned monstrous offspring their own class, order, genus, species, and subspecies classifications, distinct from and unrelated to their parents' classification in organismal taxonomies. This practice conferred upon the physician the epistemological authority to assess ontological kind and the nominal ability to elide nineteenth-century distinctions of race: for instance, by classifying the offspring of racially unlike mothers as like-subspecies of monstrosity. Yet even as the taxonomic practices of teratology appeared to supersede categories of human race, teratological frameworks ultimately also relied on and fortified particular nineteenth-century logics of human racial hierarchy.

The chapter's first opening vignette offered a concrete example of how teratological taxonomy could seem to overwrite concurrent distinctions of race. A comparison of two other case reports from the 1860s provides further illustration. One, from 1864, involved a woman of European descent in Rhode Island. The woman was young and had never given birth before. Her labor was reportedly uneventful up until the delivery of a stillborn "anencephalous foetus," which her physician sent to the prominent Harvard physician Jeffries Wyman as a specimen for collection. The second report centered on an infant born to a woman of African descent in South Carolina in 1866, just one year after the abolition of racial slavery in the state. When the physician A. A. Moore arrived late at night, the twenty-five-year-old woman had been in labor for close to forty hours and was experiencing intense and unrelenting pain, her breathing short and her pulse feeble. Four more hours passed before she delivered her child, a stillborn infant the physician described as "an *Anencephalus*."[27]

In identifying anencephaly, the physicians were not just diagnosing a medical condition but also explicitly designating a species of being: more particularly, a species belonging to Class I, Order I, Genus III of the human monstrosities in Saint-Hilaire's widely disseminated taxonomy. Notably, mid-nineteenth-century physicians engaged in the classification of human as well as monstrous species. Both Wyman and Moore had professional connections to leading proponents of polygenesis, the theory of separate racial origins that was sometimes invoked to defend racial slavery and segregation.[28] Under the precepts of polygenesis, the two women from these case reports—one of Western European descent and the other of African descent—would be classified as belonging to different species from one another. Yet, remarkably, they bore offspring classified as belonging to the same species.

Existing within an alternate taxonomic world, monstrous offspring sometimes appeared untethered from the orderings of human difference so central to nineteenth-century racial science and to the nineteenth-century institutions of imperialism and slavery that from time to time surfaced explicitly in the case literature on monstrosity. Indeed, the very definition of monstrosity as "departures" or "deviations" from "the type of the [parental] species" appeared to flout the dictum of "like begets like."[29] This dictum, initially posited by Aristotle as a principle of animal generation, had come to undergird the influential hereditarian conception of race as an inviolable trait transmitted from mother to offspring, powerfully codified in laws defining hereditary racial slavery in the Atlantic World.[30] The monstrous offspring of women could seemingly contravene this "natural law" of racial descent: born to racially categorized women but classified as members of their own species apart.

In addition to unsettling categorical boundaries of race, monstrous bodies could also elude the categories of binary sex. Case histories from across the century frequently described the sex indeterminacy of monstrous bodies, reflecting a constellation of present and/or absent anatomical structures that resisted an unequivocal assignation of *male* or *female*. The case literature on monstrous birth brimmed with explicit designations of nonbinary sex, which included "not a male, neither was it a female," "of neither sex," "sex doubtful," "sex is somewhat doubtful," "sex rendered extremely doubtful," "sex could not be determined," and "bilateral hermaphrodite."[31] In the early nineteenth century, some practitioners even categorized "hermaphroditism"—which referred to mixed or ambiguous characteristics of sex—as itself constituting a type of monstrosity.[32]

Seeming to defy the conventional taxonomies of race and binary sex used to order human bodies, monsters instead demanded their own system of classification. As discussed, US medical practitioners drew heavily on Saint-Hilaire's work for this purpose. Leading US practitioners glossed Saint-Hilaire's teratological taxonomy in medical reference works and used his system to organize catalogs of monstrous specimens in medical museums; physicians across the country invoked his nomenclature to diagnose individual infants in clinical cases and presentations.[33]

US physicians did not just passively adopt taxonomic systems from European scientists—they actively elaborated and revised them. In 1866, the New York physician George Fisher proposed a more detailed and rigorous "scientific system of nomenclature and classification" to distinguish the varied anatomical forms of conjoined twins, explaining that so-called "double monsters" had as yet received inadequate attention in taxonomic literature. Aspiring to "conformity with the scientific principles required in botanical and zoological systems," Fisher enumerated three orders, nine genera, and thirty-two distinct species, with an additional twenty subspecies varieties, in the larger class of "double monsters."[34] Medical museums used some of this nomenclature to classify their growing anatomical collections, and in case reports US physicians proudly noted that the terminology was created by "one of our own countrymen."[35]

In the late nineteenth century, the University of Pennsylvania Medical School professors Barton Cooke Hirst and George Piersol also sought to update Saint-Hilaire's teratological taxonomy in their four-volume series *Human Monstrosities*, a reference work deemed "one of the masterpieces of American medical literature" by the *Journal of the American Medical Association* in an 1893 review.[36] The series' first volume opened with a two-page taxonomic chart designating the varieties of human monstrosities. As shown in figure 5.1, the chart was visually organized as a *cladogram*—a branching scientific diagram used to map out evolutionary relationships among species. It retained the Linnaean system used by Saint-Hilaire: "Class 1: Single Monsters" contained two "orders" of monstrosity; each order branched off horizontally into two to four "genuses" of monstrosity; each genus branched off into one to three "species" of monstrosity; and each "species" branched off into three to six "subspecies."[37]

Like Fisher, Hirst and Piersol explicitly positioned their classification system as akin to those used in the fields of botany and zoology: Where botanists enumerated species of plants and zoologists

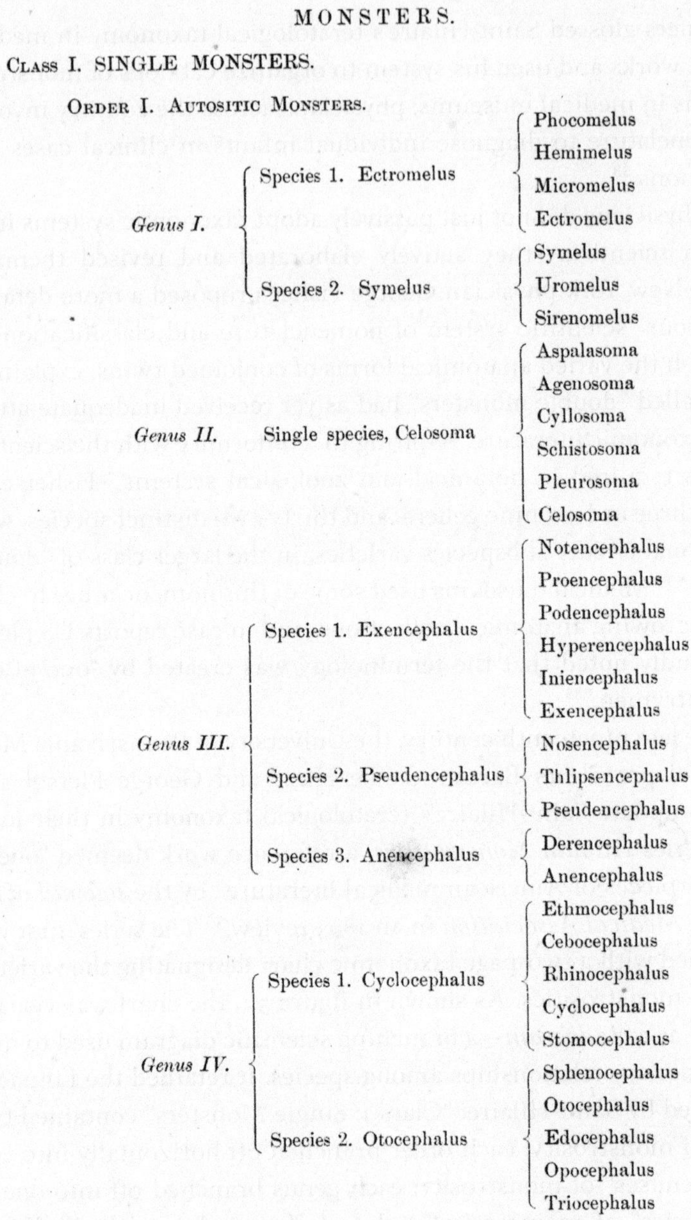

MONSTERS.

CLASS I. SINGLE MONSTERS.

ORDER I. AUTOSITIC MONSTERS.

- *Genus I.*
  - Species 1. Ectromelus
    - Phocomelus
    - Hemimelus
    - Micromelus
    - Ectromelus
  - Species 2. Symelus
    - Symelus
    - Uromelus
    - Sirenomelus
- *Genus II.* Single species, Celosoma
  - Aspalasoma
  - Agenosoma
  - Cyllosoma
  - Schistosoma
  - Pleurosoma
  - Celosoma
- *Genus III.*
  - Species 1. Exencephalus
    - Notencephalus
    - Proencephalus
    - Podencephalus
    - Hyperencephalus
    - Iniencephalus
    - Exencephalus
  - Species 2. Pseudencephalus
    - Nosencephalus
    - Thlipsencephalus
    - Pseudencephalus
  - Species 3. Anencephalus
    - Derencephalus
    - Anencephalus
- *Genus IV.*
  - Species 1. Cyclocephalus
    - Ethmocephalus
    - Cebocephalus
    - Rhinocephalus
    - Cyclocephalus
    - Stomocephalus
  - Species 2. Otocephalus
    - Sphenocephalus
    - Otocephalus
    - Edocephalus
    - Opocephalus
    - Triocephalus

FIGURE 5.1 Taxonomic diagram listing genera and species within the order of "Autositic Monsters," printed in Barton Cooke Hirst and George Piersol, *Human Monstrosities*, 4 vols. (Lea Brothers, 1891–1893), 1:11. *Source*: Courtesy of the Truman G. Blocker Jr. History of Medicine Collections, Moody Medical Library, University of Texas Medical Branch at Galveston.

enumerated species of animals, teratologists enumerated species of monstrosity.[38] This positioning aligned teratological classification with taxonomies of natural kinds, which classified types of beings, and distanced it from taxonomies of medical conditions, which classified morbidities, pathologies, and diseases.[39] Indeed, in case reports, some physicians saw no contradiction in describing an infant as both "a monstrosity" and as "perfectly healthy."[40] Though anencephaly arose through "morbid" and "pathological" processes of embryological development, the teratological designation *anencephalus* was not just a diagnosis of pathology. It was also a designation of a "distinct species," located within a taxonomy not of morbidities but of biological kinds.[41] To diagnose disease was to delineate what was not healthy in the human body; to diagnose monstrosity was to delineate what was not characteristic in the human race.

This authority was not an exclusively abstracted one. A teratological taxonomy was not a free-floating conceptual construct but one actively applied by the physician at the site of an embodied, interpersonal encounter. Hirst and Piersol explicitly intended their taxonomic system to be used in the context of clinical medical practice, presenting *Human Monstrosities* as a guide "for the physician who may meet malformations and monsters in his practice, and may desire to locate and name them."[42]

In this work of teratological classification, a medical practitioner arbitrated the species membership and human status of patients' offspring, not just theoretically but on an applied, case-by-case basis. Emphasizing the real-life stakes of this ontological categorization, an 1873 medical jurisprudence manual argued for the necessity of limiting classificatory authority to expert physicians: "If a liberty of judging what was monstrous and what not were conceded to any ignorant nurse, children simply deformed might be put to death on this pretence." In rhetoric that likewise underscored both the critical stakes of categorizing monstrosity and the special authority of medical expertise, a midcentury physician suggested that a variety of legal cases involving monstrosity could "call forth, in an especial manner, the wisdom of the medical jurist"—for instance, to determine whether an acephalous fetus counted as sufficiently human for the purposes of prosecuting a late-term abortion or whether "a pseudencephalus monster" counted as sufficiently human to have legal standing as an heir.[43] The medical ability to sort and classify monsters entailed an authority to ascertain not only the health and sickness of bodies but also the "humanness" of their shape, their biological rank in the order of life-forms, and even their legal and moral standing. Beyond the authority of assessing disease, this ability entailed the authority of assessing ontological kind.

Yet even as teratological taxonomy rendered monstrous difference as a distinction of ontological kinds, it also conceptualized monstrosity as a difference of degree, ordered along a temporal continuum. This was another paradox at the heart of monstrosity: While the category of monstrosity entailed divisions of separate kinds, it also entailed an explicitly relational form of difference—graded by continuous increments with respect not just to anatomical form but also to the temporality of development.

FRAMEWORKS OF DEVELOPMENT

Scientific theories of development undergirded the nineteenth-century field of teratology.[44] In lauding their new modern understanding of monstrosity, American physicians cited the work of French and German scientists such as Isidore Geoffroy Saint-Hilaire and his father, Étienne Geoffroy Saint-Hilaire, as well as Étienne Serres and Johann Friedrich Meckel, describing their advances in knowledge of human generation and development. In the eighteenth century, these topics had been the subjects of fierce scientific debate. Preformationists held that offspring were generated through the enlargement of prefigured parts, which existed in fully formed miniature inside an egg or sperm. By contrast, proponents of epigenesis posited that generation was a process of development: An organism did not merely enlarge but rather moved through a series of different and increasingly specialized embryological forms.[45]

Scientific teratology was premised on the latter idea. The field was predicated on an understanding of monstrosity as fundamentally developmental: That is, it was a condition produced in the course of embryological gestation, which was the sole period of an organism's life cycle during which monstrosity could arise. More specifically, "the immense majority" of monstrosities were produced through an *arrest* of development: an interruption of the embryo's progression at a critical point in its trajectory.[46] Indeed, this theory of arrested development, as exemplified in the arrested brain and skull development of anencephaly, constituted the "guiding principle in teratology" as laid out by Saint-Hilaire.[47]

In Saint-Hilaire's early nineteenth-century system, different "species" or "grades" of monstrosity corresponded to the relative timing of the arrest in the course of gestation. Glossing Saint-Hilaire's work for an American audience soon after its publication, the *American Cyclopedia of Practical Medicine* of 1834 explained that for each "grade of monstrosity, the process of evolution has advanced further before its acts became arrested, than in the [lower] grade."[48] (In this pre-Darwinian context, the word *evolution* was used interchangeably with *development*.) For instance, as described in an 1850 case report, the "thlipsencephalus species" originated with an arrest of head development in "about the third month" of pregnancy, while the slightly more developed "nosencephalus species" originated with an arrest "in about the fourth month."[49]

The taxonomic cladogram that later opened *Human Monstrosities* visually encoded this logic of temporal hierarchy, placing species and subspecies of monstrosity in relation to one another based on the timing of their descent—the order in which they emerged in the chronological sequence of development. Thus, the listing for *nosencephalus* was visually positioned above the comparatively more "primitive" *thlipsencephalus*, as shown in figure 5.1. Both were positioned above *anencephalus*, the least "evolved" subtype of all, whose arrest of head development occurred earlier in gestation (around the "fourth week") than for any other in that species or genus.[50]

In this schematic, the deviance of monstrous species was an explicitly temporal deviance: Monstrous development was development arrested in *time*. As one nineteenth-century practitioner explained, monsters "are unnatural *and out of place, because they are out of time*."[51] In US medical literature, physicians advanced the teratological precept that "monsters from arrest of development may be considered as permanent embryos," retaining "at the end of their intra-uterine life some of the organs in the simple state in which they were first formed."[52] The monster from arrest of development disrupted the continuity of the passage from unborn (embryo) to born (fully formed infant), freezing the orderly developmental progression of past into future. The birthed "permanent embryo" was a temporal dislocation: "Primitive" and "incompletely evolved," the monster was a present organism stuck in its past.[53]

The trajectory of an organism's development was structured not only by the passage of time but also by progressive improvement. Nineteenth-century physicians conceptualized and described development not merely as an increase in size and complexity but as a movement toward increasing perfection of form along a graduated continuum of attainment. A nineteenth-century American obstetrics textbook explained how an embryo "developed from this rudimentary imperfect formation, through all the stages of foetal existence, to that of the perfect child."[54] Conversely, a monster was "imperfectly developed" and "imperfectly formed."[55] Defined with respect to perfection, these conceptions of development encoded a logic of value and hierarchy. The developmental understanding of monstrosities positioned their existence within a scheme of progressive—but, significantly, degradable—physical perfectibility, a ranking of worth inscribed in the material formation of the body and mapped onto a temporal scale.

The "imperfection" of the monster was further defined by locating it within orders of animal kinds. The notion of the "Great Chain of Being"—which placed all species along a hierarchical continuum, ordered from lowest to highest—had existed since antiquity.[56] In the eighteenth century, the influential French naturalist Georges-Louis Leclerc, Comte de Buffon, drew on this concept to arrange human races in a "natural" hierarchy, placing Europeans at the top of the scale.[57] Early nineteenth-century theorists applied the concept to ascendent theories of embryology, asserting that the process of embryological development "recapitulated" the natural hierarchy of animal kinds. Formulated by Meckel and Serres, this early nineteenth-century idea was espoused by leading US scientists as well: Louis Agassiz, famous Harvard scientist and infamous proponent of scientific racism, explained in 1849 that developing embryos passed through a series of stages resembling each of the "lower" species in the hierarchy before reaching the "perfect" form of their parents.[58]

In this telling, monsters—halted at an earlier stage in the series—could illuminate the graduated relationship between humans and the "lower orders" of animals. As one Philadelphia physician averred in 1858, "The embryonic condition of a superior animal resembles, in a more or less striking manner, the permanent condition of another animal less elevated in the series." Thus, a human-born monstrous infant, arrested at this "embryonic" or "primitive" stage of development, recalled the final form of a species from "the inferior degrees of the animal scale."[59]

Teratological discourse of this period, then, invoked a doubled series or continuum: the continuum of individual development, from undifferentiated embryo to fully developed organism; and the continuum of ranked animal species, from the lowest orders of beings to the highest. This early nineteenth-century discourse imparted a temporalized aspect to the understanding of the relationships between species of being, linking a hierarchical "series of animals" to the ontogenetic time of embryological development. Embryogenesis was an explicitly chronological process: The "stages of foetal existence" corresponded to the passage of defined units of time. Thus, when "an animal less elevated in the series" was analogized to the "embryonic condition" of a "superior animal," its location within the hierarchy of beings was temporalized: It was halted at a moment in developmental time that the animals ranked above it had moved beyond. Rendered within this framework of development, the series of animal species was organized along an axis of temporality.

Already theorized with respect to a temporal continuum of development, the posited relationship between embryological development and the animal series was not so much revolutionized as it was amplified by the later nineteenth-century dissemination of Darwinian evolutionary theory.[60] This post-1859 reworking was encapsulated in the phrase "ontogeny recapitulates phylogeny," popularized by the German biologist Ernst Haeckel in the 1860s. In this explicitly Darwinian formulation, the phrase conveyed that an individual's embryological development in utero (ontogeny) retraced the evolutionary stages in the ancestral development of the tribe, race, or species (phylogeny).[61] Not all medical-scientific experts in this period accepted "ontogeny recapitulates phylogeny" as literal truth. However, they widely agreed on the general premise that in the course of intrauterine development an individual passed through stages resembling the forms of its evolutionary forebears.

This was a modification of earlier theories that purported to explain the embryo's recapitulation of the "order" or "natural series" of animals rather than the ancestral evolution of the species. The post-Darwinian category of phylogeny—the relational descent of organisms in deep evolutionary time—was temporalized independently of the category of ontogeny in a way that earlier nineteenth-century understandings of the "animal scale" and the "natural series in the animal kingdom" were not. Within this doubly temporalized configuration of "ontogeny recapitulates phylogeny," monstrosity could be powerfully articulated as a condition of "reversion": a living throwback to a more primitive ancestral race within the parental species' evolutionary descent. A Pennsylvania physician invoked Darwin's theories in 1872 to discuss how "certain deformities" might be attributed to a "*reversion* to primitive forms," while a Louisiana physician wrote in 1879 that anomalies and monstrosities "represent anatomical structures habitually found in lower forms of life, hence constitute what evolutionists term—reversions."[62]

This developmental framework of teratology thus located monstrosity not just within the time scale of embryological development but also within the time scale of animal evolution. The signal "monster by arrest of development" was both a being arrested at a "primitive" stage of embryological development and a being arrested at a "primitive" stage in the descent of species, situated within a temporalized hierarchy of animal kinds.

DEVELOPMENTAL LOGICS OF SEX, RACE, AND DISABILITY

Through this framework of temporalized animal hierarchy, US medical literature intimately linked monstrosity to broader nineteenth-century discourses of embodied human difference. More particularly, practitioners configured the nature of monstrous development with explicit reference to developmental hierarchies of sex and race as well as implicit reference to disability. Mapping the continuum of development onto a ranked series of species, they cast sex, race, and disability as interlocking forms of temporalized difference that located certain human bodies as "monstrous" through their closer proximity to the "lower orders" of animal kinds.

In nineteenth-century case reports on monstrosity, coexisting discourses of biological sex difference invoked frameworks of development in at least two distinct ways. First, they posited an ontogenetic continuum from female body to male body, casting the male body as the most advanced and perfectly developed form of the human individual. Second, they posited a phylogenetic continuum from sexually indeterminate "primitive" species to sharply sexually differentiated "higher" species, presenting binary sex difference as a marker of advanced evolutionary development.[63]

Notions of progressive development scaffolded theories of gendered sex difference in classical antiquity, which described women as less perfect, less complete, or less developed versions of men. The historian Thomas Laqueur argues that this older model of sex difference—casting men and women as gendered variations of a single kind of body, of greater or lesser degree of metaphysical perfection—was superseded in the post-Enlightenment world by a hegemonic two-sex model, which conceptualized male and female bodies as categorically distinct biological entities.[64] However, in the nineteenth-century United States, multiple and often contradictory models of sex difference existed simultaneously.[65] Even as Anglo-American physicians in this period often wrote about sex as a categorical difference in type, they also mobilized understandings of sex difference as relative and developmental in order to link monstrosity to nonmale sex.

Multiple case reports observed that conditions such as anencephaly occurred more frequently in female than male infants. To explain this pattern, some physicians explicitly asserted a common origin in arrested development for both monstrosity and femaleness. In 1837, two Southern US physicians, citing the theories of a prominent German scientist, wrote that "the observations of *Meckel* have proved the 'genital organs of the two sexes are formed primitively in the same model, and that they should be considered only as a modification of the same fundamental type'; and that the embryo is, *in all cases, primarily of the female sex*." In other words, "female" characterized the sex type of all embryos in the earliest stages of development, with some progressing into "male" types only at a later stage of gestation. The physicians invoked the work of a French medical theorist to explain that "the imperfect formation [of anencephaly] thus occurring more frequently in females has been supposed by *Georget* to be owing to a feebler energy of the formative or organic powers in the female than in the male."[66] In this, they positioned both monsters and females as less perfect versions of the more fully developed male.

Another case report from the 1830s, written by an Ohio physician, expressed similar ideas. This report not only linked monstrous development to femaleness but also used this linkage to locate the monster within a larger hierarchy of animal species, explaining that "the excessive proportion of female monsters seems to depend on the circumstance, that during the earlier period of the evolution of the foetus, *as in the lowest classes of the animal kingdom,* there is only one sex, namely, the female." From this, it followed that "when we say that the greater number of monsters are of the female sex, we only state in other terms that in the greater proportion of monstrous formations . . . the genital organs are arrested at an early period of their development."[67] In these renderings, practitioners invoked renowned scientific theorists to interpret both monsters and females as "primitive" and "imperfect" variations of a "perfected" male type—reflecting their common arrest at an earlier stage of human embryological development and their shared degradation in a hierarchy of natural kinds.

This second example shows how nineteenth-century teratological discourse could map the development of sexual difference both onto an individual continuum from female to male and onto a species continuum from sexually undifferentiated to sharply sexually dimorphic. As explored earlier, many monstrous infants were identified as being neither male *nor* female. In these cases, monsters' sexual ambiguity could align them with "lower" animal species that lacked the "higher" distinctions of binary sex. In an 1856 case report, a Missouri physician noted that "sexual distinction is absent in the early periods of foetal development," explaining that sexual organs "are anatomically alike in both sexes during the early stages of foetal growth." He explained that this temporary embryological condition in the "higher orders" of animals also characterized the "permanent condition" in the "lower" animal orders—and sometimes the permanent condition of human monstrosities, whose early arrests of embryological development could freeze them in a primitive state of undifferentiated sex. The report went on to analogize some of the genital configurations seen in monstrous human infants to the "normal structure" of genitals in other animal species.[68]

Accounts of monstrous infants' ambiguous genitalia also invoked the enduring discourse of females as less developed versions of males, with physicians describing "rudimentary" and incompletely developed "organs of male generation" as akin to "female organs." An 1835 report explained that sex was sometimes "rendered extremely doubtful" in cases of monstrous birth due to the fact that male genitalia halted in an early stage of development bore such compelling resemblance to typical female genitalia. A much later case history, in 1894, drew on a similar notion to describe an infant's sex organ as a "very rudimentary" penis that resembled "an enlarged clitoris" owing to the newborn's general condition of "arrested development."[69] Even as a substantial percentage of monstrous bodies seemed to elude traditional sex categorization, nineteenth-century practitioners still mobilized teratological discourse to affirm a hierarchy of sex that upheld the developmental supremacy of maleness.

Located within a developmental hierarchy of human bodies, teratological monstrosity implicated concepts of racial as well as sexed difference. Indeed, the two categories were inextricably entwined in a nineteenth-century discourse that positioned the development of binary sex—and sharp gendered divisions of men's and women's roles in society—as constituent of white racial progress.[70] Theorists mobilized concepts of development to underwrite a vision of white supremacy, elaborating the imagined continuum of animal kinds to include a ranking of human racial groups. In this explicitly racist rendering of developmental progress, "savage" dark-skinned peoples were located closest to the bestial species below humanity, representing the earliest and most primitive developmental stage of human existence. By contrast, "civilized" white Anglo-Americans were located at the top, representing the apex of human cultural and evolutionary development.[71]

The developmental discourse of race that came to predominate in the late nineteenth-century United States has often been described as arising in the wake of Darwinian evolutionary theory.[72] However, such discourse also bore pronounced continuities with earlier nineteenth-century teratological discourse. Late nineteenth-century theorizations of racial difference in disciplines such as ethnology, anatomy, and psychology directly invoked teratological frameworks of arrested, imperfect development. In *Races and Peoples: Lectures on the Science of Ethnography,* published in 1890, the ethnologist and physician Daniel Brinton wrote that "it is essentially on arrested or imperfect, in contrast to completed, development that the differences of races depend" and discussed the "arrested or retarded development" of the "lower races." To explain racial difference, experts such as Brinton invoked the exact language of "imperfect" and "arrested development" that underwrote the category of teratological monstrosity. In a section entitled "Criteria of Racial Superiority," Brinton defined the "higher races," which he specified as "the European or white races," as those possessing the traits most "true to the type of the species." This formulation located the racial superiority of whiteness in contradistinction to the degradation of teratological monstrosity, which was conversely defined through its severe deviation from the true "type" of the species.[73] Positioning racial inferiority as a state of arrested development, Brinton articulated a truism of late nineteenth-century racial science that the "lower races" retained "more numerous fetal, infantile, or simian traits" in their adulthood, making them "unquestionably inferior to him whose development has progressed beyond them, nearer to the ideal form of the species."[74] Brinton and other nineteenth-century race scientists thus used a common framework of development to position the "lower races" as constituting a kind of monstrosity: beings halted in a state of primitive and imperfect development on the temporal scale of descent, marked by their failure to progress to the "ideal form" of the human species.

Medical-scientific discourse configured both the monstrosity of the racial other and the racial alterity of the monster. In individual case reports of monstrous birth, Anglo-American practitioners concretized the racial Otherness of anencephalic infants in a variety of ways. In some instances, they explicitly referred to the features of non-European peoples as a way to describe and categorize the bodies of infants born to European-descended parents. In one set of examples, elite Boston physicians described "monstrous" anencephalic skulls in the Harvard Warren Anatomical Museum collection as like those of the "Caribs," Indigenous American inhabitants of northern South America and the Caribbean Islands. The catalog entries for these preserved specimens, from infants born to white parents in the 1860s, note that "from the very low and retreating forehead, the cranium somewhat resembles that of the Caribs" and that the "cranium is flattened, like a Carib's."[75]

In these references to "Caribs," the analogy of monstrosity to a racial other likely drew on understandings of figural racial traits as environmentally produced. Nineteenth-century medical literature reported that Caribs engaged in practices of "cranial deformation," intentionally flattening children's skulls by binding or securing them to cradleboards throughout their infancy, which was probably what the Boston physicians were alluding to when they described a cranial specimen as "flattened, like a Carib's." However, the physicians may also have encountered European travel literature that referred to "endemic microcephaly" in parts of the Caribbean.[76] In any case, many midcentury understandings of heredity and race—which often allowed for the heritability of environmentally acquired traits—blurred any neat distinction between cultural and congenital racial attributes.

Across case histories, physicians summoned a widely geographically varied set of non-European races to characterize the "monstrosity" of anomalous white infants. In an 1861 case, a physician in Missouri wrote that "the low, narrow, sloping forehead, the angular face with its oval malformation, made the child look more like the offspring of an Australian aboriginal than the issue of Anglo-Saxon parents." This infant was born to a "lady in the northern part of the city," who recounted an unexpected encounter with a pet bear chained to a tree while visiting a "suburban beer garden" in her fifth month of pregnancy. She had stayed in bed for two days after, fearing she would miscarry from the shock she had felt. In describing her offspring, the physician paired his invocation of racial alterity with an affect of marked horror and repugnance, characterizing the infant's face as "the most frightful physiognomy I had ever witnessed. The forehead was very low and narrow . . . the nose a tremendous 'pug' with very wide nostrils; the mouth was so hideous and unseemly as to baffle description." The mother tried to nurse the infant but found "that it could not suck, or even swallow anything from a spoon." The child's breathing became noisy and labored, and their face turned a livid blue-tinged color. They died about fifteen hours after birth.[77]

In addition to comparatively referencing Indigenous peoples of the Americas and Australia, physicians also invoked the bodies of

African-descended people to describe the features of white infants with anencephaly. In an 1864 birth in Adamsburg, Pennsylvania, the mother, a white woman, told the physician she had fainted early in her pregnancy after being approached by a Black soldier who came to her door and asked her for an axe. As discussed in chapter 1, the woman in this case described the soldier as "the worst featured and most disgusting human being she had ever beheld." Her child, born about six months later with anencephaly, was described by the physician as "precisely the color of a mulatto," with a nose "very broad and very flat."[78]

In an 1870 case, the physician was called to the house of "Mrs. K" a few miles out from Maysville, Wisconsin, on "a wild and stormy morning" in January. Mrs. K's labor had already lasted fifteen hours when the physician arrived, and she had been in great pain for the last ten of those. She was attended by an old woman who repeatedly assured her all was well and exhorted her to keep pushing. Following the delivery, the physician reported that the newborn's "ears and nose were rather larger than natural, especially the latter, which was flattened at its base, so that it bore some resemblance to that of a negro." He also noted that "the eyes were closed, like those of a newly-born pup"—a series of analogies that linked Blackness, animality, and monstrosity together in the medically narrated body of the infant.[79]

As later nineteenth-century discourses of race increasingly emphasized congenital rather than environmental origins of racial traits, leading biomedical experts concretized the linkage between monstrosity and attributes of racial inferiority by specifying a common mechanism of production. In an 1892 lecture, the prominent biologist Henry Fairfield Osborn described features of cranial development as markers of difference between "races which are in different stages of evolution." He asserted that in "white races" the typical "features of skull development are primarily the increase of the cranium and the late closure of the cranial sutures." By contrast, he claimed that "the early closure and arrest of brain development" in the "black races" was "well known." Casting racial difference as a hierarchy of developmental progress, Osborn explained that an arrest of cranial development that constituted "an anomaly in the white" was "normal in the black."[80] Through a common framework of development, white-supremacist concepts of race and monstrosity were bound together in very specific ways: The characters of "inferior" races were defined in scientific terms as "monstrous"—produced through an arrest of physiological development. This definition, in some sense, went beyond just simile or analogy. In Osborn's late nineteenth-century racial and teratological discourse, a "monstrous" white child's head did not just look *like* a Black child's head but was generated through the same mechanism, the material product of the same biological phenomenon of arrested development.

These developmental discourses of monstrosity helped produce and mobilize the entanglement of mutually defining imaginaries of race and *disability* (a word used here as an analytic term to refer to contingent social and cultural conceptions of othered embodiment and variant physical form). Indeed, critical attention to teratological monstrosity elucidates the nexus of disability, race, and sex as formative historical constructions of difference. The historian Douglas Baynton notes that the idea of disability has been invoked throughout US history to explain the nature of racial and sexual difference, describing how disability has been cast "as a sign of and justification for" racial and gender inequality.[81] The history of teratological monstrosity further exposes this entwinement by showing how medical discourse defined and stabilized imaginaries of sex and racial hierarchy with reference to notions of bodily deformity and defective development. The category of medical monstrosity linked and concretized cultural imaginaries of bestial species, female and nonbinary sexes, nonwhite races, and anomalous bodies through a framework of temporalized biological hierarchy, anchored and given corporeal culmination in the "imperfectly evolved" anatomy of the newborn monster.[82] In this figure of monstrous embodiment, social hierarchies of sex, race, and disability were given common grounding in the biological processes of gestational development, mediating between and merging the meanings of social and biological difference.

MONSTROUS DESCENT AS RACIAL DEGENERATION

Even as "monstrous" bodies anchored a biological imaginary of hierarchy and social order, they also threatened that order. Nineteenth-century medical discourses positioned monsters not just as icons of racial alterity but also as literal embodiments of "racial degeneration." This term referred to a condition of organic degradation or regression to which all human beings—even, and especially, white Anglo-American ones—appeared vulnerable. In materially merging the figure of the "racial other" and the "racial degenerate," monsters suggested an uneasy insight into the instability of the imagined racial-sexual order, foregrounding the porosity of the boundaries between racial types, the fragility of racial inheritance, and the liabilities of women's reproductive bodies.

Disrupting the racial dictum of "like begets like," teratological monstrosity provided a way to imagine relations of evolutionary descent among different species and types: a path through which one kind of being could produce an unlike kind. For this reason, the phenomenon of monstrosity long appealed to scientists as a potential mechanism for evolution. In the late eighteenth and early nineteenth century, Étienne Geoffroy Saint-Hilaire was enthralled with the idea of monstrosity as key to understanding the "transmutation of species," positioning "monsters as the harbingers of evolutionary change"; Charles Darwin recorded Richard Owen's suggestion to him that "the production of monsters . . . presents an analogy to the production of species." In Richard Goldschmidt's twentieth-century theory of "the hopeful monster," monstrosity was again posited as an evolutionary mechanism.[83]

While the "hopeful monster" was proposed to explain the generation of new species, the nineteenth-century "monsters by arrest of development" more obviously marked out a path of evolutionary regression than of evolutionary novelty. Stuck in an earlier era of developmental time, they represented a slide backward down the scale of animal beings to a more primitive and imperfect form. This interpretation positioned monstrous newborns not only as analogues of "lower races" but also as embodiments of racial degeneration.

In linking degeneration to concepts of racial difference, nineteenth-century clinicians participated in an intellectual tradition that extended back to early modern Europe. In the eighteenth century, Buffon claimed that the "inferior climate" of the New World caused degeneration, which he connected to characteristics such as smallness, weakness, and nonwhite skin. The eighteenth- and early nineteenth-century German naturalist Johann Friedrich Blumenbach similarly held that human racial varieties were produced through environmentally induced "degeneration" away from an original Caucasian form. Later, a more typological view of racial difference prevailed but still cast certain races as in and of themselves "degenerate types."[84] These ideas contextualized medical theorizations of race in the nineteenth-century United States, even as those theorizations were also shaped and refigured by new social, political, and interpersonal clinical contexts.

Discourses of degeneration structured US physicians' interpretations and representations of teratological monstrosity across the course of the nineteenth century. In the text (and, as shown in the previous chapter, the illustrations) of clinical case histories, physicians described monstrous infants as a degenerated or typologically degraded form of humanity—a literal embodiment of a slide back down the scale of animal kinds toward a less perfect form. As discussed, practitioners linked the ontogenetic continuum of individual development to the phylogenetic continuum of animal kinds, interpreting monsters as stuck in a stage of primitive development that their human parents had progressed far beyond.[85]

In the later nineteenth century, anxieties about racial degeneration among European and European-descended populations became increasingly pervasive.[86] This anxiety was a fear of both biological and social decline: a concern that the (white) human body would devolve into a degraded state—imagined, now through an explicitly Darwinian evolutionary framework, as a regress to the "phylogenetically less mature types" of evolutionary forebears—and that the moorings of society would concomitantly deteriorate.[87] Cultural historians of the United States have identified intensifying fears of "degeneration and racial decline" beginning in the late nineteenth century, expressed in the work of experts such as the American psychologist and educator G. Stanley Hall, who, explicitly influenced by Haeckel's recapitulation theory, worried about white American children's failure to progress through the epochal stages of their proper racial development.[88]

In the US context, later nineteenth-century fears of racial degeneration were entwined with contingent imperatives to reassert and maintain racial hierarchy and boundaries in the wake of Emancipation and the end of chattel slavery—an institution that had been centrally involved in defining and structuring US categories of race—as well as with new anxieties surrounding immigration and overseas imperial expansion late in the century.[89] Claims about the degeneration of the "American race" underwrote late nineteenth-century efforts to restrict immigration on the basis of individual physical or mental "defect" as well as of racial and national origin, emphasizing how ideas about racial degeneration intimately implicated categories of disability.[90] The overseas expansion of US empire after the Spanish-American War in 1898 also amplified discourses of racial degeneration, which were marshalled to express anxieties about white "racial deterioration" in newly US-occupied territories such as the Philippines.[91]

Amid these changing contexts, later nineteenth-century case reports continued to invoke previously established teratologic logics of degradation and decline to primitive forms, while also beginning to refer explicitly to "racial degeneration" in addition to "degradation of the organism" and to frame their fears of organismal regress in Darwinian evolutionary terms. Lamenting "the forces which are only too plainly working toward racial degeneration and disintegration," a Georgia physician wrote in 1897 that obstetric practitioners were in a special position to see these "forces at work." As discussed earlier, late nineteenth-century physicians began to identify the characters of monstrosities as "evolutionary reversions," casting the production of monstrosity as a retreat to a more primitive order of beings along a Darwinian scale of evolution.[92]

Situated in new contexts of social and political attention to the notion of racial degeneration, the medical category of monstrosity—which theorized and concretized the degradation of type at the level of the individual organism—assumed an even more charged cultural resonance. Embodying the mechanism of racial degeneration, the biological figure of the monster also articulated its threat, suggesting the instability of the racial order (and, especially, of whiteness) by revealing the insecurity of racial reproduction.

In case histories of monstrous birth, the offspring that physicians spoke of as stuck in a "primitive state of formation," akin to "the lower orders of animals" and "the inferior classes of animals," were generally born to specific women who, as far as the physicians had noted, bore no obvious flaws. Nineteenth-century case histories instead frequently noted that the women who gave birth to monsters were "well formed" or "well-developed."[93] True, some "monsters" were born to women already marginalized or demonized in nineteenth-century medical discourse, as in the case of enslaved Black women who bore "monstrous" offspring within a violent regime of slavery that both inscribed and was predicated on the assignation of racial inferiority.[94] Indeed, a significant number of "monstrous specimens" were birthed by women already deemed suspect or inferior by virtue of race, religion, ethnicity and immigration status, or transgression of sexual or gender norms—which might include being "masculine," being unmarried, and/or being suspected of sexual promiscuity.[95]

But many of the monsters in American medical collections were the progeny of women described as "respectable ladies," a phrase typically reserved for married, middle- and upper-class, Protestant, Anglo-American white women: women who were wives to white, "able-bodied" Protestant men and mothers to "well-formed" and "healthy" and "perfect" American children. They were women introduced in case reports as "a highly respectable and intelligent lady of my neighborhood" or "a happy wife and mother, with all the comforts of an elegant home."[96] In these cases of monstrous birth, refined women with no obvious signs of racial, sexual, social, or bodily deviance produced "degenerated" children, interpreted by physicians as a slide down an imagined scale of worth toward a more imperfect form.

That these women gave birth to monsters presented, then, a concern for Anglo-American biomedical elites. If the offspring of such women were not guaranteed to form in those ways which in "natural state are destined," then no one's racial reproduction was secure: The destiny of descent could be thwarted in the perilous stage of development.[97] At a time when Anglo-American racial science sought to establish increasingly hardened and immutable biological boundaries between the races, the birth of monsters bluntly exposed the biological instability of a social order predicated on racial inheritance.[98]

Although monstrous births occurred in all races of women, nineteenth-century developmental discourses on race and monstrosity presented white women as particularly vulnerable. Early nineteenth-century teratologists taught that "monstrosity is much more frequent in the higher than the lower" orders of animal kinds. They explained this by asserting that "the more complicated the organization, the more stages of development the various organs have to pass through, and the more likely, therefore is their development to be interfered with from various causes, than in the simply organized."[99] Mapped onto the developmental hierarchy of human races that proliferated in nineteenth-century US medical discourse, a logic emerged in which the "complexly developed" white race was more prone than the "simpler" races to monstrous deviations from the course of their more intricate racial development. At the same time that practitioners conjured imaginaries of Black and Indigenous bodies to describe the nature of anomalous white infants, they simultaneously positioned Black and Indigenous populations themselves as less liable to congenital anomalies.

This discourse appeared in a variety of late nineteenth-century sources. An 1887 presentation on comparative disease in "white and colored races" at the American Surgical Association asserted that "congenital deformities are rarer in negroes than in whites."[100] After the presentation, multiple colleagues averred that this was a truism in medical and surgical practice. A report in the *American Journal of the Medical Sciences* made claims about the rarity of "congenital deformity" among an Indigenous people in South America, who allegedly never experienced "a case of monstrosity or other irregularity in birth."[101] Although concurrent and seemingly contradictory discourses actively linked "congenital deformities" to Indigenous peoples—as in the pervasive trope that associated microcephaly with Aztecs or Caribbean peoples—they cast these conditions as "typical" racial traits in nonwhite populations and as "anomalies" or "deviations from type" only when they appeared in white populations.

In its intersection with nineteenth-century teratology, the developmental discourse of white supremacy—that is, of the white race as the most civilized, evolutionarily advanced, and complex of the races—thus positioned developing white offspring as most imperiled by the threat of monstrous deviation. In this context, the category of monstrosity signified not just racial alterity but also a specific kind of racial vulnerability: a heightened potential for degeneration and decline that inhered in the childbearing bodies of women from the most "advanced" racial groups, exposing the precariousness of whiteness by threatening to disrupt its orderly reproduction.

In the early twentieth century, fears about degeneration, racial decline, and the vulnerabilities of white reproduction would be deployed to justify and rally the powerful US eugenics movement.[102] By revealing how nineteenth-century teratology linked race to reproduction through the idiom of monstrous degradation, the history of biological monstrosity both elucidates nineteenth-century racial logics and highlights continuities with later reproductive regimes.

PARADOX AND THE FIGURE OF THE MONSTER IN THE RACIAL IMAGINARY

Suffused with ambiguities and inconsistencies, the multiple racial-reproductive logics of monstrosity offer insight into how practitioners navigated the tensions inherent in their racial imaginary. Earlier chapters have discussed the paradoxes at the heart of the category of monstrosity, showing how monstrosity embodied a relation of difference that entailed simultaneous kinship and alienation—both like and unlike, both family and stranger, both human and not human. Attention to the multiple racial logics of monstrosity continues to expose these paradoxes, revealing how monstrosity was rendered as a difference of separate kinds and simultaneously as a difference of degree or gradation; as simultaneously ontological (a type of being) and nosological (a type of morbidity); and as a classification system that seemed to overwrite taxonomic distinctions of human race yet also was mobilized to articulate and affirm them. Underscoring both the categorical and developmental logics of human racial hierarchy, the contradictions and paradoxes of teratological monstrosity echoed but also provided a means to navigate the many contradictions in concepts of race.

The historian Jennifer Morgan writes that early modern racial hierarchies emerged in "a space of corporeal contradiction": a logic of reproductive bodies, foundational to racial slavery, that implicitly recognized "sameness" even as it insisted on "fundamental difference."[103] This paradox continued to animate nineteenth-century hierarchies of race. Across the nineteenth century, categories of race were conceptualized as increasingly distinct from one another, the boundaries between them theorized as more and more impermeable: from an earlier nineteenth-century vision of racial difference as environmentally malleable, arising from the climate and contingencies of geographic place, to late nineteenth-century notions of fixed, totalizing racial difference that inhered immutably in the biological body.[104] Yet the very commitments and anxieties of racial science belied this firm conceptual separation of the races. The relatedness of human bodies was tacitly affirmed in the very practices of the fields that effaced it. Black patients' bodies were experimented on to learn things about white patients; anxieties over racial contamination, miscegenation, and racial ambiguity implicitly acknowledged the porosity of racial boundaries.

In the mid–nineteenth century, competing schools of thought in Anglo-American racial science were divided between those who believed that all humans belonged to the same species (monogenesis) and those who believed that different races had been created as separate species (polygenesis). The ascendance of Darwinian evolutionist thinking in the later nineteenth century seemed to resolve this debate, asserting that all races (indeed, all species) were related to each other through common histories of ancestral descent. Yet late nineteenth-century evolutionists continued to promote the idea of deep racial difference; as the scholar George Stocking argues, they simply replaced the "synchronic" hierarchy of polygenism with a "diachronic framework" for racial hierarchy that assigned racial groups to different places along "a temporal evolutionary continuum of physical and cultural development."[105] Rather than emphasizing human relatedness, evolutionist discourse worked hard to shore up a racial imaginary predicated on the separateness of racial groups, in this case by locating them along a hierarchy of development that temporalized their disunion.

Early and mid-nineteenth-century evolutionary thinking broadly associated with the French naturalist Jean-Baptiste Lamarck held that traits acquired in a person's lifetime (for instance, an environmentally induced change in skin color or head shape) could be inherited by offspring, potentially allowing for so-called racial characteristics to change rapidly in the course of a generation. By contrast, Darwinian evolutionism laid out a much lengthier time scale of adaptation. The increased temporal scale of Darwinian evolution allowed late nineteenth-century theorists to cast "the differences between races as so deeply rooted in time as to be almost primordial," even while claiming to regard "mankind as ultimately unified."[106] This occurred during a period of US history when major political projects—including the suppression of Black claims to social and civic equality following Reconstruction, the restriction of immigration and citizenship eligibility, and the expansion of US empire—depended on the assertion of a secure racial hierarchy. In this context, many Anglo-American theorists were deeply motivated to affirm the fixity of racial difference. Even if all humans ultimately descended from a common ancestor, they argued, the temporalized distance between races—the deep Darwinian evolutionary time separating them—was so vast as to be untraversable.

Yet astride a doubled temporal continuum of ontogenic and phylogenic development, monsters could in a sense collapse this time scale of racial descent. Monsters, merging the figures of the "racial other" and the "racial degenerate," revealed the potential in every human to conceive progeny that declined, in the parent's own lifetime, to an earlier and "lower" racial form. As both analogue of an "inferior race" and embodiment of a "racial degenerate," monstrosity theorized a particular relationship among races: one that was developmental, hierarchical, temporalized, and fraught with reproductive danger. But even as it exposed this reproductive instability of the racial order, the category of monstrosity also promised to smooth over the foundational contradiction between "sameness" and "fundamental difference" that plagued imaginaries of race, offering a way to acknowledge the biological relatedness of "inferior" kin while still placing them outside the "true type" of the human species. In these capacities, medical discourse on monstrosity became a potent way for nineteenth-century physicians both to elaborate concepts of biological racial hierarchy and to negotiate their paradoxes.

The nineteenth-century medical engagement with monstrosity also powerfully illuminates linkages of race, sex, and disability in emerging biomedical discourse. Configuring the racial and sexual difference of nonwhite and nonmale bodies as deviations of biological development, medical discourses of monstrosity conceived a racial-sexual order both predicated on and imperiled by imaginaries of congenital disability. In this formulation, the category of monstrosity foregrounded pregnancy and women's reproduction as sites of particular racial vulnerability, positioning gestation as a critical window in which racial inheritance could either be perfectly realized or monstrously degraded in the offspring's bodily form. Binding together potent cultural anxieties over racial, reproductive, and bodily deviance, the figure of the monster suggested and affirmed a protoeugenic imperative to intervene on "defective" reproduction for the protection of racial integrity.

CHAPTER SIX

Monstrous Legacies

Eugenic Afterlives of Monstrosity

Mrs. L's 1924 letter to Charles Davenport was penned tidily in black ink, each of the ten pages carefully hand-numbered at the top. Davenport was not the first or even second expert that Mrs. L had consulted about her predicament. She had first turned to her own doctor, "one of the finest obstetricians" in her city, but his reassuring platitudes failed to satisfy her. Next, she approached a professor on the science faculty at a nearby university, but he likewise proved unable to assuage her concerns. Now, she reached out to Davenport—academic biologist, director of the Eugenics Record Office in New York State, and key architect of the national US eugenics movement. For Mrs. L, the "calamity" of her first birthing experience demanded an explanation to make sense of, and she was determined to get a robustly scientific one.[1]

In an era marked by the elaboration of "scientific motherhood"—the notion that childbearing and child-rearing should be guided by expert medical and scientific advice—middle-class women like Mrs. L took an increasingly active role in seeking out and applying biomedical expertise on matters of maternity.[2] Mrs. L's involvement in soliciting and helping to configure a scientific explanation for her birth experience reflects how ascendent biomedical discourses circulated between lay and professional spheres in the early twentieth century, intimately interacting with lived reproductive experiences. By the 1920s, the field of eugenics, defined by proponents as "the science of improvement of the human race by better breeding," constituted an influential source of biomedical expertise.[3] Offering an enticingly simple biological explanation for the United States' wide-ranging social and economic ills, eugenicists promised a solution that hinged on the control and management of sexual reproduction. It was in this context that Mrs. L turned to Davenport, a professional biologist she had never spoken to or met, for advice on the most intimate aspects of her fertility and familial life.

In her letter to Davenport, Mrs. L described the stressful circumstances leading up to her first experience of childbirth. She had felt unready for marriage at the time of her wedding two years earlier to her husband, a World War I veteran who had been badly wounded in France. In particular, she was "quite ignorant of matters pertaining to sex," and her initial reactions to the expectations of matrimony "were of a highly nervous order." After eight months of struggling to "accomplish sexual intercourse naturally," she visited a medical specialist who performed a "slight operation." While this eased the physical difficulty of the act for her, she still felt an overwhelming sense of discomfort and anxiety surrounding sex with her husband, which persisted at the time of conception two months later.[4]

The birth was devastating. She had initially felt proud of herself for being "able to give birth to my child without the use of instruments," which she felt reflected well on her health and physical constitution. But then she and her husband received "a most terrible shock." Upon delivery, it was discovered that the stillborn infant's "head was abnormal": "Twice the size of the head of a normal boy baby," it "extended towards the back in an egg-shaped manner." Mrs. L presented the birth as a source of everlasting parental shame: "I am sure that I do not need to tell you how carefully my husband and I guard our terrible secret," she wrote to Davenport.[5]

Mrs. L deeply wanted children, and she had worked hard to fortify herself for healthy motherhood. "I am at present a very healthy woman, much healthier than I have ever been," she wrote to Davenport. Yet before she and her husband could even contemplate having another child, she needed to know: What was the "possibility of such a thing recurring"? "Not to have children would be an absolute tragedy for both of us, but, naturally, that tragedy would be infinitely preferable to a worse one," she wrote.[6]

For Mrs. L, this tragedy seemed to constitute both the grief of losing a longed-for child and the shame of failing at eugenic motherhood—the imperative to birth and raise "sound" and "fit" offspring for the good of the family, the nation, and the race.[7] The details Mrs. L offered in her letter suggested the inculcation of a worldview predicated on a deep moralization of biological health, bodies, and reproduction. Her husband had been able to survive septicemia following a war wound only because of his "athletically trained and morally clean body."[8] Her ability to give birth without complications proudly demonstrated her fitness for motherhood. Delivering a biologically "abnormal" child then seemed to impugn that fitness, constituting a "terrible secret" to hide in furtive shame.

To help Davenport make the requested assessment, Mrs. L presented and elaborated on a range of possible biological explanations, rooted in understandings of physiology and genetic heredity. Neither her husband's body nor her own escaped scrutiny for potential blame. Could her husband's "germ cells have been poisoned" by his bout of septicemia during the war, resulting in damaged sperm? Could her nervousness have had "an upsetting effect" on her "glandular secretions" during conception and gestation? Most pressingly, Mrs. L wished to know if the trait was genetically inherited. She first offered for Davenport's consideration a summary of her and her husband's "family history for four generations back," suggesting her detailed familiarity with Davenport's research methods.[9]

Davenport served as director of the Eugenics Record Office (ERO), established in 1910 in Cold Spring Harbor, New York, as the premier center for eugenic research in the United States. At the ERO, researchers collected US family histories and filled teeming rows of cabinet files with pedigree charts, which they used to identify and trace the transmission of "desirable" and "undesirable" traits across generations. Their methods rested on a foundational understanding of human value as hereditarily determined—dictated by the content of chromosomes and genes at the moment of conception. To improve the nation and the human race, they believed, America simply needed to promote the transmission of "fit" genes and prevent the transmission of "unfit" genes to future generations.[10]

Making clear the applied political implications of this deterministic hereditary doctrine, the ERO promised to help US state and local governments "locate the centers in which their defectives and delinquents are being bred" and take "steps that will diminish such reproduction."[11] The category of "defective" persons implicated wide-ranging conditions of poverty, social marginality, and physical and intellectual disability—all construed as fixed hereditary traits that menaced the country's social and economic future. While promising benefit for the whole nation and indeed all of humanity, the ERO's agenda was heavily predicated on an imaginary of a white, Christian, middle-class America that needed to be purged of disability from within and protected from racial "contamination" from without.[12]

To advance their mission, ERO eugenicists advocated targeted immigration bans, marital restrictions, the coercive confinement and sterilization of "defectives" in state institutions, and, most subtly, the cultivation of a "quickened eugenic sentiment" in the hearts and minds of everyday people like Mrs. L. This cultivated eugenic sentiment would then guide laypeople's personal conduct in their reproductive lives, inspiring those of "superior" stock to marry and raise large families with similarly "superior" partners and pressuring those likely to produce "inferior" offspring to refrain from conceiving children.[13]

Given her apparent familiarity with Davenport's emphasis on the genetic inheritance of defect, Mrs. L may have been surprised by the answer she received. In a typewritten reply to Mrs. L, Davenport reported there was "little evidence" that the condition she described "depends, to any important degree, upon hereditary factors." He advised her to "be careful to avoid undue nervous excitation during gestation," explaining "there is a possibility of disturbance in endocrine secretions which might in turn influence the development of the child." Ultimately, however, he assured her that "it does not seem probable that a second child would be abnormally developed in the same way."[14]

While Davenport's de-emphasis on hereditary factors may have seemed out of character, it was perhaps not so surprising that he would give a woman like Mrs. L his blessing to conceive again. While eugenic advocates claimed that their movement transcended social prejudice, focusing only on the unbiased facts of genetics, in practice they showed themselves concerned primarily with limiting the reproduction of those already socially marginalized in relation to class, disability, race, ethnicity, citizenship status, gender-role conformity, and sexuality. In the case of the white, well-educated, middle-class, and respectably married Mrs. L., Davenport was inclined to see an instance of birth anomaly as a tragic one-time accident rather than as evidence of innately defective genetic stock. Yet for Mrs. L herself, steeped in imperatives of eugenic motherhood that enjoined her to bring forth "well born" children as her gendered duty to the nation and the race, the birth remained a source of furtive and fearful shame.[15]

Moving into the twentieth century, this chapter traces changes, contractions, and paradoxical expansions in the biomedical engagement with monstrosity—which, in this era, now centrally implicated professional academic biologists and eugenicists as well as physicians and laypeople. The chapter begins by surveying the shifting landscape of US medical and scientific attention to monstrous births in the early twentieth century. This attention continued to include medically attended births and scientific specimen collection, shaped by new institutional and political contexts of life in the early twentieth-century United States. At the beginning of the century, a brief surge of academic scientific interest in teratology centered the influence of environment on embryological development. In this period, scientists, laypeople, physicians, and social reformers alike engaged in increasingly fraught conversations surrounding the relative importance of environment and heredity in human development. As a hereditarian focus increasingly came to dominate, biomedical attention shifted away from major teratological monstrosity and toward the slighter but far more ubiquitous "hereditary defects" of greatest interest to the ascendent US eugenics movement.

Yet in other critical ways the legacies of teratological monstrosity persisted in the eugenics era, continuing to animate biomedical logics of defect, race, and reproduction. As the previous chapter argued, nineteenth-century medical practitioners invoked monstrosity to theorize racial difference as both biologically hierarchical and vulnerable to the dangers of defective descent, laying the groundwork for an imperative to intervene on biological reproduction for the preservation of the racial order. In the early twentieth century, the imperative of racialized reproductive control took powerful and unprecedented political forms. Even as eugenicists foregrounded far subtler conditions of hereditary "defect," the specter of the biological monster continued to haunt imaginaries of racial and reproductive deviance. Significations of nineteenth-century teratological monstrosity lived on in scientific, political, and popular discourse, surfacing in both experts' and laywomen's frameworks for understanding bodies, birth, disability, and human value.

TERATOLOGY IN THE EARLY TWENTIETH CENTURY

Mrs. V's history with pregnancy was a troubled one. Her first pregnancy, in 1911 when she was twenty-seven, ended in a miscarriage. She underwent two medical procedures afterward to clean out tissue from her womb, both performed without anesthesia, and subsequently suffered from a persistent uterine infection. She had been "unusually healthy and strong" while growing up, but after this experience her vigor seemed to dwindle. She conceived again two years later. It was a medically difficult pregnancy, marked by symptoms of kidney disease in the last month. Her arduous labor, attended by medical practitioners who used forceps and other instruments to hasten delivery, resulted in the birth of a stillborn son.[16] The escalating use of medical interventions during pregnancy and childbearing typified broader national trends in this period—as did the high rates of morbidity and mortality associated with these obstetric practices, which frequently entailed aggressive use of instruments and scant attention to infection control during delivery.[17]

Now, at age thirty, Mrs. V was pregnant again. The pregnancy had not begun auspiciously. In the earliest weeks, Mrs. V was "subjected to nervous shock" when her parents arrived unexpectedly from out of town to stay with her at her home in Mount Vernon, Washington. Affective tensions did not resolve during the course of this surprise visit, as Mrs. V bristled against her parents' "considerable worry on account of changes in temperament incidental to her pregnancy and misunderstood by her guests."[18]

Like many of her nineteenth-century predecessors discussed in chapter 1, Mrs. V experienced sustained physical unease throughout her pregnancy. At first, the discomfort was persistent but manageable. She drank laxative doses of bottled mineral water every day to ease her constipation. She eventually began to feel fetal movement, though only in the form of sporadic "sudden kicking." Toward the end of the pregnancy, her discomfort burgeoned. In the final week, her belly swelled rapidly, bringing new heights of discomfort. The pressure from the immense distension made it feel impossible to comfortably fill her lungs with air, and the tension on her back produced spasms of pain. She began to sleep sitting up at night because lying down in this state felt intolerable.[19]

Mrs. V gave birth in November 1914. Though the delivery occurred at home, it was heavily shaped and directed by obstetric interventions—an increasingly common experience for white middle-class women like Mrs. V in this period, as twentieth-century US physicians began to consolidate practical and cultural authority (no longer just aspirational) over childbirth.[20] Mrs. V's physician, George Ritter Smith, conducted a vaginal examination and then "ruptured the membranes" to induce labor. He and his assistant administered anesthesia to Mrs. V for the pain of her contractions and used forceps to deliver her child, a stillborn infant described by Smith as an anencephalic "monster."[21]

In a published case report, Smith discussed a variety of potential causes of monstrosities, beginning with "heredity"—a category of explanation that began to routinely appear in the case literature on monstrosity in the late nineteenth and early twentieth centuries. The rest of the possible explanations on the list, however, focused on environmental factors during pregnancy. Like nineteenth-century predecessors, Smith discussed the potential role of maternal emotions in disrupting prenatal development, citing the work of experts who believed that "shock, worry, deprivation, etc., may produce vascular and nutritional disturbances in the endometrium which may seriously affect the growth of the ovum." In her narration of significant events during her pregnancy, Mrs. V also positioned the relevance of the emotional distress she had endured during her parents' visit. In addition to maternal emotions, Smith mentioned that exposure to "chemical poisons circulating in the maternal blood may affect the young embryo," showing himself conversant with the latest laboratory research in the linked fields of embryology and teratology. He explained that "experiments have proved that lithium, sodium, and potassium produced characteristic monsters"; noting the work of American as well as German biologists, he described how "Stockard and Lewis produced monsters from the eggs of the common minnow by treating them with solutions of magnesium chloride."[22]

Smith's appeal to the laboratory findings of prominent US scientists such as Charles Stockard marked a change from earlier case literature. When Smith's nineteenth-century predecessors discussed experimental research in teratology, they cited work being done in continental Europe.[23] In the early twentieth century, however, the United States emerged as a center of experimental embryological science, which entailed a surge in research on anomalous (i.e., teratological) as well as typical embryological development.[24] In 1908, leading American embryologist Franklin Paine Mall, who went on to found the Carnegie Institution's renowned Department of Embryology at Johns Hopkins, released "A Study of the Causes Underlying the Origin of Human Monsters." In narrating the renaissance of institutional interest in embryology in the United States, Mall and colleagues accorded a significant place to this teratological work, highlighting its release as a moment that "marked the conversion of our studies of embryology from a local to a national enterprise."[25] The broader rise of academic biology in US universities produced a distinct class of professionals who now, along with physicians, studied and exercised authority over the scientific knowledge of monstrosity. In "Origin of Human Monsters," Mall praised "the masterful strokes of American teratologists" who conducted their own experimental research on anomalous embryological development in laboratory animal species.[26]

The rising prominence of embryological research in the study of monstrosity also occasioned a new focus on acquiring embryos as well as fetuses and infants for specimen collections, an endeavor that jointly engaged biologists, physicians, and childbearing patients. Spearheading a national embryo-collection project based at Johns Hopkins, Mall and his colleague Arthur Meyer enjoined physicians to send embryological specimens of miscarried "monsters" from their patients. As in nineteenth-century collection, these patients came from heterogeneous class backgrounds: Mall and Meyer noted that they received a large amount of "embryological material" from "physicians practising among the poorer classes, as well as from gynecologists and obstetricians practising among the wealthier."[27]

New social and political contexts of the early twentieth century also shaped this collection. The expansion of the United States as an imperial power with overseas colonial holdings—following the 1898 acquisition and subsequent occupation of the Philippines, Guam, and Puerto Rico—enabled new sites of extractive acquisition. Mall and Meyer called attention to "the large number of specimens emanating from a single hospital in Manila," facilitated by the American graduates of Hopkins Medical School who staffed this hospital in the US-occupied Philippines. (Mall and Meyer explained that these Hopkins-trained physicians "responded loyally to our request for Filipino embryos for a study of racial embryology," suggesting how an investment in concepts of biological racial difference remained entangled in medical activity and studies of development.) The Progressive Era elaboration of government oversight and regulation could also engender novel avenues for collection. Mall and Meyer noted that a new city law in Baltimore requiring physicians to register their patients' miscarriages and stillbirths proved to be "of great advantage" to the embryo-collection project, allowing the scientists to enroll the city- and state-run Departments of Health in efforts to acquire specimens.[28]

Physicians participated in embryological research activity not only by sending in miscarried embryos from their patients but also, like Mrs. V's physician, by keeping abreast of new experimental research on the effects of teratogens on laboratory animal species. Biomedical attention to *teratogens*—specific environmental agents that disrupt embryological development—is typically dated to much later in the century, associated with rising awareness of the prenatal effects of the drug thalidomide and the viral disease rubella in the 1960s. The emergence of teratology as an organized US research discipline is often dated to the 1960s as well, with the founding of the first research journal and professional society dedicated exclusively to teratology as a distinct academic field.[29]

However, the medical and scientific literature on monstrosity reflects much earlier study and discussion of teratogens (i.e., specific chemical and physical agents capable of disrupting embryological development) in both academic biological research and clinical obstetric practice. The early twentieth-century "American teratologists" praised by Mall conducted research not only on invertebrate and fish species, whose developing eggs were more obviously exposed to the external environment, but also on mammalian species who gestated their young inside the womb. In addition to treating the developing eggs of fish species with various chemical solutions, the biologist Stockard also conducted research with collaborator Dorothy Craig on the influence of alcohol on guinea pigs' embryological development.[30] By the early 1920s, researchers at US universities were studying the effects of trans-species blood infusions on rabbits' embryological development as well as the effects of radiation exposure on rats' embryological development.[31] In these experimental studies, academic scientists exposed pregnant laboratory animals to specific chemical or physical agents, producing teratological "monstrosities" in the developing offspring.

Clinical medical practitioners took note of these activities. In a 1913 medical journal article, a prominent Philadelphia physician described recent studies and relayed their conclusions that monstrosity arose as a result of "external influences" that created "an unfavorable environment" for embryological development. A case report by a Boston physician from the early 1910s likewise discussed the newest findings of research in "experimental teratology" conducted "upon chicks, sea urchins, and the like." Some early twentieth-century physicians also applied the concept of teratogenic exposure more directly to consideration of human patients. For instance, a 1923 case history of an "anencephalic monster" born to a nineteen-year-old Jewish immigrant from Russia ruled out potential causes by noting that the patient, Rose F., "had no unusual illness, surgical operations, or X-ray exposure previous to delivery," positioning disease and exposure to a specific physical agent (radiation) as possible etiologies of monstrous development.[32]

Mall presented advances in experimental teratology as a climactic moment in long-standing debates of broad significance to humanity. In his introduction to the "Origin of Human Monsters," he wrote that "from the earliest ages of the world's history the study of monsters, and the causes which produce them, has been one of the capital problems in anatomy, medicine and natural history." He claimed that all this discussion could be reduced to a single question: " 'Are the conditions which produce a monster germinal and therefore hereditary, or are they produced from normal germs by external influences?' " New laboratory research in teratology, he wrote, now offered a definitive answer. Monstrosity was not determined at the time of conception, traceable to preexisting defects in the parents' egg and sperm; rather, it was contingently produced, emerging from the operation of "external influences which act upon the egg after fertilization."[33] Framing monstrous development as a question of heredity versus environment, Mall proclaimed the latter to be the cause.

THE POLITICAL STAKES OF ENVIRONMENT VERSUS HEREDITY

In 1916, Mrs. C. L. H. of Harrisonville, Missouri, wrote to the US Children's Bureau to inquire if they might help her with "a debate concerning heredity and environment."[34] The Children's Bureau, a federal agency created in 1912 to address the health and well-being of US children and families, reflected a broader early twentieth-century investment in the development of social welfare services and the expanding capacities of government. Although the bureau, like other Progressive Era institutions, lauded the possibilities for circulating and applying scientific knowledge to social problems, it proved hesitant to wade into the debate on biological determinants of human development. In response to another letter of inquiry on the subject, bureau chief Julia Lathrop averred that "the Bureau would not care to be drawn into the controversy as to the relative influence of heredity vs environment." As her correspondent was "doubtless aware," Lathrop wrote, academics and policymakers were currently "divided into hostile camps" on the matter.[35] In an era of increasing state and expert involvement in matters of public welfare, the debate over the importance of heredity versus environment implicated fiercely contested visions for how to best manage and improve the health of the American body politic.

Yet the conceptual separation and opposition—indeed, antagonism—between the categories "heredity" and "environment" had not always appeared so self-evident. Indeed, for much of the nineteenth century a sharp conceptual cleavage between "heredity" and "environment" did not exist. In these more capacious earlier renderings of heredity, the content of what parents transmitted to offspring was understood as a composite resulting from the mutable convergence of the parents' cumulative life experiences, circumstances, and "original constitutional endowments."[36] This constitutional inheritance entailed tendencies or predispositions, which then interacted with and could be reshaped by new environmental conditions and life experiences. Nineteenth-century discourse on the cause of monstrosity, which sometimes suggested that a mother's "nervous temperament" or constitution predisposed her to strong emotional impressions from external events during pregnancy, reflected this characteristic blurring of environmental and constitutional factors in explaining human development.[37]

In the late nineteenth century, however, a dichotomy between internal hereditary and external environmental determinants of development began to sharpen. The understanding of internal determinants was often articulated with reference to a new theory of the "germ plasm," which posited that the factors determining development were contained in and transmitted to offspring exclusively through the parental germ cells (sperm and egg).[38] In the most rigid renderings of genetic heredity, the course of an individual's development was locked in at the time of conception, impermeable to any later interaction with the environment.

Some late nineteenth-century US physicians began to incorporate the concept of "germ plasm" and ideas of genetic heredity in their speculative discussions of monstrous etiology, though these ideas still largely took a backstage to the focus on other potential causes. In 1896, when a thirty-year-old working-class woman called Mrs. M gave birth to an infant with anencephaly in an obstetric clinic at Rush Medical College, the supervising physician Frank Stahl considered that "the ovum may have inherited a tendency to abnormal growth." Ultimately, however, both Stahl and Mrs. M identified external influences during gestation as the major cause of her infant's condition. Mrs. M recounted a harrowing moment she experienced during the third month of her pregnancy, when she witnessed a Chicago streetcar collide with a small boy. Powerless to stop the unfolding tragedy, Mrs. M watched in horror as the car ran over the child, crushing and mangling his body. Stahl proposed that a pregnant woman's physiological reaction to a severe emotional shock of this kind could affect the physical processes of development inside her womb. He relayed that these kinds of "disturbing influences from without" generally played "a far more important role than heredity" in the genesis of monstrosity.[39]

By the first decades of the twentieth century, the relative influence of internal hereditary versus external environmental factors on development had become a hotly contested and politically charged controversy. The topic engaged not only scientists and physicians but also public-health officials, policymakers, and laypeople. Diverse childbearing women, ranging from working-class white women who wrote in to the Children's Bureau to the largely middle-class membership of the Black women's club movement, were keenly interested in determining which factors mattered most in ensuring the "healthy," "perfect," or "normal" development of their offspring.[40] As new cultures of motherhood encouraged women to take up expert guidance on pregnancy and maternity, including from recently established state institutions such as the Children's Bureau or from local community uplift organizations, some early twentieth-century women directly documented their concerns and ideas in advice-seeking correspondence and newsletters.

These sources suggest how childbearing laywomen participated in and sometimes expanded or redefined the terms of discourse on determinants of development. When early twentieth-century biologists such as Mall discussed "external factors" that could influence development, they described exposure to discrete physical and chemical agents such as mechanical agitation, radiation, temperature extremes, atmospheric pressure, lithium, and alcohol.[41] However, in advice-seeking letters written to the Children's Bureau in the 1910s and 1920s, childbearing laywomen identified more complex external conditions that they worried might affect offspring's prenatal development. They described their concerns about disabling environments of economic deprivation, overwork, inadequate access to medical care, untreated disease, violence and cruelty from husbands, and lack of familial support during pregnancy.[42] A woman from Georgia who introduced herself as a "farmer's wife" asked about possible effects of the intensive manual labor she needed to perform while pregnant. A working-class woman in Illinois, nearing the end of her pregnancy, wrote an agonized letter disclosing the conditions of poverty, hunger, and domestic abuse that she "had to suffer and endure these eight months." She implored the Children's Bureau to "if possible start an association to protect mothers who are to give birth," emphasizing the significance of external environmental conditions for both her own well-being and her offspring's development. When she birthed the child she now carried, she wrote, she would be "afraid to look upon its little face. How can it be human and a perfect child after all that I have been through?"[43] In these accounts, laywomen offered a more capacious and socially situated framing of potential environmental influences on gestation than did biomedical experts (even as they tended to reproduce the same language that denigrated "abnormal" infants as "imperfect" or less than "human").

While the Children's Bureau refrained from taking an official position in "the controversy as to the relative influence of heredity vs environment" on human development, the agency largely sought to implement social reforms focused on improving environmental living conditions, including access to health care, nutrition, education, and social services during and after pregnancy. This was also the approach taken by some nongovernmental community organizations. As one major example, early twentieth-century Black women's clubs advocated prenatal care reforms within the purview of their efforts toward "racial uplift." Sadie Black Hamilton, writing for the Child Welfare Department of the National Association of Colored Women's Clubs (NACWC) in 1924, enjoined Black communities to "Begin with Pre-natal Care. Clinics and visiting nurse services. Extended visiting nurse services at birth." A NACWC report listing community uplift actions to be taken by club women included an injunction for them to work toward instituting local prenatal clinics. The NACWC's news magazine extolled community outreach efforts that included education "on the care of all parts of the body, the treatment of diseases, the regulation of diet, the value of fresh air, adequate sleep, and the minimum standard of pre-natal care."[44] These efforts emphasized the significance of maternal health and environment for prenatal development.

Early twentieth-century researchers in teratology, now convinced of the centrality of environmental influence on development, also voiced their support for social interventions aimed at improving environmental conditions in the prenatal period. The biologist Stockard reasoned that "it is possible to control embryonic development to such an extent as to produce abnormal structures. May not the proposition be reversed and unfavorable environments be treated in such a manner as to render them favorable to normal development?" He argued that to improve "the quality of offspring" in the American population, the "hygienic reform" of mothers' living conditions "is most important, and must precede, or go before, the selective mating of human beings or the eugenics movement."[45] Though Stockard agreed with eugenicists' contention that interventions were needed to "improve the quality of offspring" in the nation, he offered a substantially different opinion on what those interventions should be.

As Stockard alluded, leaders of the US eugenics movement at this time vehemently rejected an emphasis on interventions designed to improve environmental and community living conditions. They instead drew on a rigidly deterministic vision of heredity to establish the interlocking research and policy agenda of their increasingly powerful movement, which touted "race improvement" through "better breeding." Eugenicists promised to protect America from a burgeoning class of "hereditary defectives"—prominently including "the feeble-minded," "the insane," "the criminalistic," and immigrants from areas other than Western Europe—who, they claimed, were overdrawing the resources, unraveling the social fabric, and contaminating the "racial stock" of the nation.

The sinister implications of this eugenic program, which called for "securing the best blood for future generations" and "eliminating defective blood" from "future American stocks," may appear obvious to present-day readers.[46] Yet it is difficult to overstate the sweeping popularity and influence the movement once enjoyed in the early twentieth-century United States. In this period, a vast array of politicians, academics, religious leaders, community organizations, and laypeople enthusiastically championed the eugenic cause. While mainstream formulations typically centered an ideal of white Christian middle-class America, the movement's philosophy found favor across a striking range of seemingly unlikely populations, including examples of Black American and Jewish American communities who explicitly embraced eugenic tenets. State fairs hosted eugenic exhibits and events, including "better baby" and "fitter family" contests; churches across the country participated in a eugenic sermon-writing competition; and educational institutions from primary schools to colleges introduced the topic of eugenics into their course curricula.[47] Members of the institutional elite explicitly strategized to promote popular enthusiasm for eugenics, noting privately that "eugenics can never amount to anything practically" unless it became "a popular movement with a certain amount of religious flavor in it." (In a letter to Davenport, the prominent eugenicist and Yale economics professor Irving Fisher proposed tapping into existing anti-immigration sentiment as a "good lever by which to interest Americans in eugenics," describing the push for immigration restriction as "a golden opportunity to get people in general to talk eugenics.")[48]

While recognizing the diffuse and decentralized nature of American eugenics as a historical phenomenon, it is remarkable to note the prominence of academic scientists in theorizing, legitimizing, and often successfully codifying the movement's programmatic agenda. Signature policy goals drew on doctrines from the ascendent field of genetics and specifically from an interpretation of biological heredity in which discrete, quantifiable traits were fixed in and transmitted through the inviolable and all-determinative "germ plasm" or "proto-plasm" (the genetic material of sperm and egg cells). Insisting that "all men are created *bound* by their protoplasmic makeup," leading eugenic scientists—prominently including those at the ERO, the research institute Mrs. L wrote to—mobilized theories of genetic determinism to design, advocate, and justify interventions to prevent the propagation of "hereditary defectives."[49] Harry Laughlin, the ERO superintendent, proudly declared that a burgeoning number of state laws allowing involuntary sterilization "have been based upon the researches of the ERO" and wrote of the ERO's continued involvement in "the legislative, judicial, and administrative aspects of eugenical sterilization" in the 1920s. In his capacity as expert consultant to a special congressional committee on immigration, Laughlin advocated for immigration bans on the basis of national origins. Laughlin advised national legislators that unchecked immigration from areas other than Northern and Western Europe would result in "the contamination of future American stocks by the permanent introduction of excessive amounts of defective alien germ-plasm," demonstrating how ERO researchers deployed hereditarian biological terms and theories to underwrite and advance the movement's legal and policy aims.[50]

Not all eugenic advocates agreed with the approach taken by the ERO. There was considerable political diversity among the vast swathe of Americans professing to support eugenics in the early twentieth century, and those who proposed a focus on environment in conjunction with heredity often condemned ERO-backed policies such as eugenic sterilization laws. Notably, some local enactments of eugenic reform emphasized both environmental and hereditary improvement as complementary rather than conflicting imperatives for community uplift.[51] Yet this orientation increasingly went against the prevailing dogma of the movement's formal institutions. National leaders of the US eugenics movement confidently proclaimed the centrality of heredity—configured in explicit opposition to environment—as the foundation of the eugenic agenda.[52]

Fiercely advocating a set of interventions designed "by sterilization or segregation, [to] prevent the reproduction of the socially inadequate," movement leaders insisted that efforts to improve environment were futile because a person's inherent quality was already fixed and "locked" at the moment of conception. Davenport declared that "from the fate that is thus determined at the moment of fertilization of the egg, no individual can escape himself or be redeemed by others through any efforts made subsequently by changing the environment."[53]

In correspondence with the Yale professor and eugenicist Fisher, Davenport reacted with obvious irritation to the suggestion that eugenic researchers should investigate the validity of recent teratological research about the influence of environmental factors on reproduction. Although the issue was framed as an intellectual one, the political stakes of the concern were evident. Explicitly making the connection to their movement's policy agenda, Fisher wrote to Davenport that "it seems to me from the practical standpoint of eugenics important that there shall be no question" on the insignificance of environmental influence. He stressed that "in particular it makes a difference as to our attitude toward hygiene and our utilization of the hygiene movement." In other words, if environmental factors substantially affected development and heredity, then perhaps eugenic policymakers should focus on improving community living and public-health conditions rather than concentrating more exclusively on identifying and preventing genetically undesirable conceptions as a way to better the nation's future generations. Davenport, firmly committed to the latter course of action, ridiculed and witheringly rejected Fisher's proposal, insisting that such research should not be dignified with further attention.[54] In this context, scientific questions about determinants of development simultaneously constituted overtly political provocations about the means and justification for managing the quality and descent of human populations.

THE ECLIPSE AND PARADOXICAL EXPANSION OF SCIENTIFIC INTEREST IN MONSTROSITY

In the early twentieth-century debate between environmental and hereditary determinants of human development, the latter ultimately seemed to prevail in US biomedical discourse. In an otherwise laudatory biography of the embryologist Franklin Paine Mall published in 1934, the physician and biologist Florence Sabin suggested that Mall "went too far in his stressing of the environment as the cause of all pathologic ova," assuring her readers that if Mall, who died in 1917, had "lived ten years longer, he would certainly have modified this emphasis."[55] By the 1930s, attention to environmental influences on development had become largely subordinated in US scientific research, replaced by a focus on genetic sources of human variation. The eugenics movement's emphatic focus on genetic over environmental determinants—at a moment when teratological research firmly foregrounded the latter—contextualized a waning biomedical focus on monstrous birth.[56]

It was not that eugenic researchers professed total disinterest in teratology or the birth of infants with conditions such as anencephaly. Even as they proclaimed that genetics superseded other ways of studying human development and descent, ERO researchers explicitly listed teratology as one of the half-dozen fields they drew on to compile their guiding catalog of human traits.[57] In his capacity as director of the ERO, Davenport personally reached out in 1915 to physicians and superintendents at local maternity wards and social agencies that primarily served a population of lower-class childbearing women. He asked them to report the birth of infants with major congenital anomalies so that ERO field-workers could record details and take the parents' family histories, providing data for the ERO's larger project of inventorying the nation's genetic stock and mapping out its sources of degeneracy.[58]

Davenport's request was enthusiastically received by a number of New York physicians. One, Robert Dickinson, exulted that "it gives me sincere pleasure to be of use. Your writings and studies are of the keenest interest and I wish you all the success in the world." Another, Joshua Ronsheim, lamented that "at the present writing my obstetric practice & that in the hospital is 'disgustingly' normal," but promised to inform Davenport "of the first case that comes under my observation." A third New York physician, Herbert Allen, reported that he had secured permission for ERO field-workers to enter the hospital where he did his obstetrical work, "so that from now on when anything interesting occurs I shall be glad to send you word." By contrast, Julia Lathrop, chief of the US Children's Bureau, rebuffed Davenport's request to have bureau case workers report anomalous births to the ERO, informing him that "inquiry is confidential and the mothers are especially assured that no personal connection will be made with the information they furnish."[59]

The ERO ended up filing several sparse case reports of anencephaly from hospitals, including the Lying-In Hospital of the City of New York and the Jewish Maternity Hospital. The physician Elizabeth Muncey, in her capacity as an ERO field-worker, visited the Lying-In Hospital to collect parental family histories relating to a 1917 birth. She reported, however, that "I was not allowed to question the mother as she knew nothing of the deformity"—suggesting how practices of concealing infant bodies from mothers, widely noted in nineteenth-century case reports, continued into the twentieth century.[60]

Eugenicists' interest in conditions such as anencephaly, however, paled in comparison to their interest in new, far subtler categories of human defect—including deviations so imperceptible that they could be identified only through expert eugenic analysis. Of greatest concern were invisible, widespread conditions such as "feeble-mindedness" and "hereditary criminality," which eugenicists framed as discrete transmissible traits that were proliferating unchecked in America's gene pool, posing an enormous social and economic "burden" on the nation.[61] By contrast, a condition such as anencephaly constituted a less compelling focus for eugenic intervention. Anencephaly was comparatively rare; it did not appear to be hereditary; its dramatic, highly visible morphological presentation required no eugenic acumen to identify. Those affected did not survive past early infancy, making it difficult for eugenicists to portray the condition as a major financial drain on US state and institutional resources. The linked ascendance of genetics and eugenics thus marked a broad transition in emphasis within the biomedical study of "congenital abnormalities," seeming to shift attention away from the specimens of teratological monstrosity that had filled nineteenth-century cabinets and display cases.

On closer inspection, however, there is far more to the story than a simple narrative of eugenic defect replacing or displacing teratological monstrosity as a focus of scientific study. From the start, nineteenth-century teratology had positioned the relation of monstrous anomaly to minor anomaly as simply one of degree: In the words of the philosopher Michel Foucault, "The monster is the major model of every little deviation. It is the principle of intelligibility of all the forms that circulate as the small change of abnormality."[62] In the late nineteenth-century reference work *Human Monstrosities*, the medical professors Barton Hirst and George Piersol wrote that "it is necessary to study systematically anomalies of development as a whole, for many monsters are but exaggerations of abnormal conditions frequently seen and of slight degree." In teratological work of this period, the increasingly elaborated categories of "hemiterata" or "minor terata" bridged the difference between gross monstrosity and more minor deviations of the sort that would become deeply significant to early twentieth-century eugenicists.[63]

Human Monstrosities defined the category of "hemiterata" to "include all human bodies with anything unusual in development, not grave enough to be called monstrous." The authors acknowledged that "the difficulty of drawing a sharply dividing line between hemiterata and monsters in all cases is obvious," given that "the difference is simply one of degree." However, they reassured their physician readership that "one can almost always decide, to his own satisfaction at least, whether the degree is marked enough to constitute a monstrosity." Yet as a graduated category predicated on a developmental continuum, teratological monstrosity contained an inexorable potential for slippage and category expansion. Monstrosities, Hirst and Piersol wrote, were "the climax of anomalies in development," representing "the most radical departures from normal development presented by the offspring of man."[64] However, located along a developmental continuum with no clear breaks, "radical" departures began to shade into subtler and subtler departures from this defined "normal"—a word that increasingly supplemented or replaced the language of "perfection" that had earlier been used to define the point from which monstrosity departed.

By the twentieth century, the category of "normality," tracing origins in both medical and mathematical discourse, had come to be closely tied to numerical and statistical measurements of deviance. This period saw an increasing emphasis on describing and quantifying human norms and measuring the extent to which individual bodies deviated from them.[65] In teratological literature, the study of monstrosity increasingly became a way to index this "normality" through the delineation of its boundaries: the numericized contours of the "normal" versus "monstrous" body. In "a quantitative study in human teratology," the anatomist Charles Mead in 1930 sought "to present a quantitative method for the numerical and graphic analysis of abnormal human development as illustrated by its application to two widely diverse forms of human monstrosity." His report included figures that superimposed the silhouettes of "normal" fetuses and neonates over "monstrous" ones, graphically instantiating the meaning of monstrosity as its quantified departure from the reference point of the "normal."[66]

In this way, teratological frameworks allowed for ever subtler departures from this normative body to be understood and configured as a form of monstrous production—with all that affectively entailed. Thus, even as attention to the traditional category of teratological monstrosity dwindled, in other ways the category of monstrosity expanded as eugenicists identified more and more traits as distinguishable deviations from a eugenic norm. As a larger and larger group of smaller and smaller deviations came to be understood as nation-threatening degeneracy, the logics and affective significations of teratological monstrosity were in some respects conferred onto these more widely distributed categories of eugenic defect.

This "conferral" of monstrous signification was accomplished in specific ways. My argument is not just that eugenicists thought of defect as "monstrous" in some vague and generic sense. Rather, they invoked defined frameworks of teratological development to theorize particular concepts of human defect, racial hierarchy, and moral-biological deviance. Further, laypeople who internalized eugenic logics sometimes came to talk about and conceptualize childbearing and congenital disability in ways that reproduced affective meanings configured within nineteenth-century teratological discourses of monstrosity.

MONSTROSITY IN EUGENIC THEORIES OF DEFECT AND RACE

The eugenic focus on slighter and slighter measurements of defect and deviation played out not only in scientific publications and study at elite research institutes but also in popular gatherings across the American heartland and beyond. In Better Babies contests held at state fairs, judges enthusiastically ranked human infants using the same methods developed to assess livestock. At the 1911 Iowa State Fair, the winners of the Better Babies contest "provided the climax in the million-dollar parade of prize stock and other agricultural products, as they rode in an automobile with a runner on the side proclaiming them to be 'Iowa's Best Crop.'" By the 1920s, parents could submit both their children and themselves for eugenic scrutiny in Fitter Families competitions. Aligning even more robustly with the eugenic focus on family heredity, these competitions worked to "give the Better Baby a pedigree" by requiring that "the Better Baby be supported by a Family, fit both in their inheritance and in the development of their mental, moral, and physical traits."[67]

At the Kansas Free Fair in Topeka, Fitter Families contestants entered the fair's "Eugenics Building" for examination. The floor plan for the Eugenics Building included eight rooms: a room for the examination of infants; a room containing the eye, ear, nose, and throat examination station and the dental examination station; rooms for the psychological and psychiatric examinations; and sex-segregated rooms for the "medical" and "structural" examinations of men and women. Examiners carefully noted any defects or deficiencies, duly recorded as red marks on the family scorecard.[68]

The anatomical or structural categories of "defects" measured in Better Babies and Fitter Families contests encompassed the kind of conditions that late nineteenth-century teratologists defined as "hemiterata"—the kind of anomaly that could be "detected only by minute anatomical examination" and that, unlike anencephaly and the "major monstrosities," were often considered to be "hereditary" in tendency.[69] No one brought an infant with anencephaly to be judged in a Better Babies contest. The contests instead focused on identifying subtle defects and deviations in the anatomy of ostensibly "normal" offspring.

In addition to their focus on minute anatomical deviations, eugenicists were deeply interested in detecting putative mental defects such as "feeble-mindedness," which they further divided into three classes—"idiots," "imbeciles," and "morons"—based on perceived severity.[70] Like the historical category of monstrosity, the historical category of feeble-mindedness does not map precisely onto any single diagnostic category in present-day use, though it tended to encompass conditions today described as intellectual disabilities.[71] Significantly, eugenicists centrally conceptualized feeble-mindedness not just as a condition of cognitive deficit but also as one of social and moral degradation. Early twentieth-century eugenic leaders often claimed that the reproduction of feeble-minded people posed a particularly grave threat to the nation's economic well-being, framing the expenses of institutional care as an unacceptable "burden" on state and local governments.[72] A growing literature in disability history now explores the experiences of people, largely from poor and working-class communities, who were diagnosed as "feeble-minded," confined in medical and carceral institutions, and/or subjected to eugenic sterilization in the early twentieth century.[73]

Whether performed at clinics, research centers, agricultural fairs, or state-run institutions of confinement, eugenic examinations exposed individuals to a form of scrutiny that sought to characterize their every deviation from a posited eugenic norm. These kinds of practices drew on and elaborated a late nineteenth and early twentieth-century biomedical literature that conceived and enumerated a vast list of potential departures from a normative body, seeking to quantify deviance through measurement of everything from "length of acromion" to "girth of ankle" to "shape of the teeth" to "distance from the external angle of the eye to the angle of mouth."[74]

Yet even as the locus of biomedical interest in human anomaly shifted to categories of more and more minor deviations, the figure of the "major monstrosity" continued to haunt eugenic imaginaries of defect. In one particularly explicit example, an "anencephalic monster" appeared in a cautionary ERO pedigree designed to "illustrate the hovel source of defectives." This pedigree chart, shown in figure 6.1, was presented as an exemplar at the First International Eugenics Conference in 1912 and published in such periodicals as the *Journal of Mental and Nervous Disease*.[75] As a way of mapping ancestry and descent, such pedigrees were intended to demonstrate the hereditary nature of defect and graphically communicate the dangers of allowing "defective types" to reproduce unchecked. The pedigree in question purported to represent several generations of an impoverished rural family begotten by a "feeble-minded" and morally stunted patriarch. Among the profusion of "defective" descendants, one of the branching lines included an offspring identified as an "anencephalic monster." Telegraphing the significance of this monstrous birth, the caption offered the commentary that "the empty germ plasm yields only emptiness."[76] Here, the "anencephalic monster" was positioned as the ultimate endpoint in the racial degeneration of human stock, signifying the defective—literally the "monstrous"—nature of the hereditary material transmitted by the progenitor. Intimately connecting conditions of mental and moral degeneracy to the figure of biological monstrosity, the appearance of the "anencephalic monster" on the pedigree chart helped advance a eugenic logic in which any form of defect represented a menacing social-biological threat that had to be cast out from the national and human family.

Biomedical sources of this period explicitly theorized the relationship between anencephaly and "feeble-mindedness," locating the conditions along the same causal continuum and explaining their common origins in arrested physiological processes of development. For instance, a 1925 medical journal article cited by ERO scientists discussed failures of brain development in utero by referring to cases "whereby the process may be arrested altogether, as in anencephaly, or partially arrested, as in the brain of the idiot or low grade imbecile."[77] Davenport, in his own published writing on development and heredity, likewise placed anencephaly and idiocy on the same spectrum of development, writing that in processes of embryogenesis, "the head may develop so badly that the neural tube does not close and there is practically no brain at all. Or the

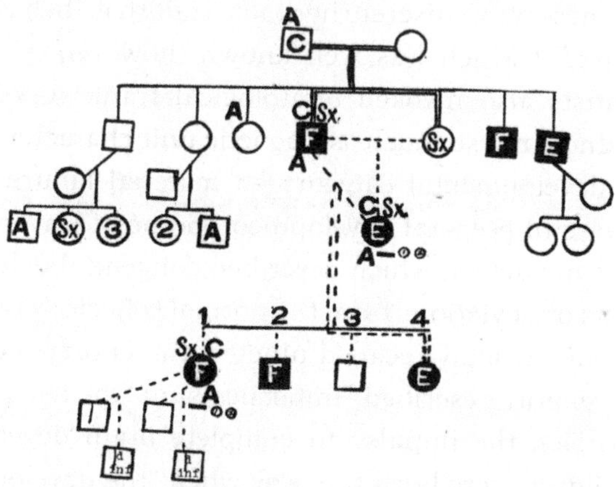

FIG. 4. This chart illustrates the *hovel source of defectives.* A feeble-minded man had by his defective sister an epileptic daughter with criminal instincts; then by this daughter he had four children, two feeble-minded, one epileptic and the fourth an anencephalic monster who died directly after birth. The empty germ plasm yields only emptiness. These things were done in a little hut in the woods until it burned down and now mother and eldest daughter, when not in the county jail or the Monmouth County almshouse, live in a cellar in town. The man is dead; but some of his protoplasm is living and at large. Case 3165.

FIGURE 6.1 Pedigree chart created by the Eugenics Record Office to illustrate the "hovel source of defectives," including "an anencephalic monster," printed in Charles Benedict Davenport and David Weeks, "A First Study of Inheritance of Epilepsy," *Journal of Nervous and Mental Disease* 38, no. 11 (1911): 646. *Source*: Courtesy of the Truman G. Blocker Jr. History of Medicine Collections, Moody Medical Library, University of Texas Medical Branch at Galveston.

brain may close and the child become a microcephalic idiot."[78] These invocations of anencephaly—placing it on a physiological continuum with "idiocy" and "imbecility"—suggest how categories denoting mental and moral inferiority were physicalized and biologized in eugenic understandings. That is, placing "idiocy" on the same spectrum as anencephaly suggested an understanding of "feeble-mindedness" as rooted in the physiology and anatomy of the body along a continuum of neural development.

Historians of eugenics have written extensively about how eugenicists invoked Mendelian genetics to describe the nature and transmission of "defects" such as "feeble-mindedness."[79] Indeed, eugenic scientists published studies explicitly purporting to show that feeble-mindedness was a discrete heritable trait that "behaves as a Mendelian recessive."[80] Much less well known, however, is the fact that eugenic scientists also invoked teratological frameworks to describe feeble-mindedness not so much as a genetic unit character but rather as an explicitly developmental category—a material failure to complete crucial pathways of prenatal development. Some of Davenport's explanations of eugenic defect, which described congenital deformity as the result of arrests or deviations from the normal trajectory of embryological development, strongly recalled nineteenth-century models of teratogenesis. Davenport described "imbeciles" and "the feeble-minded" as "persons who lack the impulse to complete brain development." He wrote that children were born this way when "the development of certain association fibres of the brain is stopped at an early stage through the running out of the proper developmental sensitiveness or responsiveness" during gestation.[81]

While Davenport was perhaps the most explicit in elaborating on embryological processes, he was not unique among his colleagues in invoking a developmental frame of defect. Other prominent American eugenicists, including the psychologist Henry Goddard and the geneticist William Castle, characterized feeble-mindedness as a condition of "arrested development," described the feeble-minded as "individuals of arrested or undeveloped mentality," and wrote that "the low grade (idiot) has not only a disturbed brain formation but his entire organism is disarranged and growth processes upset."[82] In this discourse, the medical framework of monstrosity—as an arrest or disturbance of physical development—was invoked to specify a bodily developmental basis for eugenic inferiority.

Previous chapters have suggested how nineteenth-century teratological monstrosity was configured as a transfer point between social and biological meanings of difference, providing a way to ground social hierarchies of race and kinds in the embodied biological processes of development and reproduction. Positioned as the common origin of anencephaly and imbecility, the mechanism of monstrous development worked very similarly in this context, articulating both the physiological and social/moral monstrousness of the "feeble-minded" in the eugenic worldview. In this way, the frameworks and significations of nineteenth-century monstrosity were mobilized to advance a central project of the eugenics movement: to establish a biological basis for social and moral hierarchies of human worth.

Classic scholarship on the history of monstrosity emphasizes a distinction between concepts of bodily monstrosity and concepts of moral monstrosity, portraying a chronological shift from the former to the latter.[83] According to Foucault, in the modern period the locus of monstrosity transferred out of the physical body and into the behavior or soul of an individual. Now purely a designation of moral and behavioral deviance, monstrosity no longer belonged to the "domain of somatic and natural disorder."[84] Yet the teratological-eugenic understanding of defect described earlier blurs this averred modern dichotomy between moral and somatic manifestations of monstrosity. In these theories by prominent eugenic scientists, the moral and behavioral "monstrosity" of feeble-mindedness was conceptualized as arising through the same material processes as bodily monstrosity. Significantly, eugenicists invoked frameworks of teratological development to bind together conceptualizations of both physical defect and mental defect, of both biological degradation and moral degradation.

American eugenicists further engaged frameworks of monstrous development to articulate interlocking concepts of racial hierarchy and racial degeneration and to link together racial and reproductive deviance.[85] Invoking the racialized embryological framework of nineteenth-century teratology—in which arrests of development constituted racial degeneration—eugenic scientists such as Davenport identified "defectives" as those who materially failed to attain the highest racial type. Like nineteenth-century teratological monsters (who displayed "the normal conditions of the first ages of the life of the embryo" as well as of "lower forms" on the animal scale), Davenport's eugenic defectives were beings arrested in developmental time.[86] In his work *Heredity in Relation to Eugenics* (1911), he wrote that "the traits of the feeble-minded and the criminalistic are normal traits for infants and for an earlier stage in man's evolution." Explicitly referencing nineteenth-century frameworks of development, he explained that "there is an aphorism that biologists use which is apt here—ontogeny recapitulates phylogeny. This means that the individual in its development passes through stages like those the race has traversed in its evolution"; elsewhere, he wrote that "the human child reveals in its development the past history of the race."[87]

This framing imbued developmental disruption with a racialized meaning, configuring arrest of prenatal development as arrest at a less evolved racial stage—and revealing compelling continuities with the history of nineteenth-century teratological discourse explored in the previous chapter. Likewise echoing these nineteenth-century discourses, Davenport reciprocally described racial difference as arrested development. For example, in *Race Crossing in Jamaica* (1929), Davenport and his colleague Morris Steggerda alleged the mental inferiority of African-descended people and speculated it was owing to an underdevelopment of the brain's associational fibers—the same developmental mechanism Davenport assigned to general feeble-mindedness.[88]

In these examples, Davenport used a biological-developmental framework to specify a mutually constitutive relationship between human defect and racial hierarchy, linking eugenic imaginaries of disability and race. Nor was he the only prominent eugenicist to do so. In an overtly teratological framing of racial hierarchy, an article in a 1924 volume of the *Eugenical News* (the ERO's official publication) claimed that "every Caucasian passes through a mongoloid stage in intra-uterine development." Addressing its presumptively Caucasian readership, the article directly conflated categories of racial difference and intellectual disability, explaining that "most of us outgrew the Mongolian state which remains 'in our midst' but among the imbeciles one finds cases where the Mongolian condition is not in the midst but on the surface." Invoking the signature teratological concept of arrested embryological development, the article continued, "Such have remained foetuses grown large but not differentiated. They are the Mongolian idiots."[89] ERO eugenicists thus invoked classic teratological frameworks in a deeply derogatory formulation of disability and race—one that configured the formal "monstrosity" of both non-Caucasians and individuals born with what is now called Down syndrome or Trisomy 21.[90]

Anglo-American eugenicists used frameworks of monstrous production to articulate not only the "defective" nature of racial difference but also the putative dangers of racial hybridity. The University of Chicago biologist Horatio Hackett Newman, for example, invoked teratogenesis to warn against the dangers of interracial reproduction. Newman claimed that new experimental results suggested that the "intercrossing of human races" could result in the production of "a considerable proportion of defective and monstrous types" and posited the production of monstrosity as "a possible new source of danger incident to miscegenation."[91]

Mobilized to theorize the nature and communicate the threat of racial degeneration and racial admixture, teratological frameworks underscored the eugenic imperative to intervene in biological reproduction for the securement of racial quality. Thus, even as the frequency of the terms *monster* and *monstrosity* in biomedical case literature began to dwindle, frameworks of monstrous development structured and conditioned eugenic discourse that linked together imaginaries of race and disability as biological-reproductive defect.

CHILDBEARING WOMEN, EUGENIC MOTHERHOOD, AND MONSTROUS LEGACIES

In these ways, then, frameworks of monstrosity found new life in the work of leading eugenic scientists. Eugenic discourse, however, far exceeded the rarified realm of scientific research publications. For one, laws that authorized involuntary sterilization, mandated institutionalization, restricted marriage, and banned immigration to the United States had direct and concrete impacts on affected people's lives. Further, movement leaders explicitly aimed to enact their agenda not just through legal dictates but also by inculcating what they called a "quickened eugenic sentiment" in the populace—by getting everyday people on board with and excited about the eugenic program, prompting them to reshape their most intimate desires and everyday conduct in accordance with eugenic principles.[92]

It is challenging and perhaps impossible for a historian to quantify precisely or prove definitively the extent to which the eugenics movement did or did not succeed at genuinely reshaping people's intimate desires. But it seems fair to say that many Americans internalized eugenic logics in a variety of meaningful ways—for instance, as expressed in how they communicated and made choices about their own reproductive lives and futures.[93] How, then, might the frameworks and significations of biological monstrosity have also conditioned the way that laypeople thought about and experienced their bodies and reproduction in this era?

One possible source of insight into this question is offered in the content of advice-seeking letters written by laywomen from the 1910s through the 1930s. During an era of rising emphasis on the relevance and necessity of seeking biomedical guidance on motherhood, laywomen wrote to new organizations, from research institutes such as the Eugenics Record Office (founded in 1910) to government welfare agencies such as the federal Children's Bureau (founded in 1912), for scientific advice on managing their own fertility and childbearing.[94] Women from varied backgrounds solicited opinions on whether they should have children or on how to best care for themselves during pregnancy, laying out intimate details of their hopes, fears, and day-to-day lives.

Given that mainstream presentations of eugenic motherhood typically emphasized ideals of the white middle-class American family, it is perhaps unsurprising that the women who wrote in to prominent eugenic organizations such as the ERO and the Eugenics Research Association tended to be white and middle class.[95] Many women outside the white middle class similarly sought expert guidance on fertility and reproduction in this period, though they were likelier to turn to other venues for advice. The Children's Bureau received a substantial number of inquiries from white rural and working-class women, while early twentieth-century magazines aimed at an elite and middle-class African American readership printed letters from Black women.[96]

In many cases, women discussed the prospect of giving birth to children with congenital disabilities in language deeply steeped in the logics and imperatives of eugenic reproduction, seeming to reflect intimately internalized assumptions about hierarchies of biological and social worth. The chapter began with the story of Mrs. L, who wrote in 1924 to Davenport at the ERO for advice some months after delivering her first child, an infant with anomalous head development who died before or shortly after delivery. Mrs. L framed the import of her experience in terms of a calculation of future risk and her desire to fulfill personal imperatives of eugenic motherhood. She described herself as "a very healthy woman" and her husband as "morally clean," but she expressed a fear that there might have been other such births concealed in the far branches of one of their family trees. What if her first birth did not reflect a mere "accident," as her obstetrician had supposed, but rather an inescapable defect that lurked deep in their biological bodies, contaminating their germ cells and the whole family line?

Mrs. L ended her letter with an enjoinder to protect her carefully guarded secret, expressing a sense of deep shame and social isolation surrounding her experience.[97] This shame and secrecy emerged within a worldview predicated on a profound moralization of health, bodies, and reproduction; a severe stigmatization of disability; and a conflation of social and biological imaginaries of worth. If eugenic motherhood—the birthing and raising of "well-born children" for the good of the family, the nation, and the race—was a biological/social/moral imperative, then producing such a severely "defective" child was a biological/social/moral failure. It constituted not just a "shock" and a "tragedy" but also a "terrible secret," one that threatened to expose Mrs. L's own unfitness and unworthiness for reproduction and maternity.

An affective rhetoric centering on a desired "normal child," indexed and haunted by the monstrous specter of the deformed or defective one, animated the letters of women seeking expert advice on reproduction from a wide variety of backgrounds, even those who did not turn to eugenic organizations for guidance. A married white woman in Chicago wrote in to the Children's Bureau in 1916 during her pregnancy to request information on correct prenatal care and diet, explaining that she was "so anxious" to have a "normal child." A working-class New York woman writing in to the bureau in 1920 shared that "I have a sister (just a young woman) who has recently become pregnant. She has confided in me and I find that she is constantly depressed with the fear that her child will not be normal."[98]

Anxiety about giving birth to babies with "defects" can also be found in writings from middle-class and elite Black women in this period, often phrased in the context of concerns over the "vitality of future generations" in African American communities. In this context, expressions of concern about defective reproduction were often explicitly situated within the imperatives for racial uplift espoused by Black social reform movements of this period, reflecting in part a class politics of respectability forged amid conditions of both pervasive anti-Black racism and intra-racial class inequality. At times, this discourse veered into directly eugenic appeals. For instance, one member of the Black women's club movement—a network of community organizations focused on social and political change—averred that members should work to "diminish the number of poorly born, poorly bred and deformed children."[99]

The mainly middle-class white advice seekers, like Mrs. L, who wrote in to institutions such as the ERO were particularly explicit in their invocation of eugenic rhetoric. Young people from around the country wrote to biomedical experts to inquire about their personal probability of producing "defective" versus "normal" offspring, explaining that they would use this information to determine whether they would plan to have future children. Many addressed these inquiries directly to the nation's leading eugenic researchers at the ERO. One woman opened her letter to the "Eugenics Laboratory" by explaining, "Inasmuch as I have heard of the wonderful work you have done in the improvement of the health of future generations, I have decided to appeal to you for advice." Others noted that they wrote at the advice of their physicians. In some cases, advice seekers contacted medical research institutions such as the Rockefeller Institute for Medical Research and the New York Academy of Medicine, who then forwarded their inquiries on to the ERO.[100]

Mrs. L's infant's condition had not been compatible with life past early infancy—more akin to nineteenth-century categories of "nonviable" teratological monstrosity than the eugenic categories of hereditary defect. But other advice seekers wrote in to inquire about far subtler variations of form—the kind of "minor anomalies" described as "hemiterata" in late nineteenth-century teratological literature.[101] Letter writers likewise configured these conditions as forbidding specters of defect that could foreclose to them the possibility of future children. One advice-seeking letter from Colorado opened by explaining, "I have a double hare-lip and a double cleft-palate." The letter continued: "The question I would like to ask is this: Is my handicap hereditary? Would my children run the risk of having similar physical deformities? The fact as to whether or not I will ever have children depends wholly on your answer. . . . If your answer is to the negative I would merely accept sterilization as a matter of course." In this letter, the twenty-one-year-old writer described living a "very happy and normal life."[102] Yet at the same time the writer treated the prospect of reproducing children with the same bodily "defects"—of even taking the risk of doing so—as a precluded possibility, an unconscionable outcome to be averted at all costs. The letter concluded with a query about the nearest state that permitted sterilization.

Letter writers centrally scrutinized not just themselves but also their family trees for evidence of "inferior" characteristics. Letters from the 1920s and 1930s bundled together a broad array of traits in these imaginaries of defective reproduction, including anomalies of bodily development traditionally studied under the remit of teratology as well as a range of what might be termed cognitive, psychological, neurological, sensory, social, or behavioral attributes. Refracted through an internalized hereditarian eugenic framework, each of these attributes became a biological defect suspected to inhere in letter writers' physical bodies—in the material chromosomes of every cell—and in their deviant reproductive capacities. On this level, the eugenic era's increasing focus on invisible defects, prominently including mental or moral deviations, did not diverge as much as it might seem from the older teratological focus on bodily deviations. Instead, as these women's letters underscored, eugenic logics rendered a host of attributes as congenital defects of the physical biological body, implicitly conjuring and expanding the specter of teratological monstrosity.

One young mother, whose first child had recently "been diagnosed as feeble-minded" at the Clinic of Child Development at Yale University, wrote in for information about "the probable cost of an investigation of the family heredity" to determine "whether it is reasonably safe to have other children." Another woman, having recently learned of "three, and possibly four cases of insanity in my family," wrote that she and her husband now felt "very hesitant about having children." In a third inquiry, a woman assiduously listed the "normal healthy" members of her family for reassurance that it would be acceptable for her and her husband to reproduce. She then disclosed with shame the existence of a family member with epilepsy and intellectual disabilities "who was supposed to have been born a normal child," casting this as "an uneugenic factor in my inheritance" that made her "hesitate" to fulfill her dream of motherhood.[103]

Letters expressed the felt imperatives of eugenic motherhood in strongly affective terms, linking it to emotional and personal fulfillment as well as to broader gendered duties to society. One advice seeker, twenty-six-year-old Marie H., wrote in immediately after becoming engaged to be married. She explained, "Since I became of an age when I could understand the real happiness of a woman, I have had my heart set on having a home with a husband and children." Linking her affective as well as reproductive capacities to a eugenic logic of biological hierarchy, she wrote: "Above everything in this world I want to be the mother of well-born children! I could not be happy if my offspring were inferior."[104]

Another letter writer in the 1930s, twenty-year-old Margaret C., explained that "my greatest hope is to marry sometime not too far into the future" (though she noted parenthetically that, "incidentally, I haven't any prospects thus far"). Most of all, she wished to "have a family of my own for I adore children." However, she wrote, she was "very much afraid of passing on to my children" undesirable traits that she feared might be heritable. On behalf of herself and all her siblings, she enjoined the ERO researchers to tell her the "probable outcome" of their future reproduction: "Would it be safe for us to marry and can we expect normal offspring and to what degree?"[105]

In her lengthy letter, Margaret laid out in vivid detail anything that might constitute a concerning heritable trait in her family members or herself, subsuming a wide-ranging array of disabilities, disorders, behaviors, personality traits, and life circumstances under the sweeping eugenic category of suspected hereditary defect. Her father's mother, she had been told, was "a very temperamental woman" with "periods of imbalance" and had "extreme deafness" in later years. Her paternal uncle, who had been "considered sickly and never required to work as the other boys were" in adolescence, was "completely insane in the worst stages" and lived a "hideous existence." Another uncle, though not "seriously deficient mentally," was "given to periods of wanderlust when he would run away taking large sums of money with him." A third uncle, despite a Cornell education, had "become a habitual drunkard and spends about one week from each month in a perpetual wretched state of drunkenness."[106]

Margaret's own father had been diagnosed with epilepsy ten years earlier, after experiencing a seizure that left him unconscious for several hours. Margaret, ten years old at the time, had been terrified when her father "suddenly toppled over at the supper table." She had watched helplessly as he "grew rigid and livid in color," his muscles convulsing until he lapsed into unconsciousness. These seizures, which now occurred weekly, rendered her father unable to work. Margaret had begun studying to be a teacher so that she could bring in income to alleviate her father's financial worries for the family. If it turned out that she was unfit to have children, she wrote, she took some comfort in the idea that she could contribute to her family in this way. She described her siblings as "perfectly normal," with the exception of the youngest sister, who was "slightly deaf."[107]

Even as Margaret consigned her father and youngest sister to the category of "defective or inferior" relatives (as ERO superintendent Laughlin explicitly called them in his reply), she also seemed compelled to defend her family members from the ERO eugenicists' anticipated judgment. She emphasized that her father had, until the seizures began, seemed to her "the most well-adjusted man in the world"; she described how he now rallied to "fight off" impending seizures and worried for the well-being of his family. Her "slightly deaf" youngest sister, she wrote, had recently enrolled in a state school for deaf children and "enjoys it very much." She stressed that the sister was "mentally sound" and "of average intelligence, her auditory defect alone holding her back."[108]

Margaret likewise appraised her own physical and mental attributes through this moralizing calculus of social-biological value and defect, inventorying both her redemptive ("normal") and her incriminating ("defective") traits as biological hereditary qualities. While on the whole she described herself as "mentally sound," she also identified a number of traits she considered to be concerning psychological flaws. She had "a slight inferiority complex contracted in high school which consists mainly in a fear to appear before a group when speaking" and "used to have states of depression" (after her mother "helped me to see that these do no good," she was "gradually learning to take things more calmly").[109]

Surveying her physical health and body, Margaret wrote, "I am small like my mother, but have lots of vitality and am never ill, except that I am subject to severe attacks of hay-fever." This had not alarmed her, she explained, until "recently when my Health Protection teacher told the class that epilepsy is often caused by the same factors in some that cause hay fever in others." She recalled that she knew a family "where one member was afflicted with hay-fever and another epilepsy" and wondered now about the connection with her father's epilepsy. Did her own body carry the same defect that caused her father's seizures, and would she in turn transmit this "degeneracy" to her own children?[110]

Margaret C. and her five younger siblings were "all ambitious," she wrote; they had "big plans for the future." She had long hoped for a future that included children of her own, but now, consumed by thoughts of "the degeneracy so prevalent on my father's side," she could not shake the fear that she would not have "normal offspring." She wrote that her mother, a great believer in the power of education, "tries to convince me that whatever hereditary tendencies appear in the children I hope to have could be corrected by proper training from birth." Yet, she confessed, visions of children born with inherited defect "appear like a specter before me."[111]

The people who wrote these letters expressed their strong desires to have children, to be mothers. Mrs. L wrote that "not to have children would be an absolute tragedy"; Marie H. described longing for the "real happiness" of motherhood "above everything else in this world"; Margaret C. wrote of her great hope "to have a family of my own for I adore children." Yet despite this strong desire for children, letter writers were prepared to reshape their aspirations, relationships, and the trajectories of their futures to avoid the risk of contributing "inferior" offspring—children whose bodies and minds they feared would be "defective" in the same ways they castigated their kin's and sometimes their own for being.

While advice seekers rarely used the words *monster* and *monstrosity* in their letters, in some significant respects their eugenic valuations of congenital disability and defect were suffused with logics of monstrous deviance. The language they used affectively positioned giving birth to "defective" and "abnormal" offspring as a shame to be concealed, to be turned away from, to be hidden from the broader social community—as in the "terrible secret" that Mrs. L could not talk about or acknowledge to anyone outside of the biomedical experts she confided in. The formulations in their letters linked their reproductive capacities to an affective hierarchy of social and biological value: "I could not be happy if my offspring were inferior." The prospect of congenital defect, which appeared "like a specter" before them, disrupted imperatives of motherhood and projected reproductive futures, cutting them off from access to the "real happiness of a woman" in maternal love. Occupying terrain marked by the legacy of teratological monstrosity, this far broader eugenic category of defective reproduction continued to serve as a transfer point among notions of biological, social, and affective degradation.

In taking up eugenic teachings, women were engaging with the cutting-edge scientific discourse of their time; they were attempting to think about and order their reproductive lives in rational, scientific ways. Yet this application of scientific thinking did not designify the fearsome cultural meanings of anomalous childbearing, as nineteenth-century practitioners had promised it would. It instead conferred these fearsome meanings onto their own reproductive bodies and onto slighter and slighter "deviations" of the human form.

Attention to "teratological afterlives" in the eugenics era thus further underscores how scientific discourse on monstrosity served to produce and mobilize rather than demystify and strip away moral and cultural meanings. In his classic essay "Monstrosity and the Monstrous," the philosopher Georges Canguilhem described how scientific teratology served to separate the physical phenomenon of "monstrosity" from the moral and social transgression signified by "the monstrous," asserting that "the transparency of monstrosity to scientific thought cuts monstrosity off from any relation to the monstrous" starting in the nineteenth century.[112]

Yet this history reveals how modern scientific attention, far from "cutting off" moral signification, instead capacitated the figure of the teratological monster—the "hideous" progeny dislocated in developmental time—as a transfer point between biological and social meanings of human alterity. In mapping the presence of an "anencephalic monstrosity" onto a eugenic pedigree of defective descent, ERO eugenicists invoked the bodily abjection of curtailed development to convey the social inferiority of a "defective" class. In describing the common origins of anencephaly and imbecility, the mechanism of monstrous development articulated both the physical and the moral degradation of the "feeble-minded" in the eugenic worldview. In seeking and internalizing eugenic guidance on their reproductive lives, childbearing women located congenital disability within conflated imaginaries of social, moral, and biological deviance. Even as the formal scientific category of "monstrous birth" waned and faded away, its legacies and its imprints persisted.

Epilogue

According to the precepts of scientific teratology, birth marked the intractable endpoint of a monster's development: Monstrosity was, by definition, formed in utero, the result of physiological processes that occurred exclusively during gestation. Yet, as this book has shown, birth marked just the beginning of a newborn's development into a biological monster.

Across interwoven and multisensory domains of medical meaning making, infants transformed into scientific specimens of monstrosity. The preceding chapters have explored how emerging practices of US medical science configured the "monstrosity" of anomalous bodies, producing a biological category that linked and materialized concepts of racial, reproductive, and bodily defect. These multimodal historical practices shaped monstrosity in diffuse ways. Narratives of monstrous pregnancy located the meanings of monstrosity within disruptions of familial, racial, and human–animal boundaries. Affective interactions with living newborns established monstrosity as a conflicted and ambivalent state of simultaneous kinship and alienation, at once like and unlike a human child. Visual representation located monsters both within and outside of racialized imaginaries of the human and orders of animal kinds. Taxonomic classifications rendered the nature of monstrous difference as simultaneously categorical and continuous, entailing both ontological separation and a relation of graduated degree. Teratological theories of development cast race, sex, and disability as temporalized, biologically hierarchical, and rooted in women's deviant reproduction. Though the focus on major teratological monstrosity waned in the early twentieth-century eugenics era as attention shifted to far slighter deviations of human form, the category of biological monstrosity paradoxically also expanded. As teratological frameworks were applied to ever-subtler and slighter imperfections of the human form, significations of biological monstrosity were conferred onto a widening swathe of newly visible deviations from "normality."

Configured in these ways, the biomedical category of monstrosity reflected and engendered potent cultural meanings of human difference, articulating a racial-sexual order both defined and perpetually imperiled by conceptions of disability and deviant reproduction. Positioned as a state of concurrent kinship and alienation, monstrosity could shore up contradictions of unstable racial imaginaries—offering a way to acknowledge the biological relatedness of "deviant" kin while still placing them outside the social, affective, and taxonomic boundaries of the human. Rendered as the embodied endpoint of racial degeneracy, monstrosity could establish the political stakes of reproduction as an area of eugenic intervention and control. Mediating between and merging the meanings of social and biological alterity, monstrosity could offer a biodevelopmental basis for a social order predicated on hierarchies of race, sex, and disability.

By 1963, encountering the term *monster* in the *Journal of the American Medical Association* had become startling, even shocking, to a practitioner such as Dr. Hulda Thelander. Thelander regarded the word as so incongruous with modern medical science that she initially assumed its appearance must have been a mistake.[1] However, as these chapters have shown, monstrosity was not an accidental vestige from a prescientific past. It was instead an enduring category that intimately engaged and shaped formative discourses of reproduction and human difference in modern US medical science.

The ubiquity of monstrosity as a clinical medical term increasingly declined in the decades after 1930, although it still occasionally surfaced in US medical journals for many years.[2] Scientific interest in teratology as an area of research dwindled during this time as well, as mid-twentieth-century biomedical researchers focused more heavily on genetics and heredity. In the 1960s, however, teratology experienced a resurgence in the United States as an organized academic discipline.[3] This coincided with widespread national attention to the prenatal effects of the drug thalidomide as well as to the rubella epidemic, catalyzing new awareness of *teratogens*—a term popularized in this period to describe environmental agents capable of disrupting prenatal development.[4]

This renewal of interest in teratology occasioned expressions of discomfort over the term's etymology, which embeds the Greek word *teras*, "monster."[5] The words *monster* and *monstrosity* encountered increasingly vehement critique in the later twentieth century during a period of rising public discourse and organized activism around disability rights.[6] Late twentieth-century disability activists and scholars emphatically condemned the "association of monsters and disabilities." In 1985, Paul Longmore cited the use of the word *monster* to describe physical disability as a particularly glaring example of the "linguistic reinforcement of prejudice," an application of language that conferred stigma by conveying that disabled people "are less human than the rest."[7]

Of course, the recognition that the term *monstrosity* conferred stigma was not a novel late twentieth-century proposition. Even nineteenth-century medical practitioners had sometimes had to acknowledge the word's stigmatizing connotations. Recall that in 1842 a widely used obstetrics textbook cautioned physicians not to classify a child with only "minor deformities" as a monster, "for the very word conveys a horrible, or at least an unpleasant, impression." Thelander, in her letter written more than a century later, pointed out how the word also stigmatized those who conceived and bore children denigrated as "monstrous."[8] With the burgeoning of the disability rights movements and scholarship in the later twentieth century and the rise of what Longmore called "a new social and political self-consciousness" among disabled people, critiques of the stigmatization of disability gained new sharpness and traction.[9] Today, classifying a human being as a "monstrosity" is understood to be so obviously and outrageously stigmatizing that many readers will be shocked to learn the term appeared in a leading American medical journal as late as 1983.[10]

Though monstrosity no longer delimits a biomedical category, it continues to convey the often entangled meanings of race, sex, and disability in public and popular discourse more broadly. In 2014, to justify his killing of the Black teenager Michael Brown, the police officer Darren Wilson portrayed him as "a monster with terrible resilience and incredible strength."[11] In 2024, to impugn the womanhood of the Algerian boxer Imane Khelif, a competitor shared an image of her as a horned, muscle-bound "monster" confronting a slim white woman with straight, flowing hair. In films and novels, long-standing tropes persist in linking supernatural monstrosity to real-life physical disabilities.[12]

Although now linguistically decoupled from the fictive and metaphorical monsters that proliferate in popular culture, the biological conditions formerly described as monstrosities also continue to exist. The birth of infants with anencephaly—the condition most frequently described in the nineteenth-century clinical literature on monstrosity—still occurs today, albeit at a substantially lower rate than in the past. A dramatic drop in national incidence can be traced to a public-health intervention starting in 1998: the mandatory fortification of the national grain supply with folic acid, a nutrient that supports neural tube development during early pregnancy.[13] Increasing use of prenatal diagnostic technologies paired with access to abortion care have also contributed to this decline.

Across changing historical contexts, the birth of infants with anencephaly has remained fraught with social and political meanings. In the early 1990s, two infants with anencephaly were at the center of a pair of landmark legal cases related to organ donation and the allocation of medical resources, posing dilemmas that hinge on still-contested definitions of death, life, and personhood.[14] Contemporary experiences of anencephalic birth continue to elicit intense and widely varying emotions for parents and families, something that highly medicalized settings are rarely designed to make space for. In one anonymized example shared with me, a mother of a newborn with anencephaly yearned to nurse and be with her newborn at home for the duration of the infant's short life—a desire that she found clashed with the medicalized imperatives of the institution in which she gave birth.

In the twenty-first century, as in the past, anencephaly has also become enrolled in attempts to exert control over pregnancy and women's reproduction. Contemporary antiabortion groups deploy poignant personal narratives of anencephalic birth as a way to communicate the virtues of eschewing abortion. The website for one such organization, which advocates total abortion bans with no exceptions for "perceived threat to the mother's health or life," includes a personal testimonial page that movingly recounts the gestation, birth, and death of an infant with anencephaly. The post ends with a heartfelt exhortation by the infant's grandmother for others to similarly "choose life."

Recent legal changes have further reshaped meanings, narratives, and experiences of anencephalic pregnancy and birth. In the wake of the Supreme Court decision in *Dobbs v. Jackson Women's Health Organization* (597 U.S. 215 [2022]), state legislatures criminalized abortion care in large swathes of the United States, including Texas, the state where I live and work. After her prenatal screening revealed anencephaly, Houston resident Samantha Casiano recalled her doctor saying, "Well, because of the new law, you don't have any options. You have to go on with your pregnancy."[15] Casiano described her pain and anger at being forced against her will to carry the pregnancy to term and endure a harrowing labor, all the while tormented by the certain knowledge that the child she birthed would imminently die. In 2024, the Texas Supreme Court rejected a lawsuit brought by Casiano and other women denied abortion care in Texas. The court also refused in this ruling to clarify the "medical exception" to Texas's abortion ban, leaving physicians vulnerable to lifetime imprisonment—up to ninety-nine years—should the state retroactively deem their patient to have been insufficiently close to death at the time they intervened to save her. Women in Texas have developed sepsis, hemorrhaged, and even died as hospitals delay or deny care for pregnancy loss to comply with the new state law.[16]

Much has changed about the position of physicians and medical associations since the history this book chronicles. Although the American Medical Association once led the nineteenth-century campaign to outlaw abortion, in 2022 the organization vehemently condemned the "egregious" Supreme Court decision to recriminalize it—describing the revocation of abortion access as "an assault on reproductive health" and "a brazen violation of patients' rights to evidence-based reproductive health services."[17] (In another notable departure from the nineteenth century, the contemporary American Medical Association no longer restricts its membership to white male physicians alone.) Yet while there are substantial differences, today's world also bears troubling continuities with an earlier era in which patriarchal institutions sought to assert authority over pregnancy and women's reproductive bodies.[18]

In protesting the *Journal of the American Medical Association*'s use of the word *monster*, Dr. Thelander concluded her 1963 letter by expressing her hope that "the word will disappear from the medical literature."[19] In some notable ways, Thelander's wish has finally come true. To be sure, the Greek word *teras* persists in the etymology of contemporary biomedical terms. A *teratogen* refers to an environmental agent capable of disrupting prenatal development. A *teratoma* refers to a germ-cell tumor containing multiple types of mature tissue. The field of teratology still exists (although its eponymous academic journal has been renamed *Birth Defects Research*). But teratology is now described as the scientific study of abnormalities of development, not the scientific study of monstrosity. Medical journals such as the *Journal of the American Medical Association* no longer identify infants with anatomical differences as monsters. Indeed, no word exists in today's clinical nomenclature that denotes the precise set of referents that the term *monster* once did. In this sense, then, *monstrosity* has indeed disappeared from the medical lexicon.

But the disappearance of the term *monstrosity* did not expunge the influence of the concepts that the category once materialized: the protean and persistent logics of social and biological alterity, of "defective" and "deviant" bodies, of sexual and racial orders of human kinds. The term's disappearance did not negate the broader cultural interest in controlling women's reproduction, nor did it dispel the hierarchical renderings of human difference that the monster had linked and embodied.

As this book has shown, the medical engagement with monstrosity can be located within a larger history of practices that generated, circulated, and entrenched conceptions of innate biological difference and hierarchy, especially of race, sex, and disability. Deep-rooted investments in biological understandings of difference persist today, sometimes in subtle ways. For example, in medicine, notions of innate difference have endured in practices such as race-corrected clinical algorithms and race-coded pharmacogenomics, which invoke presumptively categorical divisions of race as a proxy for biological risk in clinical decision-making.[20]

Conceptions of innate biological difference also persist in some not-so-subtle ways. Overt claims about a hierarchy of biological human value—the notion that some people are innately worth more than others because of their putatively superior biological makeup—have surfaced in mid-2020s discourse on US social policy, immigration restriction, and a resurgent pronatalist movement.[21] And there is nothing remotely subtle about the federal government's recent attempts to recuperate by decree the idea of race and sex as "biological reality." A 2025 presidential executive order on sex categories aims to establish an "immutable biological classification" that is fixed "at conception"—a rigid biological determinism that echoes the eugenicist Charles Davenport's insistence on "the fate that is thus determined at the moment of fertilization."[22] Another 2025 order formally rebukes a Smithsonian exhibit for promoting "the view that race is not a biological reality but a social construct."[23]

Notably, at the same time that political authorities seek to revive the central premise of nineteenth-century race science, they work to bar the teaching of its history.[24] Perhaps they recognize that honest historical inquiry poses a powerful challenge to conceptions of innate difference, revealing the contingency and instability of racial and gendered categories as historically created—rather than natural biological—constructions. Rigorous examination of these histories illuminates the social, political, economic, legal, and institutional practices that have produced, maintained, and entrenched categories of difference and inequity over the course of generations. Further, such examination can allow us to recognize how and why the residues of a monstrous past live on.

Knowing about this history does not in and of itself change the legacies of the past in the present world. Historical knowledge is not prescriptive, and it is not inherently curative. But historical knowledge can be powerful—a fact tacitly acknowledged today in political edicts that seek to suppress and censor its teaching. By exposing and exploring the past processes that produced constrictive meanings of bodies, reproduction, and human difference, history can open up the room to imagine how it might be otherwise.

Acknowledgments

I have relied on many people over the years of researching and writing this book. This project owes much to wonderful advisers. Evelynn Hammonds's wisdom and incisive insight guided me in thinking through complex histories. David Jones's mentorship provided a model of dedication, integrity, and generosity that I aspire to. Allan Brandt continues to buoy me with his inimitable care and compassion: He is the kind of mentor who sees and believes in the very best version of you and inspires you to believe in it too.

I began this research as a graduate student at Harvard University, where I also received excellent guidance from Sarah Richardson and other History of Science Department and History Department faculty such as Nancy Cott, Anne Harrington, Evelyn Brooks Higginbotham, Walter Johnson, Katharine Park, Scott Podolsky, Janet Browne, Naomi Oreskes, Gabriela Soto Laveaga, Rebecca Lemov, and Sophia Roosth. Fellow graduate students shared thoughtful feedback and talked through ideas with me, including Marc Aidinoff, Leena Akhtar, Katie Baca, Erik Baker, Alyssa Botelho, Stephanie Dick, Cara Fallon, Nayanika Ghosh, Shireen Hamza, Emily Harrison, Lisa Haushofer, Jordan Howell, Andrew Inkpen, Dani Inkpen, Devin Kennedy, Max Kenner, Gustave Lester, Wythe Marschall, Allyssa Metzger, Eli Nelson, Kat Poje, Christopher Rudeen, Mashaal Sohail, Liat Spiro, Alexis Turner, Maddie

Williams, and Che Yeun. Special thanks to Udodiri Okwandu, my terrific senior thesis advisee turned graduate school friend turned fellow professor.

I am grateful to the archivists, curators, and librarians who helped with the research for this book: Clare Clark at Cold Spring Harbor Laboratory, Cornelia King at the Library Company of Philadelphia, Brian Spatola and Elizabeth Lockett at the National Museum of Health and Medicine, Beth Lander at the College of Physicians of Philadelphia, Jack Eckert and Jessica Murphy at Countway Library, Kelly Caldwell and Alison Hansen at Moody Medical Library, and Paula Summerly at the Old Red Medical Museum. Dominic Hall at the Warren Museum offered exceptionally generous and enthusiastic assistance throughout. Research funding was provided by the Charles Warren Center for Studies in American History at Harvard University; the Genentech Center for the History of Microbiology and Biotechnology at Cold Spring Harbor Laboratory; the American Philosophical Society; the Consortium for the History of Science, Medicine, and Technology; and the Library Company of Philadelphia.

As a lecturer at Yale University, I benefited greatly from the sage insight and generosity of John Harley Warner, Naomi Rogers, and Joanna Radin in the History of Medicine Section. Emily Wang, Lisa Puglisi, the SEICHE Center for Health and Justice, and the students of the US Health Justice Course Initiative encouraged me to connect historical scholarship to urgent problems of health inequity in the present day. My phenomenal undergraduate students were a constant source of energy and inspiration. Angélica Clayton, Deborah Coen, Melissa Grafe, Kathleen Keenan, Megann Licskai, Carolyn Roberts, Jason Schwartz, and many others warmly welcomed me into the History of Science and Medicine Program. Matthew Graham, Casey Kogut, Dani Lee, Darius Longarino, Madison Needham, and Di Wu enriched my time in New Haven.

In the Dartmouth Society of Fellows, I received wonderfully attentive and energetic mentorship from Leslie Butler. Fellow postdocs Bench Ansfield, Curt Gambetta, rl Goldberg, Jorge Ramirez-Lopez, Whitney Barlow Robles, Aanchal Saraf, Amy Schiller, Danielle Simon, Natalie Teale, Monique Ulysses, Kasia Warburton, and Yiren Zheng provided rich conversation and warm camaraderie through frosty Upper Valley winters. History Department faculty Annelise Orleck, Soyoung Suh, Bethany Moreton, Pamela Voekel, Jennie Miller, and Darrin McMahon offered insightful comments on my work. Myles Blencowe, Laura McDaniel, and Emily Walton shared advice and support. Heartfelt thanks are owed to Sa Whitley and Tory Jeffay, whose extraordinary generosity enabled me to find a home in New Hampshire.

I completed this book at the Institute for Bioethics and Health Humanities at the University of Texas Medical Branch. It has been an honor to join a community of scholars committed to the pursuit of health equity at a moment when that commitment requires real conviction and courage. I thank Lisa Campo-Engelstein and Kristen Peek for their support, integrity, and heartening leadership in troubled times. I am proud of our brave graduate students' refusal to be cowed in their work toward health justice. I feel fortunate to have excellent colleagues such as Alberto Aparicio, Matty Hemming, Jarrel de Matas, Rachel McClere, Stephen Molldrem, Maile Young, and Xiang Yu. I thank Trevor Engel for nuanced conversations about interconnected histories of disability, race, and medicine. I am so grateful to Elise Smith for her endless thoughtfulness and encouragement. Special thanks to Jacob Moses, who has been a wise and profoundly insightful interlocuter for many years.

Thanks are owed to many great PhD students who aided in checking citations, helped compile the bibliography, and/or read and discussed a draft of the introduction chapter for their Reproductive Ethics seminar: Hannah Carpenter, Grayson Jackson, Mikaela Kim, Ginika Oguagha, Vishnu Subrahmanyam, Peyton Swanson, Lorenah Vásquez, Francis Amuzu, Carmen Haynes, and Susan Lee. Georgia Loutrianakis adeptly helped decipher historical handwriting. Evelyn Lamb provided outstanding assistance and enthusiasm in the final stages of manuscript preparation.

I thank the Columbia University Press editors Stephen Wesley and Alex Gupta and series editors Samuel Kelton Roberts and Michael Yudell for their generous support of this project, the anonymous peer reviewers for their stimulating comments, Annie Barva for her skillful and attentive copyediting, and Jennifer Quincey for her thoughtful reading of the manuscript. A version of chapter 1 first appeared as "Conceiving Monsters: Women, Knowledge, and Anomalous Births in the

Nineteenth-Century United States," *Bulletin of the History of Medicine* 99, no. 2 (Summer 2025): 316–46, copyright © Johns Hopkins University Press. A version of chapter 5 first appeared as "Monstrosity in Medical Science: Race-Making and Teratology in the Nineteenth-Century United States," *Isis: A Journal of the History of Science Society* 114, no. 3 (September 2023): 513–36, copyright © History of Science Society, published by the University of Chicago Press. I thank both journals for permission to publish revised versions.

I am indebted to Wangui Muigai for her brilliant, careful, and immensely generative feedback on drafts of every chapter (sometimes multiple versions) over the past few years and for her indispensable camaraderie. Laura Briggs, Deirdre Cooper Owens, Sharla Fett, and Sasha Turner provided invaluable comments on the manuscript at different stages of its writing. Pablo Gómez offered incredibly helpful guidance on the introduction and the revision process. Scott Gilbert supported this project in so many ways, not least by modeling for me a form of exuberant intellectual inquiry unconstrained by rigid disciplinary boundaries. Bruce Dorsey taught me to approach the study of history with imagination, rigor, and empathy. For their continually energizing insights and all-around generosity, I am grateful to Kelsey Henry, Lilla Orr, Marco Ramos, Aaron van Neste, Beans Velocci, and Kathryn Wataha.

I have moved many times while writing this book, from densely populated East Coast cities to a tiny northern Appalachian town to a barrier island off the Texas Gulf Coast. I cherish the friendships and communities that have sustained me wherever I am and the spaces that have allowed me to pursue joyful and creative movement practices in fellowship with others. James Maguire and Kelsie Lopez filled day-to-day life with revitalizing warmth and laughter. I am grateful for the memory of Nina and Jason. I thank my aunts, uncles, and cousins for their loving encouragement; John Gee for his unwavering support; and Elizabeth and Graciela for their constant care and companionship. Endless love and gratitude to Malcolm, Lise, Abigail, and Rebecca. And to Bernie, Esther, June, and Samuel—may their memory be for a blessing.

Notes

INTRODUCTION

1. J. B. S. Jackson, "Case of Monstrosity—(Siren)," *Boston Medical and Surgical Journal* 3, no. 3 (1869): 35.
2. Jackson, "Case of Monstrosity—(Siren)," 35.
3. J. B. S. Jackson, *Descriptive Catalogue of the Warren Anatomical Museum* (A. Williams, 1870), 112–13.
4. Joseph L. Roberge, "Sympodia in Identical Twins: Report of a Case," *Journal of the American Medical Association* 186, no. 7 (1963): 728.
5. H. E. Thelander, "Use of the Term 'Monster,'" *Journal of the American Medical Association* 187, no. 8 (1964): 621.
6. Lorraine Daston and Katharine Park, *Wonders and the Order of Nature, 1150–1750* (Zone, 1998), 173–214; Marie-Hélène Huet, *Monstrous Imagination* (Harvard University Press, 1993), 1–78; Mary Fissell, *Vernacular Bodies: The Politics of Reproduction in Early Modern England* (Oxford University Press, 2004), 64–69, 157–95.
7. Georges Canguilhem, "Monstrosity and the Monstrous," trans. Therese Jaeger, *Diogenes* 10, no. 40 (1962): 27–42, retranslated in *Knowledge of Life*, ed. Paola Marrati and Todd Meyers, trans. Stefanos Geroulanos and Daniela Ginsburg (Fordham University Press, 2008), 134–48.
8. Although the term *biomedical* dates to the twentieth century, I use the term more broadly to also encompass nineteenth-century medical discourse that engaged life sciences such as anatomy, physiology, embryology, histology, pathology, and zoology to interpret and intervene on the human body.

9. Aristotle, *Generation of Animals, with an English Translation by A. L. Peck* (Harvard University Press, 1902), 401, 417.

10. W. W., "Monstrosities," *Western Medical and Physical Journal* 3, no. 3 (1835): 413; Barton Hirst, "Two Recent Additions to the Teratological Collection in the Wistar and Horner Museum," *University of Pennsylvania Medical Magazine* 4, no. 10 (1892): 693.

11. Isidore Geoffroy Saint-Hilaire, *Histoire générale et particulière des anomalies de l'organisation chez l'homme et les animaux, ou, Traité de tératologie*, 3 vols. (J-B. Baillière, 1832–1837). On teratology in early nineteenth-century France, see Bertrand Nouailles, *Le monstre, la vie, l'écart: La tératologie d'Étienne et d'Isidore Geoffroy Saint-Hilaire* (Classiques Garnier, 2017); and Peter Cryle and Elizabeth Stephens, *Normality: A Critical Genealogy* (University of Chicago Press, 2017), 23–62.

12. See, e.g., P. C. Simpson et al., "The Intrauterine Treatment of Fetal Cardiac Failure in a Twin Pregnancy with an Acardiac, Acephalic Monster," *American Journal of Obstetrics and Gynecology* 147, no. 7 (1983): 842–44.

13. For examples of relevant work in the history of science and medicine, see Daston and Park, *Wonders and the Order of Nature*; Lorraine Daston, "What Can Be a Scientific Object? Reflections on Monsters and Meteors," *Bulletin of the Academy of Arts and Sciences* 52, no. 2 (1998): 35–50; Michael Hagner, "Enlightened Monsters," in *The Sciences in Enlightened Europe*, ed. William Clark et al. (University of Chicago Press, 1999), 175–218; and Sara Ray, "From Monsters to Malformations: Anatomical Preparations as Objects of Evidence for a Developmental Paradigm of Embryology, 1770–1850," *Journal of the History of Biology* 55, no. 1 (2022): 35–57. In disability studies and disability history, see Robert Bogdan, *Freak Show: Presenting Human Oddities for Amusement and Profit* (University of Chicago Press, 1988); Rosemarie Garland-Thomson, ed., *Freakery: Cultural Spectacles of the Extraordinary Body* (New York University Press, 1996); Ellen Samuels, "Examining Millie and Christine McKoy: Where Enslavement and Enfreakment Meet," *Signs* 37, no. 1 (2011): 53–81; and Cynthia Wu, *Chang and Eng Reconnected: The Original Siamese Twins in American Culture* (Temple University Press, 2012).

14. See, e.g., Jeffrey Jerome Cohen, ed., *Monster Theory: Reading Culture* (University of Minnesota Press, 1996); Julie Crawford, *Marvelous Protestantism: Monstrous Births in Post-Reformation England* (Johns Hopkins University Press, 2005); Martha Few, "Atlantic World Monsters: Monstrous Births and the Politics of Pregnancy in Colonial Guatemala," in *Women, Religion, and the Atlantic World*, ed. Lisa Vollendorf and Daniella J. Kostroun (University of Toronto Press, 2009), 205–22; Asa Simon Mittman and Peter J. Dendle, eds., *The Ashgate Research Companion to Monsters and the Monstrous* (Routledge, 2012);

and Caroline Joan Picart and John Edgar Browning, eds., *Speaking of Monsters: A Teratological Anthology* (Palgrave Macmillan, 2012). On racialized imaginaries of monstrosity in histories of slavery and colonialism, see Jennifer Morgan, "'Some Could Suckle Over Their Shoulder': Male Travelers, Female Bodies, and the Gendering of Racial Ideology, 1500–1770," *William and Mary Quarterly* 54, no. 1 (1997): 167–92; Stefanie Hunt-Kennedy, "Imagining Africa, Inheriting Monstrosity: Gender, Blackness, and Capitalism in the Early Atlantic World," in *Between Fitness and Death: Disability and Slavery in the Caribbean* (University of Illinois Press, 2020), 13–38; Surekha Davies, *Renaissance Ethnography and the Invention of the Human: New Worlds, Maps, and Monsters* (Cambridge University Press, 2016); and Ahmed Ragab, "Monsters and Patients: An Archaeology of Medicine, Islam, and Modernity," *History and Theory* 55, no. 4 (2016): 112–30.

15. Monstrous birth has received relatively little attention to date in scholarship on the modern US history of childbirth and reproduction. The most notable exceptions are several book chapters and articles that discuss the topic in the context of the social history of childbirth in antebellum slavery. See Marie Jenkins Schwartz, *Birthing a Slave: Motherhood and Medicine in the Antebellum South* (Harvard University Press, 2010), 212–26; Marli Weiner, with Mayzie Hough, *Sex, Sickness, and Slavery: Illness in the Antebellum South* (University of Illinois Press, 2012), 114–22; and Jenifer Barclay, "Bad Breeders and Monstrosities: Racializing Childlessness and Congenital Disabilities in Slavery and Freedom," *Slavery and Abolition* 38, no. 2 (2017): 287–302. Scholarship on the history of pregnancy and congenital disabilities in later US history (following the dissolution of "monstrosity" as a medical category) includes Leslie J. Reagan, *Dangerous Pregnancies: Mothers, Disabilities, and Abortion in Modern America* (University of California Press, 2010); and Janet Golden, *Message in a Bottle: The Making of Fetal Alcohol Syndrome* (Harvard University Press, 2005). For scholarship on monstrosity in relation to childbirth and reproduction in a different national context, see Nora E. Jaffary, "Monstrous Births," in *Reproduction and Its Discontents in Mexico: Childbirth and Contraception from 1750 to 1905* (University of North Carolina Press, 2016), 141–73.

16. Evelleen Richards, "A Political Anatomy of Monsters, Hopeful and Otherwise: Teratogeny, Transcendentalism, and Evolutionary Theorizing," *Isis* 85, no. 3 (1994): 377–411; Frida Gorbach, "Teratology in Mexico. 19th Century," *Medicina nei secoli* 26, no. 1 (2014): 245–67; Nora E. Jaffary, "The Monstrous Nation: The 1895 *Salon de Anomalías* in Mexico's National Museum, 1895," *Journal of Women's History* 34, no. 2 (2022): 11–30; Salim Samar Al-Gailani, "Teratology and the Clinic: Monsters, Obstetrics, and the Making of Antenatal Life in Edinburgh, c. 1900" (PhD diss., University of Cambridge, 2010).

17. Harvey Lindsly, *Medical Science and the Medical Profession in Europe and the United States: An Introductory Lecture* (P. Force, 1840), 29; Frank Stahl, "Maternal Impressions and Their Significance: With Presentation of a Case of Anencephalia et Acrania," *American Journal of Obstetrics and Diseases of Women and Children* 33, no. 4 (1896): 511; Charles Benedict Davenport, *Heredity in Relation to Eugenics* (H. Holt, 1911), 3.
18. These reports come from Alabama, Arkansas, California, Colorado, Connecticut, Delaware, Florida, Georgia, Illinois, Indiana, Iowa, Kansas, Kentucky, Louisiana, Maine, Maryland, Massachusetts, Michigan, Minnesota, Mississippi, Missouri, Nebraska, New Hampshire, New Jersey, New Mexico, New York, North Carolina, Ohio, Pennsylvania, Rhode Island, South Carolina, Tennessee, Texas, Virginia, Washington, West Virginia, and Wisconsin as well as from sites of informal US imperialism in Central America and formal US imperialism in the Philippines.
19. For classic work on the professional and institutional history of nineteenth-century US medicine, see John Harley Warner, *The Therapeutic Perspective: Medical Practice, Knowledge, and Identity in America, 1820–1885* (Princeton University Press, 1997); Charles E. Rosenberg, *The Care of Strangers: The Rise of America's Hospital System* (Johns Hopkins University Press, 1995); and Paul Starr, *The Social Transformation of American Medicine* (Basic, 1982), 30–197.
20. Aristotle, *Generation of Animals*, 417, 401.
21. Feminist and queer theorists analyze the monster as a powerful trope of difference and deviance, implicating it in the formation of racial, gendered, sexual, and corporeal subjectivities. See Rosi Braidotti, "Signs of Wonder and Traces of Doubt: On Teratology and Embodied Differences," in *Feminist Theory and the Body: A Reader*, ed. Janet Price and Margrit Shildrick (Routledge, 1999), 290–301; Christina Sharpe, *Monstrous Intimacies: Making Post-Slavery Subjects* (Duke University Press, 2010); Margrit Shildrick, *Embodying the Monster: Encounters with the Vulnerable Self* (Sage, 2002); Rosemarie Garland-Thomson, *Extraordinary Bodies: Figuring Physical Disability in American Culture and Literature* (Columbia University Press, 1997); Donna Haraway, "A Cyborg Manifesto: Science, Technology, and Socialist-Feminism in the Late Twentieth Century," in *Simians, Cyborgs, and Women: The Reinvention of Nature* (Routledge, 1991), 149–81; and Michel Foucault, *Abnormal: Lectures at the Collège de France, 1974–1975* (Picador, 2003).
22. Braidotti, "Signs of Wonder," 292; Shildrick, *Embodying the Monster*, 4–5; Garland-Thomson, *Extraordinary Bodies*, 8. For a similar point related to "abjected and delegitimated bodies," see Judith Butler, *Bodies That Matter: On the Discursive Limits of "Sex"* (Routledge, 1993), 16.
23. Braidotti, "Signs of Wonder," 292; Shildrick, *Embodying the Monster*, 17; Foucault, *Abnormal*, 63.

24. Daston and Park, *Wonders and the Order of Nature*, 173–214.

25. Barton Cooke Hirst and George Piersol, *Human Monstrosities*, 4 vols. (Lea Brothers, 1891–1893), 1:83.

26. On monstrosity as deviation from species type, see Edward Schumann, "Observations Upon the Formation of Terata," *American Journal of Obstetrics and Diseases of Women and Children* 67, no. 6 (1913): 1159; Henry Lewis, "Iniencephalus," *American Journal of Obstetrics and Diseases of Women and Children* 34, no. 1 (1897): 11; and "Monster/Monstrosity," in *Globe Encyclopaedia*, ed. John Ross (Estes & Lauriat, 1877), 305. On taxonomic orders of monstrosity, see George J. Fisher, *Diploteratology: An Essay on Compound Human Monsters* (Van Benthuysen's Steam Printing House, 1866), 3–4; and Hirst and Piersol, *Human Monstrosities*, 1:11–18.

27. Hirst and Piersol, *Human Monstrosities*, 1:11; Alfred Swaine Taylor, *A Manual of Medical Jurisprudence*, 7th American ed. (H. C. Lea, 1873), 396. See also Francis H. Ramsbotham, *The Principles and Practice of Obstetric Medicine and Surgery: In Reference to the Process of Parturition*, 1st American ed. (Lea & Blanchard, 1842), 511.

28. On dermoid cysts as "parasitic monsters," see Hirst and Piersol, *Human Monstrosities*, 1:5. On the lives and experiences of nineteenth-century conjoined twins, see Samuels, "Examining Millie and Christine McKoy"; and Wu, *Chang and Eng Reconnected*.

29. On the "impossibility" of life "for the great majority" of monstrosities, see Theophilus Parvin, "Monsters," *Medical and Surgical Reporter* 77 (1897): 5; and Charles Stolz, "Some Common Monstrosities," *Transactions of the Indiana State Medical Society* (1898): 250.

30. The prevalence of these conditions in the case literature is consistent with their far greater population incidence as compared to other conditions historically classified as monstrosities, even though the birth of infants with anencephaly did not elicit the same level of popular and commercial attention as the birth of infants with comparatively rarer conditions (such as conjoined twins). Along with *anencephalus*, closely related or synonymous nineteenth-century diagnostic terms that referred to arrests in the embryological development of brain and skull included *acephalus, acrania, derencephalus, exencephalus, iniencephalus, nosencephalus, notencephalus, paracephalus, pseudencephalus*, and *thlipsencephalus*.

31. Hirst and Piersol, *Human Monstrosities*, 2:109; Lewis, "Iniencephalus," 11. Noting that "it is partly by reason of its frequency that anencephaly has been described so often and so fully," the obstetrician John W. Ballantyne estimated its occurrence at approximately 1 in 1,500 births in 1905. Ballantyne, *Manual of Antenatal Pathology and Hygiene: The Embryo* (Wood, 1905), 334. Beginning in the late 1990s, the fortification of the national US grain supply with folic acid

played a major role in reducing the US population incidence of anencephaly. Centers for Disease Control and Prevention, "Updated Estimates of Neural Tube Defects Prevented by Mandatory Folic Acid Fortification—United States, 1995–2011," *Morbidity and Mortality Weekly Report* 64, no. 1 (2015): 1–5.

32. An authoritative early twentieth-century treatise on antenatal pathology noted that "the consideration of the theories of teratogenesis in several instances resolved itself into the consideration of the theories of the production of anencephaly. . . . In discussing teratogenesis I constantly had to refer to this monstrosity, for all the theories were made by their proposers to apply to it." Ballantyne, *Manual of Antenatal Pathology and Hygiene*, 334. On "arrest of development" as the "guiding principle" of Saint-Hilaire's teratology, see Richards, "Political Anatomy of Monsters."

33. On the significance and "privileged epistemological status" of the skull in nineteenth-century racial science, see Ricardo Roque, "Authorised Histories: Human Remains and the Economies of Credibility in the Science of Race," *Kronos*, no. 44 (2018): 70; Ann Fabian, *The Skull Collectors: Race, Science, and America's Unburied Dead* (University of Chicago Press, 2010); Christopher Willoughby, "Skull Collecting, Medical Museums, and the International Dimensions of Racial Science," in *Masters of Health: Racial Science and Slavery in U.S. Medical Schools* (University of North Carolina Press, 2022), 125–41; and Nancy Leys Stepan, *The Idea of Race in Science: Great Britain, 1800–1960* (Archon, 1982), 20–46, 83–110.

34. Scott F. Gilbert, *Developmental Biology*, 10th ed. (Sinauer, 2014), 393–97.

35. S. N. Berry et al., "The Impact of Anencephaly on Parents: A Mixed-Methods Study," *Death Studies* 46, no. 9 (2022): 2198–207; and Selena Simmons-Duffin, "A Good Friday Funeral in Texas: Baby Halo's Parents Had Few Choices in Post-Roe Texas," NPR, April 6, 2023, https://www.npr.org/sections/health-shots/2023/04/06/1168399423/a-good-friday-funeral-in-texas-baby-halos-parents-had-few-choices-in-post-roe-te.

36. Judith Walzer Leavitt, *Brought to Bed: Childbearing in America, 1750 to 1950*, 30th anniv. ed. (Oxford University Press, 2016), 12 (graph); Charlotte G. Borst, *Catching Babies: The Professionalization of Childbirth, 1870–1920* (Harvard University Press, 1995), 1–12.

37. Leavitt, *Brought to Bed*, 64–86; Borst, *Catching Babies*, 1–11; Gertrude Jacinta Fraser, *African American Midwifery in the South: Dialogues of Birth, Race, and Memory* (Harvard University Press, 1998), 139–237; Brianna Theobald, *Reproduction on the Reservation: Pregnancy, Childbirth, and Colonialism in the Long Twentieth Century* (University of North Carolina Press, 2019), 29–36.

38. Stephen C. Kenny, "The Development of Medical Museums in the Antebellum American South: Slave Bodies in Networks of Anatomical Exchange," *Bulletin*

of the History of Medicine 87, no. 1 (2013): 32–62; Daina Ramey Berry, *The Price for Their Pound of Flesh: The Value of the Enslaved, from Womb to Grave, in the Building of a Nation* (Beacon, 2017); Wendi A. Lindquist, "Stealing from the Dead: Scientists, Settlers, and Indian Burial Sites in Early-Nineteenth-Century Oregon," *Oregon Historical Quarterly* 115, no. 3 (2014): 324–43; Trevor Engel, "A 'Most Remarkable Trait': 'Flathead' Skulls, Indigenous Pathologization, and Transinstitutionalization," *Osiris* 39, no. 1 (2024): 117–34.

39. Leavitt, *Brought to Bed*, 74–77.

40. G. P. Boerstler, "Monstrosity," *Nashville Journal of Medicine and Surgery* 9 (1855): 121–22; Drs. Cohen and Durr, "Case of Monstrosity," *Charleston Medical Journal and Review* 7 (1852): 67–70; A. L. Sweet, "An Interesting Obstetric Case," *Medical Record* 16, no. 19 (1879): 439.

41. Hirst and Piersol, *Human Monstrosities*, 1:11, 83; Theresa Bannan, "A Case of Monstrosity," *Medical Record* 45, no. 25 (1894): 788.

42. Oliver Wendell Holmes, *The Poet at the Breakfast-Table: His Talks with His Fellow-Boarders and the Reader* (James R. Osgood, 1872), 263; Oliver Wendell Holmes, "Scholastic and Bedside Teaching," in *Medical Essays: 1842–1882*, Riverside ed. (Houghton, Mifflin, 1891), 279–80.

43. Canguilhem, "Monstrosity and the Monstrous," 142–43; Rosemarie Garland-Thomson et al., "Introduction: Step Right Up! A New Introduction to the Old Freak Show," in *Freak Inheritance: Eugenics and Extraordinary Bodies in Performance*, ed. Rosemarie Garland-Thomson et al. (Oxford University Press, 2024), xvi. The oppositional framing of scientific understanding and cultural understanding is common both to works that celebrate the ascendence of the former and to those that critique it. Dudley Butler Wilson charts a shift from fraught signs in the "age of superstition" to naturalized objects in the "age of science"; Stephen Asma credits European scientists and physicians with "rescuing monsters from the melodramatic arena of spiritual and moral meaning." Although Marie Jenkins Schwartz offers a decidedly less triumphalist account of medical science, she likewise presents "scientific" and "cultural" meanings as oppositional foils, contrasting nineteenth-century physicians who regarded monstrous births "as the result of faulty congenital development" with laypeople who regarded them as "a sign requiring cultural interpretation." Wilson, *Signs and Portents: Monstrous Births from the Middle Ages to the Enlightenment* (Routledge, 1993); Asma, *On Monsters: An Unnatural History of Our Worst Fears* (Oxford University Press, 2009), 143–44; Schwartz, *Birthing a Slave*, 212.

44. Dorothy E. Roberts, *Fatal Invention: How Science, Politics, and Big Business Re-Create Race in the Twenty-First Century* (New Press, 2011), 26–36; Bruce R. Dain, *A Hideous Monster of the Mind: American Race Theory in the Early Republic* (Harvard University Press, 2002), 197–226; Audrey Smedley, *Race in*

North America: Origin and Evolution of a Worldview, 4th ed. (Routledge, 2011), esp. 213–50.

45. Banu Subramaniam, *Ghost Stories for Darwin: The Science of Variation and the Politics of Diversity* (University of Illinois Press, 2014); Sandra G. Harding, ed., *The "Racial" Economy of Science: Toward a Democratic Future* (Indiana University Press, 1993), part 3: "Who Gets to Do Science?," 197–267; Todd L. Savitt, "Medical Experimentation and Demonstration on Blacks in the Old South," in *Race and Medicine in Nineteenth- and Early-Twentieth-Century America* (Kent State University Press, 2007), 77–88; Susan Reverby, "Ethical Failures and History Lessons: The U.S. Public Health Service Research Studies in Tuskegee and Guatemala," *Public Health Reviews* 34, no. 1 (2012): 1–18. On the production of health-related knowledge outside of bioscientific frameworks of legitimation, see Sharla M. Fett, *Working Cures: Healing, Health, and Power on Southern Slave Plantations* (University of North Carolina Press, 2000).
46. Natalia Molina, *Fit to Be Citizens? Public Health and Race in Los Angeles, 1879–1939* (University of California Press, 2006); Nayan Shah, *Contagious Divides: Epidemics and Race in San Francisco's Chinatown* (University of California Press, 2001); Keith Wailoo, *Dying in the City of the Blues: Sickle Cell Anemia and the Politics of Race and Health* (University of North Carolina Press, 2001); David S. Jones, *Rationalizing Epidemics: Meanings and Uses of American Indian Mortality Since 1600* (Harvard University Press, 2004); Dorothy E. Roberts, *Killing the Black Body: Race, Reproduction, and the Meaning of Liberty* (Pantheon, 1997); Samuel Kelton Roberts, *Infectious Fear: Politics, Disease, and the Health Effects of Segregation* (University of North Carolina Press, 2009).
47. D. Roberts, *Fatal Invention*; Evelynn Hammonds and Rebecca Herzig, *The Nature of Difference: Sciences of Race in the United States from Jefferson to Genomics* (MIT Press, 2008); Lundy Braun, *Breathing Race Into the Machine: The Surprising Career of the Spirometer from Plantation to Genetics* (University of Minnesota Press, 2014); Deirdre Benia Cooper Owens, *Medical Bondage: Race, Gender, and the Origins of American Gynecology* (University of Georgia Press, 2017); Rana Hogarth, *Medicalizing Blackness: Making Racial Difference in the Atlantic World, 1780–1840* (University of North Carolina Press, 2017); Warwick Anderson, *Colonial Pathologies: American Tropical Medicine, Race, and Hygiene in the Philippines* (Duke University Press, 2006); Leslie Schwalm, *Medicine, Science, and Making Race in Civil War America* (University of North Carolina Press, 2023); Michael Yudell, *Race Unmasked: Biology and Race in the Twentieth Century* (Columbia University Press, 2014).
48. Ian Haney-López, *White by Law: The Legal Construction of Race* (New York University Press, 2006); Gloria J. Browne-Marshall, *Race, Law, and American Society: 1607–Present*, 2nd ed. (Routledge, 2013).

49. Cooper Owens, *Medical Bondage*, 8, 108–22.

50. Laura Briggs, "The Race of Hysteria: 'Overcivilization' and the 'Savage' Woman in Late Nineteenth-Century Obstetrics and Gynecology," *American Quarterly* 52, no. 2 (2000): 246–73; Cooper Owens, *Medical Bondage*; Miriam Rich, "The Curse of Civilised Woman: Race, Gender, and the Pain of Childbirth in Nineteenth-Century American Medicine," *Gender & History* 28 (2016): 64–67.

51. This approach situates the topic of monstrosity within a burgeoning literature that foregrounds childbearing and reproductive medicine as constitutive of historical discourses of gender, race, and disability in the Americas. See, e.g., Laura Briggs, *Reproducing Empire: Race, Sex, Science, and U.S. Imperialism in Puerto Rico* (University of California Press, 2002); Jennifer L. Morgan, *Laboring Women: Reproduction and Gender in New World Slavery* (University of Pennsylvania Press, 2004); Reagan, *Dangerous Pregnancies*; Cooper Owens, *Medical Bondage*; Sasha Turner, *Contested Bodies: Pregnancy, Childrearing, and Slavery in Jamaica* (University of Pennsylvania Press, 2017); Katherine Paugh, *The Politics of Reproduction: Race, Disease, and Fertility in the Age of Abolition* (Oxford University Press, 2017); Nora Doyle, *Maternal Bodies: Redefining Motherhood in Early America* (University of North Carolina Press, 2018); Shannon Withycombe, *Lost: Miscarriage in Nineteenth-Century America* (Rutgers University Press, 2018); Theobald, *Reproduction on the Reservation*; Wangui Muigai, "'Something Wasn't Clean': Black Midwifery, Birth, and Postwar Medical Education in *All My Babies*," *Bulletin of the History of Medicine* 93, no. 1 (2019): 82–113; Cassia Roth, *A Miscarriage of Justice: Women's Reproductive Lives and the Law in Early Twentieth-Century Brazil* (Stanford University Press, 2020); Lara Freidenfelds, *The Myth of the Perfect Pregnancy: A History of Miscarriage in America* (Oxford University Press, 2020); Felicity Turner, *Proving Pregnancy: Gender, Law, and Medical Knowledge in Nineteenth-Century America* (University of North Carolina Press, 2022); and Elizabeth O'Brien, *Surgery and Salvation: The Roots of Reproductive Injustice in Mexico, 1770–1940* (University of North Carolina Press, 2023).

52. On developmental discourses of race in the nineteenth century, see Matthew Frye Jacobson, *Barbarian Virtues: The United States Encounters Foreign Peoples at Home and Abroad, 1876–1917* (Hill and Wang, 2000), 139–41; and George W. Stocking, *Victorian Anthropology* (Collier Macmillan, Free Press, 1987). On interlocking discourses of race, civilization, evolution, and animality, see Gail Bederman, *Manliness and Civilization: A Cultural History of Gender and Race in the United States, 1880–1917* (University of Chicago Press, 1996); Zakiyyah Iman Jackson, *Becoming Human: Matter and Meaning in an Antiblack World* (New York University Press, 2021); and Kyla Schuller, *The Biopolitics of Feeling: Race, Sex, and Science in the Nineteenth Century* (Duke University Press, 2018).

53. On the historical association of binary sexual difference with human racial evolution, see Bederman, *Manliness and Civilization*, 25–28, 121–69; and Beans Velocci, *Sex Isn't Real: The Invention of an Incoherent Binary* (Duke University Press, 2026).

54. Bederman, *Manliness and Civilization*; Briggs, "Race of Hysteria."

55. Alexandra Minna Stern, *Eugenic Nation: Faults and Frontiers of Better Breeding in Modern America* (University of California Press, 2005); Wendy Kline, *Building a Better Race: Gender, Sexuality, and Eugenics from the Turn of the Century to the Baby Boom* (University of California Press, 2001).

56. Karen Yourish, Annie Daniel, Saurabh Datar, Isaac White, and Lazaro Gamio, "These Words Are Disappearing in the New Trump Administration," *New York Times*, March 7, 2025.

57. Nancy Leys Stepan, "Race and Gender: The Role of Analogy in Science," *Isis* 77, no. 2 (1986): 261–77; Nancy Krieger and Elizabeth Fee, "Man-Made Medicine and Women's Health: The Biopolitics of Sex/Gender and Race/Ethnicity," *International Journal of Health Services* 24, no. 2 (1994): 265–83; Cooper Owens, *Medical Bondage*. I use the combined term *sex/gender* here to refer to categories of human sex difference, recognizing that these categories embed and rely for their discursive coherence on cultural imaginaries of gender. See Judith Butler, *Gender Trouble: Feminism and the Subversion of Identity* (Routledge, 1990), 1–33; and Velocci, *Sex Isn't Real*.

58. Hazel V. Carby, *Reconstructing Womanhood: The Emergence of the Afro-American Woman Novelist* (Oxford University Press, 1987); Briggs, "Race of Hysteria"; Bederman, *Manliness and Civilization*.

59. D. Roberts, *Fatal Invention*, 4; Evelynn Hammonds, "Straw Men and Their Followers: The Return of Biological Race," Social Science Research Council, 2006, http://raceandgenomics.ssrc.org/Hammonds; Nancy Leys Stepan, "Race, Gender, Science, and Citizenship," *Gender & History* 10, no. 1 (1998): 26–52. On formations and doctrines of race in US history, see Michael Omi and Howard Winant, *Racial Formation in the United States* (Routledge, 1994); and Karen E. Fields and Barbara Fields, *Racecraft: The Soul of Inequality in American Life* (Verso, 2014).

60. Garland-Thomson, *Extraordinary Bodies*, 8. On disability "as a sign of and justification for" racial and gender inequality, see Douglas Baynton, "Disability and the Justification of Inequality in American History," in *The New Disability History: American Perspectives*, ed. Paul K. Longmore and Lauri Umansky (New York University Press, 2001), 33–57.

61. M. Middleton, "Cases of Malformation: With Reflections on Congenital Abnormities," *American Journal of the Medical Sciences* 55, no. 109 (1868): 69–76; Thomas Stedman, "Influence of Maternal Impressions in the Etiology of

Congenital Deformities," *Medical Record* 31, no. 1 (1887): A4–A9; W. W., "Monstrosities"; H., "Embryotic Influences—Acephalous Child," *Boston Medical and Surgical Journal* 22, no. 23 (1840): 362–63.

62. For an example of how a late nineteenth-century medical journal used the word *disability*—in this case to refer to acquired conditions or injuries that disqualified troops from further military service—see "Report of the Surgeon General," *Cincinnati Lancet and Clinic* 15, no. 25 (1885): 782. On changing historical definitions of disability, see Sarah F. Rose, *No Right to Be Idle: The Invention of Disability, 1840s–1930s* (University of North Carolina Press, 2017).

63. Nadja Durbach, *Spectacle of Deformity: Freak Shows and Modern British Culture* (University of California Press, 2010), 14–21.

64. Garland-Thomson, *Extraordinary Bodies*, 6; Baynton, "Disability and the Justification of Inequality"; Catherine Kudlick, "Disability History: Why We Need Another 'Other,'" *American Historical Review* 108 (2003): 763–79. More recent work continues to expand the scope of *disability* as a term of analysis, transcending "a rigid codification of the meaning and definition of disability" as a fixed subject position or "identity to be claimed" and calling for disability studies scholarship that "continually revisits, reframes, rejects, reimagines the proper subject/object of its analysis." Jina B. Kim, "Disability in an Age of Fascism," *American Quarterly* 72, no. 1 (2020): 267; Kelsey Henry et al., "Origins, Objects, Orientations: New Histories and Theories of Race and Disability," *Disability Studies Quarterly* 43, no. 1 (2023), https://doi.org/10.18061/dsq.v43i1.9719.

65. This literature explores how disability is racialized and gendered as well as how racial and gendered difference are rendered as disability; the ways state violence, economic exploitation, and global inequity differentially produce disability in racialized and gendered populations; and the lived experience of disability for individuals with marginalized racial and gender identities. See, e.g., Henry et al., "Origins, Objects, Orientations"; Sami Schalk and Jina B. Kim, "Integrating Race, Transforming Feminist Disability Studies," *Signs* 46, no. 1 (2020): 31–55; Sami Schalk, *Bodyminds Reimagined: (Dis)ability, Race, and Gender in Black Women's Speculative Fiction* (Duke University Press, 2018); Ellen Samuels, *Fantasies of Identification: Disability, Gender, Race* (New York University Press, 2014); Nirmala Erevelles, *Difference and Disability in Global Contexts: Enabling a Transformative Body Politic* (Palgrave Macmillan, 2011); Jasbir Puar, *The Right to Maim: Debility, Capacity, Disability* (Duke University Press, 2017); Adria L. Imada, *An Archive of Skin, an Archive of Kin: Disability and Life-Making During Medical Incarceration* (University of California Press, 2022); Dea Boster, *African American Slavery and Disability: Bodies, Property, and Power in the Antebellum South, 1800–1860* (Routledge, 2013); Jenifer Barclay, *The Mark of Slavery: Disability, Race, and Gender in Antebellum America*

(University of Illinois Press, 2021); and Micah Khater, "No Use to the State: Phrasing Escape and a Black Radical Epistolary of Disability in Early Twentieth-Century Alabama Prisons," *Disability Studies Quarterly* 43, no. 1 (2023), https://doi.org/10.18061/dsq.v43i1.9662.

66. Rosemarie Garland-Thomson, "Disability," in *Keywords in Health Humanities*, ed. Sari Altschuler et al. (New York University Press, 2023), 58; Garland-Thomson, "Disability Studies: A Field Emerged," *American Quarterly* 65, no. 4 (2013): 916. Simi Linton writes that disability studies fundamentally offers a "challenge to the notion that disability is primarily a medical category." Linton, *Claiming Disability: Knowledge and Identity* (New York University Press, 1998), 2. However, rejecting the medical model of disability in no way precludes inquiry into medicine as an object of historical analysis. As Julie Livingston points out, "Questioning the rationale and power of medicine, its ideas, language, and practices, the way it shapes the opportunities and constraints on human beings, does not preclude one from pursuing its history; indeed, it might even motivate the desire to know." Livingston persuasively rejects the drawing of rigid disciplinary boundaries between medical and disability history, writing that "there is no need to choose camps unless we narrow our definition of each field, a prospect I find unproductive." Livingston, "Comment: On the Borderland of Medical and Disability History," *Bulletin of History of Medicine* 87 (2013): 561–62.
67. Rosemarie Garland-Thomson, "Feminist Disability Studies," *Signs* 30, no. 2 (2005): 1557; Garland-Thomson, *Extraordinary Bodies*, 6. Disability studies scholars such as Jina B. Kim, Nirmala Erevelles, and Jasbir Puar define disability "less as a static category of identity—a descriptor of what someone is—and more as a process," describing it as a contingent "historical event" rather than an ahistorical "fixed state or attribute." Kim, "Disability in an Age of Fascism," 267; Erevelles, *Disability and Difference*, 26; Puar, *Right to Maim*, xiv.
68. On how medical discourses rendered bodies socially, politically, and legally legible in particular historical contexts, see, e.g., Anderson, *Colonial Pathologies*; Shah, *Contagious Divides*; F. Turner, *Proving Pregnancy*; and Molina, *Fit to Be Citizens?*
69. Adriana Petryna, *Life Exposed: Biological Citizens After Chernobyl* (Princeton University Press, 2002); P. Brown et al., "Embodied Health Movements: New Approaches to Social Movements in Health," *Sociology of Health & Illness* 26, no. 1 (2004): 50–80; Keith Wailoo et al., eds., *Genetics and the Unsettled Past: The Collision of DNA, Race, and History* (Rutgers University Press, 2012).
70. Carolyn Roberts, "Pharmaceutical Captivity, Epistemological Rupture, and the Business Archive of the British Slave Trade," *Business History Review* 97, no. 2 (2023): 289. My methodological approach in this book draws from fields such as history of science and medicine, health humanities, gender and sexuality

studies, disability studies, African American studies, and science studies/sociology of scientific knowledge.

71. Marisa Fuentes, *Dispossessed Lives: Enslaved Women, Violence, and the Archive* (University of Pennsylvania Press, 2016), 7, 78.

72. Nirmala Erevelles and Michael Gill, "The Absent Presence of Elsie Lacks: Hauntings at the Intersection of Race, Class, Gender, and Disability," *African American Review* 50, no. 2 (2017): 123–37. For approaches to reading "scanty" or "absent" historical archives among scholars of Black studies and Atlantic World slavery, see Saidiya Hartman, *Wayward Lives, Beautiful Experiments* (Norton, 2019); and Sasha Turner, "The Nameless and the Forgotten: Maternal Grief, Sacred Protection, and the Archive of Slavery," *Slavery & Abolition* 38 (2017): 232–50. For approaches from feminist historians of medicine, see Barbara Duden, *The Woman Beneath the Skin* (Harvard University Press, 1991); and Cooper Owens, *Medical Bondage*. Another source of general methodological inspiration is the midrashic tradition, an exegetic mode that elaborates and fills in the gaps of sparse or cryptic source text.

73. Evelynn Hammonds, "Black (W)holes and the Geometry of Black Female Sexuality," *differences: A Journal of Feminist Cultural Studies* 6, nos. 2–3 (1994): 139.

74. On the "materiality" and "meaning" of bodies as mutually constituted, see Judith Butler's theorization of cultural discourse formation as "a process of materialization," in Butler, *Bodies That Matter*, 9; Saidiya Hartman on the "discursive constitution of blackness" through the "corporealization of the body and the fixation of its constituent parts as indexes of truth and racial meaning," in Hartman, *Scenes of Subjection: Terror, Slavery, and Self-Making in Nineteenth-Century America* (Oxford University Press, 1997), 57–58; Walter Johnson on processes through which "the physical coordinates of human bodies" were "made meaningful," in Johnson, *Soul by Soul: Life Inside the Antebellum Slave Market* (Harvard University Press, 1999), 161; and Margrit Shildrick on how meaning and subjectivity are actualized through the "material engagement" of bodies, in Shildrick, *Dangerous Discourses of Disability, Subjectivity, and Sexuality* (Palgrave Macmillan, 2009), 25. On experiential, socially situated, and material practices of knowledge making, see Pablo Gómez, *The Experiential Caribbean: Creating Knowledge and Healing in the Early Modern Atlantic* (University of North Carolina Press, 2017); Steven Epstein, *Impure Science: AIDS, Activism, and the Politics of Knowledge* (University of California Press, 1996); and Pamela Smith et al., *Ways of Making and Knowing: The Material Culture of Empirical Knowledge* (University of Chicago Press, 2017).

75. Sara Ahmed, "Affective Economies," *Social Text* 22, no. 2 (2004): 117–39; Shildrick, *Dangerous Discourses of Disability*, 17–38; Mel Y. Chen, *Animacies: Biopolitics, Racial Mattering, and Queer Affect* (Duke University Press, 2012).

1. MONSTROUS PREGNANCIES: WOMEN'S NARRATIVES AND MEDICAL KNOWLEDGE MAKING

1. Charles T. Hildreth, *Case of Notencephale: With Engravings* (Published for the Author, 1834); Hildreth, "Art. I—Case of Notencephale," *Medical Magazine* 3 (1834): 3–16.
2. Hildreth, *Case of Notencephale*, 4–8.
3. Hildreth, *Case of Notencephale*, 4.
4. On the history of belief in maternal impression, see Huet, *Monstrous Imagination*, 11–102; and Sarah Richardson, *The Maternal Imprint: The Contested Science of Maternal–Fetal Effects* (University of Chicago Press, 2021), 26–82.
5. Hildreth, *Case of Notencephale*, 5.
6. Hildreth, *Case of Notencephale*, 5.
7. Hildreth, *Case of Notencephale*, 5–6.
8. Charles E. Rosenberg, "The Therapeutic Revolution: Medicine, Meaning, and Social Change in Nineteenth-Century America," *Perspectives in Biology and Medicine* 20, no. 4 (1977): 485–506.
9. Hildreth, *Case of Notencephale*, 6–7.
10. Laurel Thatcher Ulrich, *A Midwife's Tale: The Life of Martha Ballard, Based on Her Diary, 1785–1812* (Knopf, 1990); Leavitt, *Brought to Bed*, 8, 36–141; Borst, *Catching Babies*, 117–60.
11. Rich, "Curse of Civilised Woman," 70; Briggs, "Race of Hysteria."
12. Leavitt, *Brought to Bed*, 116–41; Jacqueline Wolf, *Deliver Me from Pain: Anesthesia and Birth in America* (Johns Hopkins University Press, 2009), 13–42.
13. Hildreth, *Case of Notencephale*, 16, 7.
14. Hildreth, *Case of Notencephale*, 7–8. Also on *notencéphale* or *notencephalus*, see Saint-Hilaire, *Histoire générale*, 2:295–98.
15. J. B. S. Jackson, *A Descriptive Catalogue of the Monstrosities in the Cabinet of the Boston Society for Medical Improvement* (Freeman and Bolles, 1847), 27–30; Accessions 05785, 05786, and 05787 (nonextant), Warren Anatomical Museum Collection, Countway Library, Center for the History of Medicine, Harvard Medical School, Boston.
16. Hildreth, *Case of Notencephale*, 3–16; Hildreth, "Art. I—Case of Notencephale"; Saint-Hilaire, *Histoire générale*, 2:313.
17. For catalogs of nineteenth-century medical specimen collections that included "monstrosities," see J. Jackson, *Descriptive Catalogue of the Monstrosities*, and *Descriptive Catalogue of the Warren Anatomical Museum*; Wistar Institute of Anatomy and Biology, *Catalogue of the Anatomical Museum of the University of Pennsylvania* (1832; L. R. Bailey, 1850), 34–38; Robert Ray et al., *A Catalogue of*

the Pathological Cabinet of the New York Hospital (S. S. & W. Wood, 1860); Joseph J. Woodward, "Chapter VIII: Anomalies and Monstrosities," in *Catalogue of the Medical Section of the United States Army Medical Museum* (US Government Printing Office, 1867), 127–28; William Pepper, *Descriptive Catalogue of the Pathological Museum of the Pennsylvania Hospital* (Collins, 1869); James Tyson, *Catalogue of the Specimens in the Pathological Museum of the Philadelphia Hospital* (Collins, 1874); and Wood Museum of Bellevue Hospital, *Catalogue of the Wood Museum of Bellevue Hospital, New York City, Comprising a Descriptive and Classified List of Anatomical and Pathological Specimens* (Dept. Press, 1880). On collections in medical museums in the US South, see Kenny, "The Development of Medical Museums."

18. Briggs, "Race of Hysteria," 247; Cooper Owens, *Medical Bondage*; Leavitt, *Brought to Bed*, 64–86. For examples of "monstrous" births in nineteenth-century maternity hospitals and wards, see Henry Tuck and J. B. S. Jackson, "Rare Form of Monstrosity; Case of Acephalus," *Boston Medical and Surgical Journal* 94, no. 16 (1876): 439–42; and "Woman's Hospital of Philadelphia 1895 Annual Report," 1895, Woman's Hospital of Philadelphia Records, Barbara Bates Center for History of Nursing, Philadelphia, PA.
19. On physicians' authority over enslaved women and anomalous births, see Schwartz, *Birthing a Slave*, 212–26.
20. Alexander Y. Nicoll and Richard D. Arnold, "Account of an Anencephalus, or Human Monstrosity Without a Brain and Spinal Marrow," *Southern Medical and Surgical Journal* 2, no.1 (1837): 18, 12–13.
21. Nicoll and Arnold, "Account of an Anencephalus" (1837), 10.
22. On the ongoing criminalization of Black motherhood at the intersection of racial, gender, and class-based discrimination, see Michele Goodwin, *Policing the Womb: Invisible Women and the Criminalization of Motherhood* (Cambridge University Press, 2020); Dorothy E. Roberts, "Unshackling Black Motherhood," *Michigan Law Review* 95, no. 4 (1997): 938–64.
23. Deborah Gray White, *Ar'n't I a Woman? Female Slaves in the Plantation South* (Norton, 1999), 86. See also J. Morgan, *Laboring Women*; and S. Turner, *Contested Bodies*.
24. Hortense J. Spillers, "Mama's Baby, Papa's Maybe: An American Grammar Book," *Diacritics* 17, no. 2 (1987): 74.
25. White, *Ar'n't I a Woman?*, 86–90.
26. Nicoll and Arnold, "Account of an Anencephalus" (1837), 10.
27. Sharpe, *Monstrous Intimacies*, 2.
28. *Fulton v. Shaw*, 4 Rand. 597 (1827).
29. Nicoll and Arnold, "Account of an Anencephalus" (1837), 18.
30. Schuller, *The Biopolitics of Feeling*, 8, 10–15.

31. Alexander Y. Nicoll and Richard D. Arnold, "Account of an Anencephalus, or Human Monstrosity, Without a Brain and Spinal Marrow," *American Journal of the Medical Sciences* 22, no. 43 (1838): 253–57; Nicoll and Arnold, "Account of a Human Monstrosity, Which Possessed Neither a Brain nor a Spinal Marrow," *Lancet* 29, no. 740 (1837): 202–4.

32. Holmes, "Scholastic and Bedside Teaching," in *Medical Essays*, 279–80.

33. Leavitt, *Brought to Bed*, 12 (graph); Borst, *Catching Babies*, 1–12; G. Fraser, *African American Midwifery in the South*, 139–237; Theobald, *Reproduction on the Reservation*, 29–36.

34. Leavitt, *Brought to Bed*, 87–115.

35. See, e.g., G. A. Fackler, "Society Reports: Academy of Medicine," *Cincinnati Lancet and Clinic* (1885): 293–97; and J. G. Carpenter, "Report of a Case of Monstra Deficientia to the Central Kentucky Medical Association," *Missouri Medical and Surgical Journal* 37, no. 3 (1879): 281–82.

36. W. W. Pennell, "A Pseudocephaloid Infant," *Medical and Surgical Reporter* 62 (1890): 81; Samuel Purple, "A Literary, Historical, and Practical Sketch of Acrania, 'Brainless' or Pseudencephalus Monsters," *New York Journal of Medicine and Collateral Sciences* 5, no. 1 (1850): 45.

37. J. B. S. Jackson, *A Descriptive Catalogue of the Anatomical Museum of the Boston Society for Medical Improvement* (William D. Ticknor, 1847), 264; Stephen Williams, "Case of Monstrosity, with Some Remarks Upon Moles, Marks, &c," *American Journal of Medical Sciences* (1835): 88–91; Pennell, "Pseudocephaloid Infant," 81.

38. S. B. Cunningham, "A Case of Monstrosity," *Southern Medical and Surgical Journal* 1, no. 3 (1845): 121.

39. J. B. S. Jackson, "Case of Monstrosity, in Which the Brain, Heart, Lungs, Stomach, Liver, Spleen, Pancreas, and Right Kidney Were Wanting," *American Journal of the Medical Sciences* 42 (1838): 362.

40. On "the American preoccupation with empiricism" in the first half of the nineteenth century, see John Harley Warner, *Against the Spirit of System: The French Impulse in Nineteenth-Century American Medicine* (Princeton University Press, 1998), 3–16, 8.

41. John S. Billings, "On Medical Museums, with Special Reference to the Army Medical Museum at Washington," *Boston Medical and Surgical Journal* 119, no. 12 (1888): 272–73.

42. For discussions of experimental teratology in nineteenth-century obstetric case literature, see, e.g., Stahl, "Maternal Impressions"; and H. Lewis, "Iniencephalus." On nineteenth-century medical engagement with embryology, see Shannon Withycombe, "From Women's Expectations to Scientific Specimens: The Fate of Miscarriage Materials in Nineteenth-Century America," *Social History of Medicine* 28, no. 2 (2015): 245–62.

43. Rima D. Apple, *Perfect Motherhood: Science and Childrearing in America* (Rutgers University Press, 2006), 11–33.

44. F. Turner, *Proving Pregnancy*; Withycombe, *Lost*, 125–61; Judith Walzer Leavitt, "The Growth of Medical Authority: Technology and Morals in Turn-of-the-Century Obstetrics," in *Women and Health in America: Historical Readings*, ed. Judith Walzer Leavitt (University of Wisconsin Press, 1999), 636–58; Charles M. Green, "The Care of Women in Pregnancy," *Boston Medical and Surgical Journal* 126, no. 8 (1892): 186–90.

45. John Barry, "Cases of Monstrosities, with Special Reference to the Theory of Maternal Impressions," *Medical Record* 46, no. 26 (1894): 811.

46. Billings, "On Medical Museums," 271.

47. J. W. B. Garrett, "Singular Case of Monstrosity," *Western Journal of Medicine and Surgery* 6 (1850): 2; Charles Hasbrouck, "Notes of Country Obstetric Practice," *Transactions of the Medical Society of New Jersey* (1871): 208; John Fraser, "A Sternopagous Monster," *American Journal of Obstetrics and Diseases of Women and Children* 23 (1890): 841; Mark Knapp, "The Clinical History of an Anencephalous Monster," *Medical Record* 51, no. 15 (1897): 530; I. M. Shrader, "Some Incidents in the Practice of Obstetrics," *Western Medical Reformer* 57 (1897): 138.

48. For a related argument about laywomen's involvement in nineteenth-century medical interpretations of miscarriage, see Withycombe, "From Women's Expectations to Scientific Specimens."

49. Purple, "A Literary, Historical, and Practical Sketch of Acrania," 47; F. H. Getchell, "Transactions of Societies: Summary of the Transactions of the College of Physicians of Philadelphia: Case of Monstrosity," *American Journal of Medical Sciences* 106 (1867): 418.

50. On the persistence of maternal-impression theories in nineteenth-century science and medicine, see Richardson, *The Maternal Imprint*, 34–39.

51. William Morland, "Extracts from the Records of the Boston Society for Medical Improvement," *American Journal of the Medical Sciences* 50 (1853): 356–61, reprinted in *Ohio Medical and Surgical Journal* 6, no. 1 (1853): 49–59; J. Richards, "Maternal Impressions," *Philadelphia Medical Times* 19, no. 8 (1889): 340; Stahl, "Maternal Impressions," 511.

52. Stahl, "Maternal Impressions," 509. See also, e.g., N. C. Skinner, "A Singular Foetal Malformation," *Medical Examiner* 116 (1854): 461–66; W. H. Tingley, "Observations on the Above Case," *Missouri Medical and Surgical Journal* 14, no. 3 (1856): 219–36; Sandy Harrel, "An Acephalous Monstrosity," *Nashville Journal of Medicine and Surgery* 75, no. 3 (1894): 103–5; "Brief of Current Literature: Obstetrics," *American Journal of Obstetrics and Diseases of Women and Children* 37, no. 4 (1898): 551.

53. See, e.g., G. Garland, "Acephalous Monster," *Western Journal of Medicine and Surgery* 7, no. 3 (1851): 213; A. W. Lueck, "Acephalic Babe," *Medical and Surgical Reporter* 22, no. 8 (1870): 150; J. S. Haldemann, "Gleanings from Exchanges: Maternal Impressions and Acephalous Foetus," *Philadelphia Medical Times* 12, no. 22 (1882): 763.
54. L. P. S., "Influence of Maternal Feelings—Acephalous Child, &c.," *Boston Medical and Surgical Journal* 24, no. 5 (1841): 73.
55. A. A. Moore, "Anencephalic Monster," *American Journal of the Medical Sciences* 54 (1867): 281; A. A. Moore, "Anencephalic Monster," *Medical and Surgical Reporter* 47, no. 17 (1882): 461.
56. Weiner, with Hough, *Sex, Sickness, and Slavery*, 114; Barclay, "Bad Breeders and Monstrosities," 294–95.
57. On nineteenth-century discourses of "impressibility" and racialization, see Schuller, *Biopolitics of Feelings*.
58. See, e.g., Garrett, "Singular Case of Monstrosity"; George Badger, "A Rare Case of Monstrosity," *Medical Record* (1869): 166; E. J. Overend, "Maternal Impressions," *Pacific Medical Journal* 33 (1890): 70–77; T. W. Burton, "Iniencephalic Monster," *Western Medical Reformer* 57, no. 4 (1897): 209–13; William Hestle, "Obstetrics," *American Gynaecological and Obstetrical Journal* 15 (1899): 386–93; "A Monstrosity: The One Born Below Town Reported to the Medical Convention," *Austin Daily Statesman*, April 30, 1894.
59. Henry A. Riley, "Medical Cases in the Courts," *Medical Record* 32, no. 14 (1887): 452; Egbert Grandin, "Transactions of the State Medical Society," *American Gynaecological and Obstetrical Journal* 3, no. 7 (1893): 639–40.
60. On monstrous births in earlier periods, see Daston and Park, *Wonders and the Order of Nature*, 173–214; and Huet, *Monstrous Imagination*.
61. Garrett, "Singular Case of Monstrosity," 6; J. Jackson, *Descriptive Catalogue of the Warren Anatomical Museum*, 90; S. S. Oslin, "A Monstrosity," *Medical Review* 3 (1875): 199; Flint L. Keyes, "Two Cases of Monstrosity," *Medical and Surgical Reporter* 12, no. 31 (1865): 501; Drs. Lucas and Pankake, "Anencephalous Monster," *Medical and Surgical Reporter* 63, no. 25 (1890): 717; O. P. Baer, "First Causes of Structure and Character of the Embryo in Utero," *United States Medical Investigator* 7 (1878): 157.
62. George Peck, "Bureau of Obstetrics: Abstract of Discussion," *Medical Advance* 17, no. 2 (1886): 123; Hestle, "Obstetrics," 386.
63. Overend, "Maternal Impressions," 74; Dr. Hadlock, "Cincinnati Academy of Medicine: Acephalous Foetus," *Medical and Surgical Reporter* 21, no. 19 (1869): 280; D. M. Hudson, "Case of Monstrosity," *Medical Examiner* 114 (1854): 326.
64. J. Jackson, *Catalogue of the Anatomical Museum of the Boston Society for Medical Improvement*, 256–57; Barry, "Cases of Monstrosities," 813.

65. On the significance of animals in sentimental culture, see Karen Halttunen, "Humanitarianism and the Pornography of Pain in Anglo-American Culture," *American Historical Review* 100 (1995): 303–34; and Jennifer Mason, *Civilized Creatures: Urban Animals, Sentimental Culture, and American Literature, 1850–1900* (Johns Hopkins University Press, 2005).
66. On earlier iconography of "suckling as a point of intimate connection between human and beasts," see Londa Schiebinger, *Nature's Body: Gender in the Making of Modern Science* (Beacon, 1993), 53–59.
67. J. M. Stevenson, "Case of Monstrosity," *Medical and Surgical Reporter* 12 (1865): 223.
68. J. N. Snively, "Remarkable Case of Monstrosity," *Medical and Surgical Reporter* 24 (1871): 383; and Peck, "Bureau of Obstetrics," 118–21.
69. Miriam Rich, "Monstrosity in Medical Science: Race-Making and Teratology in the Nineteenth-Century United States," *Isis* 114, no. 3 (2023): 513–36.
70. Morland, "Extracts from the Records of the Boston Society for Medical Improvement," 358; Case Notebook, vol. 2, Cases and Notebooks of J. B. S. Jackson, 1836–1874, John Barnard Swett (J. B. S.) Jackson Papers, Countway Library, Center for the History of Medicine; George Courtright, "Gynecology: Monstrosities vs. Maternal Impressions," *Transactions of the Ohio State Medical Society* (1898): 319–22; Stahl, "Maternal Impressions," 506; Haldemann, "Gleanings from Exchanges," 763; Francis Minot, "Reports of Medical Societies: Extracts from the Records of the Boston Society for Medical Improvement: Anencephalous Foetus," *Boston Medical and Surgical Journal* 62 (1860): 160.
71. J. W. Underhill, "Transactions of the Obstetrical Society of Cincinnati: Maternal Impressions Affecting the Fetus in Utero," *American Journal of Obstetrics and Diseases of Women and Children* 11, no. 3 (1878): 634–35.
72. Morland, "Extracts from the Records of the Boston Society for Medical Improvement," 356, 361; J. Jackson, *Descriptive Catalogue of the Warren Anatomical Museum*, 93.
73. On nineteenth-century medical advice literature for women, see Apple, *Perfect Motherhood*, 11–33.
74. George Napheys, *The Physical Life of Woman: Advice to the Maiden, Wife, and Mother* (George MacLean, 1870), 158, 173.
75. S. R. Millen, "Effects of Maternal Impressions on the Foetus," *Medical and Surgical Reporter* 49, no. 11 (1883): 305.
76. On the late nineteenth-century medical interest in asserting authority over the prenatal period, see Green, "Care of Women in Pregnancy."
77. Elisabeth Robinson Scovil, *Preparation for Motherhood* (H. Altemus, 1896), 50.

78. E. G. Cook, *Mothers and Daughters: A Manual of Hygiene for Women and the Household* (New York Arcade, Fowler & Wells, 1884), 213–14; Seth Pancoast, *The Ladies' New Medical Guide* (J. E. Potter, 1890), 585.
79. Cook, *Mothers and Daughters*, 213; Napheys, *Physical Life of Woman*, 173; Baer, "First Causes," 154.
80. Cook, *Mothers and Daughters*, 167; Napheys, *Physical Life of Woman*, 159, 115–16.
81. Horace O. Conger and Caroline P. Crane, *Obstetrics and Womanly Beauty: A Treatise on the Physical Life of Woman, Embracing Full Information on All Important Matters for Both Mothers and Maidens* (American Publishing House, 1900), 283–84; Napheys, *Physical Life of Woman*, 115, 159.
82. Morland, "Extracts from the Records of the Boston Society for Medical Improvement," 357.
83. Barry, "Cases of Monstrosities," 813.
84. Barry, "Cases of Monstrosities," 813.
85. J. Manlove, "Remarks on a Case of an Acephalous Monster, Read Before the Medical Society of Tennessee at Its Annual Meeting," *Western Journal of Medicine and Surgery* 4, no. 5 (1845): 401; Charles D. Meigs, "Case of a Monstrous Birth," *American Journal of the Medical Sciences* 30 (1855): 13.
86. R.U. Moffat, "Medical Progress: Teratology," *Missouri Medical and Surgical Journal* 75, no. 6 (1898): 327; J. Edwards, "Case of Acephalous Monster," *Nashville Journal of Medicine and Surgery* 45, no. 6 (1890): 228.
87. Richard Wood, "An Anencephalous Monster," *Medical Record* 48, no. 25 (1895): 893; "Remarkable Monstrosity," *Medical Surgical Report* 46 (1882): 350.
88. Eugene S. Talbot, "Degeneracy and Marriage," *Alienist and Neurologist* 20 (1899): 45–54.
89. Allan Brandt, *No Magic Bullet: A Social History of Venereal Disease in the United States Since 1880*, 35th anniv. ed. (Oxford University Press, 2020), 6–57, 20–25.
90. See, e.g., Knapp, "The Clinical History of an Anencephalous Monster," 530; Burton, "Iniencephalic Monster," 213.
91. Peck, "Bureau of Obstetrics," 122. On the dispensary, see Charles E. Rosenberg, "Social Class and Medical Care in Nineteenth-Century America: The Rise and Fall of the Dispensary," *Journal of the History of Medicine and Allied Sciences* 29, no. 1 (1974): 32–54.
92. Charles Dana, "Report of a Case of Anencephaly, with a Microscopical Study Bearing on Its Relation to the Sensory and Motor Tracts," *Journal of Nervous and Mental Disease* 13, no. 1 (1888): 22; H. S. Crossen, "Transactions of the St. Louis Obstetrical and Gynecological Society: Anencephalus," *American Journal of Obstetrics and Diseases of Women and Children* 39, no. 2 (1899): 214–15.

93. L. Duncan Bulkley, "Society Proceedings: Northwestern Medical and Surgical Society of New York," *Medical News* 73, no. 5 (1898): 158, 159.
94. Bannan, "Case of Monstrosity," 789.
95. Moffat, "Medical Progress," 327.
96. Bulkley, "Society Proceedings," 157.
97. Norman Jewson, "The Disappearance of the Sick-Man from Medical Cosmology, 1770–1870," *Sociology* 10 (1976): 225–44.

2. MONSTROUS NEWBORNS: EMOTIONS, EMBODIMENT, AND SENSORY RELATION

1. Purple, "A Literary, Historical, and Practical Sketch of Acrania," 45, 41.
2. Purple, "A Literary, Historical, and Practical Sketch of Acrania," 41–42.
3. Purple, "A Literary, Historical, and Practical Sketch of Acrania," 43.
4. Purple, "A Literary, Historical, and Practical Sketch of Acrania," 43.
5. Purple, "A Literary, Historical, and Practical Sketch of Acrania," 43–44.
6. Foucault, *Abnormal*, 63.
7. James Gregory Mumford, *The Story of the Boston Society for Medical Improvement* (Darnell & Upham, 1901), 7.
8. Holmes, "Scholastic and Bedside Teaching," in *Medical Essays*, 279–80.
9. Katharine Park, *Secrets of Women: Gender, Generation, and the Origins of Human Dissection* (Zone, 2006), 22–23; Laura Gowing, *Common Bodies: Women, Touch, and Power in Seventeenth-Century England* (Yale University Press, 2003).
10. Ahmed, "Affective Economies," 126–28. See also Sara Ahmed, *The Cultural Politics of Emotion* (Edinburgh University Press, 2014); Shildrick, *Dangerous Discourses of Disability*, 17–38; and Chen, *Animacies*.
11. Daston and Park, *Wonders and the Order of Nature*, 176.
12. Meigs, "Case of a Monstrous Birth," 16–17; Billings, "On Medical Museums," 271.
13. Garrett, "Singular Case of Monstrosity," 2; Peck, "Bureau of Obstetrics," 122.
14. George Fisher, "Does Maternal Mental Influence Have Any Constructive or Destructive Power in the Production of Malformations or Monstrosities at Any Stage of Embryonic Development?," *American Journal of Insanity* 26, no. 3 (1870): 241; Meigs, "Case of a Monstrous Birth," 16–17.
15. Foucault, *Abnormal*, 63; Canguilhem, "Monstrosity and the Monstrous."
16. Hugh Lenox Hodge, "Summary of the Proceedings of the Pathological Society of Philadelphia: Pseudencephalous Foetus," *American Journal of the Medical Sciences* 84 (1861): 435.
17. Daston and Park, *Wonders and the Order of Nature*, 176.

18. Barton Cooke Hirst, "Teratologic Note," *Medical News* 64, no. 7 (1894): 184; P. Brouillette, "An Anencephalous Foetus," *The Clinic* 6, no. 20 (1874): 238; F. N. Smith, "A Case of Monstrosity," *American Medical Times* 2 (1861): 154; Billings, "On Medical Museums," 268; C. Terry, "Remarks Upon Some Recently Reported Cases of Monstrosity," *American Journal of Obstetrics and Diseases of Women and Children* 2, no. 3 (1869): 369.
19. Theophilus Parvin, "The Influence of Maternal Impressions Upon the Foetus," *International Medical Magazine* 1, no. 5 (1892): 493.
20. My analysis here is inspired by Charles E. Rosenberg's discussion of the "dramaturgic form" of the epidemic. The presaging of the reveal by ominous sensations bears similarities to the "plot line of increasing and revelatory tension" that Rosenberg identifies in his analysis of plague and outbreak narratives. Rosenberg, *Explaining Epidemics, and Other Studies in the History of Medicine* (Cambridge University Press, 1992), 279.
21. Minot, "Reports of Medical Societies," 160; Manlove, "Remarks on a Case of an Acephalous Monster," 401; Christopher Johnston, "Description of a Pseudencephalic Monster (Genus 11, Thlipsencephalus, Isidore Geoff. St. Hilaire)," *American Journal of the Medical Sciences* 44, no. 87 (1862): 96; Garland, "Acephalous Monster," 212.
22. Minot, "Reports of Medical Societies," 160–61; A. M. Jacobus, "Society Proceedings: Northwestern Medical and Surgical Society of New York," *Medical News* 73, no. 5 (1898): 159; Emil Mayer, "Acrania Monsters, with Report of a Case," *American Journal of the Medical Sciences* 83 (1882): 119.
23. G. Leibman, "Another Case of Dropsy of the Amnion.—Tapping.—Deformed Foetus (Acephalon).—Version on the Head.—Recovery," *Medical and Surgical Reporter* 23, no. 7 (1870): 141; Joseph Brettauer, "Transactions of the New York Obstetrical Society: Acrania with Anencephalia," *American Journal of Obstetrics and Diseases of Women and Children* 31, no. 2 (1895): 232; William Judkins, "Society Reports: Anencephalus Monstrosity (Dr. Withdrow)," *Cincinnati Lancet and Clinic* 24 (1890): 220. See also John Shaller, "An Anencephalous Monster," *Cincinnati Lancet and Clinic* 27, no. 9 (1891): 264; and William Hilkowitz, "Society Reports: Academy of Medicine of Cincinnati, Anencephalus," *Cincinnati Lancet and Clinic* 37, no. 22 (1896): 566–67.
24. W. G. Owen, "A Brownie Baby," *Medical News* 73, no. 11 (1898): 338; Hilkowitz, "Society Reports," 566; Robert T. Wilson, "Original Communications: A Contribution to the History of Hydramnios," *American Journal of Obstetrics and Diseases of Women and Children* 20, no. 1 (1887): A17; J. M. French, "Society Reports," *Western and Southern Medical Recorder* 24 (1890): 540.
25. H., "Embryotic Influences," 363; Garrett, "Singular Case of Monstrosity," 2.

26. Nicoll and Arnold, "Account of an Anencephalus" (1837), 18; Burton, "Inience-phalic Monster," 210.

27. Purple, "A Literary, Historical, and Practical Sketch of Acrania," 46.

28. L. P. S., "Influence of Maternal Feelings—Acephalous Child," 73; A. J. E., "Acephalous Foetus—Imperfect Spinal Column," *Boston Medical and Surgical Journal* 24, no. 8 (1841): 123–24; Garland, "Acephalous Monster," 212.

29. Manlove, "Remarks on a Case of an Acephalous Monster," 403; Garland, "Acephalous Monster," 212.

30. Ahmed, "Affective Economies," 126, 127–28.

31. Purple, "A Literary, Historical, and Practical Sketch of Acrania," 45.

32. Schuller, *Biopolitics of Feeling*, 16.

33. D. Lichliter, "An Anencephalic Monster: Original Communications," *Cincinnati Lancet and Clinic* 6, no. 22 (1881): 493; Purple, "A Literary, Historical, and Practical Sketch of Acrania," 47; Otis Johnson, "Case of Monstrosity; Closure of Both Ears; Imperforate Anus; Double Fissure of the Palate," in *Extracts from the Records of the Boston Society for Medical Improvement* (Printed for the Society for Medical Improvement, 1859), 3:244.

34. Nora Doyle, "'The Highest Pleasure of Which Woman's Nature Is Capable': Breast-Feeding and the Sentimental Maternal Ideal in America, 1750–1860," *Journal of American History* 97, no. 4 (2011): 958–73; Kathleen Brown, *Foul Bodies: Cleanliness in Early America* (Yale University Press, 2009), 193.

35. See Jan Lewis, "Mother's Love: The Construction of an Emotion in Nineteenth-Century America," in *Mothers and Motherhood: Readings in American History*, ed. Rima D. Apple and Janet Lynne Golden (Ohio State University Press, 1997), 52–71; Barbara Welter, "The Cult of True Womanhood: 1820–1860," *American Quarterly* 18, no. 2 (1966): 151–74; Nancy Cott, *The Bonds of Womanhood: "Woman's Sphere" in New England, 1780–1835*, with a new preface, 2nd ed. (Yale University Press, 1997); Carby, *Reconstructing Womanhood*; and Evelynn Hammonds, "Toward a Genealogy of Black Female Sexuality: The Problematic of Silence," in *Feminist Theory and the Body*, ed. Janet Price and Margrit Shildrick (Routledge, 1999), 93–104.

36. Lewis, "Mother's Love," 52; Doyle, *Maternal Bodies*, 86.

37. Johnston, "Description of a Pseudencephalic Monster," 96.

38. Ahmed, "Affective Economies," 127.

39. Sander Gilman, *Inscribing the Other* (University of Nebraska Press, 1991), 37, 31.

40. Simeon Kool, *Intimate Subjects: Touch and Tangibility in Britain's Cerebral Age* (University of Chicago Press, 2024); Gowing, *Common Bodies*.

41. J. Edwards, "Case of Acephalous Monster."

42. S. Birdsell, "A Monstrosity," *New Jersey Medical Reporter and Transactions of the New Jersey Medical Society* 4, no. 7 (1851): 312. See also Stahl, "Maternal

Impressions"; Crossen, "Transactions of the St. Louis Obstetrical and Gynecological Society," 208; and Edward Hamilton, "A Case of Exencephalus, with Specimen," *American Journal of Obstetrics and Diseases of Women and Children* 40, no. 4 (1899): 504–9.

43. J. Jackson, *Catalogue of the Anatomical Museum of the Boston Society for Medical Improvement*, 17; Dana, "Report of a Case of Anencephaly," 22; Charles Rea, "Prolonged Gestation, Acrania Monstrosity, and Apparent Placenta Previa in One Obstetrical Case," *Journal of the American Medical Association* 30, no. 20 (1898): 1166–67.

44. Johnston, "Description of a Pseudencephalic Monster," 96–97; J. W. Duncan, "Correspondence," *The Clinic* 2, no. 13 (1872): 150–51; J. Jackson, *Descriptive Catalogue of the Anatomical Museum of the Boston Society for Medical Improvement*, 253; Edward Tompkins, "An Anencephalous Monster," *Medical Record* 47, no. 22 (1895): 691; J. Jackson, *Descriptive Catalogue of the Warren Anatomical Museum*, 87.

45. Purple, "Literary, Historical, and Practical Sketch of Acrania," 40.

46. Shaller, "Anencephalous Monster," 264.

47. J. Jackson, *Descriptive Catalogue of the Anatomical Museum of the Boston Society for Medical Improvement*, 282. See also Birdsell, "A Monstrosity," 312.

48. Purple, "Literary, Historical, and Practical Sketch of Acrania," 43–44.

49. Purple, "Literary, Historical, and Practical Sketch of Acrania," 47, 50, 55.

50. Johnston, "Description of a Pseudencephalic Monster," 97.

51. Johnston, "Description of a Pseudencephalic Monster," 96–97.

52. Johnston, "Description of a Pseudencephalic Monster," 100.

53. Schumann, "Observations Upon the Formation of Terata," 1159.

54. J. Edwards, "Case of Acephalous Monster," 227.

55. Butler, *Bodies That Matter*, 16.

56. Skinner, "Singular Foetal Malformation," 461; Barry, "Cases of Monstrosities," 811.

57. A. Woodward, "A Case of Melancholia," *Medical Investigator* 9, no. 103 (1872): 319–20.

58. A. Woodward, "A Case of Melancholia," 319–20.

59. A. Woodward, "A Case of Melancholia," 319–20.

60. A. Woodward, "A Case of Melancholia," 319–20.

61. E.g., William Lowman, "Résumé on Maternal Impressions," *Medical Record* 36, no. 7 (1889): 176–79; Barry, "Cases of Monstrosities," 812; E. Montgomery, "Cases of Monstrosity," *Missouri Medical and Surgical Journal* 19, no. 2 (1861): 234; O. A. Battson, "Communications," *Medical and Surgical Reporter* 24 (1871): 50; Stedman, "Influence of Maternal Impressions," A6; Underhill, "Transactions of the Obstetrical Society of Cincinnati," 634; and Eugene Talbot, "Heredity and Atavism," *Alienist and Neurologist* 19, no. 4 (1898): 643.

62. Withycombe, *Lost*, 13–41; Freidenfelds, *Myth of the Perfect Pregnancy*, 47. See also Rosanne Cecil, ed., *The Anthropology of Pregnancy Loss: Comparative Studies in Miscarriage, Stillbirth, and Neonatal Death* (Berg, 1996).
63. The earliest efforts to systematically collect national data suggest that at the very end of the nineteenth century around 20 percent of children died before their fifth birthday. See Samuel H. Preston and Michael R. Haines, *Fatal Years: Child Mortality in Late Nineteenth-Century America* (Princeton University Press, 1991), 3.
64. On parental grief in historical settings with high infant mortality, see S. Turner, "The Nameless and the Forgotten," 235–36; and Lucia McMahon, "'So Truly Afflicting and Distressing to Me His Sorrowing Mother': Expressions of Maternal Grief in Eighteenth-Century Philadelphia," *Journal of the Early Republic* 32, no. 1 (2012): 27–60.
65. On changing historical understandings of "the fetus," see Sara Dubow, *Ourselves Unborn: A History of the Fetus in Modern America* (Oxford University Press, 2010).
66. Purple, "A Literary, Historical, and Practical Sketch of Acrania," 49; Pennell, "Pseudocephaloid Infant," 81; C. N. Ballard, "A Case of Exencephalia," *American Gynaecological and Obstetrical Journal* 9, no. 6 (1896): 745.
67. Tompkins, "An Anencephalous Monster," 691. See also Williams, "Case of Monstrosity," 90; Meigs, "Case of a Monstrous Birth," 16; and Thomas Cullen, "A Male Monstrosity," *Transactions of the New Jersey Medical Society* (1875): 126.
68. Baer, "First Causes," 157; Purple, "A Literary, Historical, and Practical Sketch of Acrania," 43. On infanticide in the nineteenth-century United States, see F. Turner, *Proving Pregnancy*.
69. On US physicians' organized campaigns against abortion in this period, see Leslie Reagan, *When Abortion Was a Crime: Women, Medicine, and Law in the United States, 1867–1973* (University of California Press, 1997), 1–112.
70. Millen, "Effects of Maternal Impressions on the Foetus," 306.
71. Fisher, *Diploteratology*, 16.
72. Ramsbotham, *Principles and Practice of Obstetric Medicine and Surgery*, 511.
73. Owen, "Brownie Baby," 338; Hirst, "Two Recent Additions to the Teratological Collection," 693.
74. Gould Smith, "A Few Cases from My Experience in Obstetrics," *Cincinnati Lancet and Clinic* 28, no. 26 (1892): 841.
75. Montgomery, "Cases of Monstrosity," 232; Owen, "Brownie Baby," 338; H. B. Buck, "Report on Obstetrics," *Chicago Medical Examiner* 10 (1869): 457–69; T. Shannon, "A Case of Monstrosity," *Medical and Surgical Report* 25 (1871): 180; Johnston, "Description of a Pseudencephalic Monster," 96; M. A. Koogler,

"A Report of Three Human Monstrosities," *American Journal of the Medical Sciences* 84 (1882): 129; G. L. Purdy, "Case of Monstrosity," *Western Medical Reformer* 1, no. 5 (1857): 204–6; Peck, "Bureau of Obstetrics," 119; J. Caldwell, "A Monstrosity," *Medical and Surgical Reporter* 29, no. 5 (1873): 87–88. An analysis of hundreds of case reports did not yield any examples of a recognized refusal made by a woman not of Western European descent or by a woman who gave birth in an institution for indigent patients.

76. "Notes and Comments," *Atlanta Medical and Surgical Journal* 1, no. 2 (1884): C. Hard, "A Case of Monstrosity," 126; Fackler, "Society Reports: Academy of Medicine," 294.
77. Skinner, "Singular Foetal Malformation," 461.
78. Owen, "Brownie Baby," 338; J. F. Johnson, "Correspondence: A Double Monstrosity," *Atlanta Medical and Surgical Journal* 13, no. 4 (1896): 263.
79. Shildrick, *Embodying the Monster*, 17, emphasis in original.

3. MONSTROUS SPECIMENS: MATERIAL CULTURES OF COLLECTION AND DISPLAY

1. Warren Museum Accession 05820, Warren Anatomical Museum Collection, Countway Library; J. Jackson, *Descriptive Catalogue of the Warren Anatomical Museum*, 88.
2. The Warren Anatomical Museum's collections continue to exist today as a historical education and research resource but are no longer exhibited in a dedicated medical museum.
3. Oliver Wendell Holmes, "The Dorchester Giant," in *The Complete Poetical Works of Oliver Wendell Holmes*, Cambridge ed. (Houghton Mifflin, 1895), 10.
4. J. Jackson, *Descriptive Catalogue of the Warren Anatomical Museum*, 88; Francis Minot, *Extracts from the Records of the Boston Society for Medical Improvement*, vol. 4 (Printed for the Society for Medical Improvement, 1862), 76–77. On the significance of quickening in the legal and social history of abortion, see Reagan, *When Abortion Was a Crime*, 8–13.
5. Minot, *Extracts*, 76–77.
6. Rachel N. Ponce, "'They Increase in Beauty and Elegance': Transforming Cadavers and the Epistemology of Dissection in Early Nineteenth-Century American Medical Education," *Journal of the History of Medicine and Allied Sciences* 68, no. 3 (2013): 374.
7. Oliver Wendell Holmes, "Some of My Early Teachers," in *Medical Essays*, 425.
8. Usher Parsons, *Directions for Making Anatomical Preparations* (Carey & Lea, 1831), x; William Edmonds Horner, *The United States Dissector: Or, Lessons in Practical Anatomy*, 4th ed. (Lea & Blanchard, 1846), 38; D. Freeborn,

"Transactions of the New York Obstetrical Society: Formol or Formalin," *American Journal of Obstetrics and Diseases of Women and Children* 31, no. 2 (1895): 255–56.

9. Horner, *United States Dissector*, 39, 17; Parsons, *Directions*, xii, x.
10. Minot, *Extracts*, 77.
11. Parsons, *Directions*, 51–52; Horner, *United States Dissector*, 38.
12. Minot, *Extracts*, 77; J. Jackson, *Descriptive Catalogue of the Warren Anatomical Museum*, 88.
13. See J. Jackson, *Descriptive Catalogue of the Monstrosities in the Cabinet.*
14. Holmes, *The Poet at the Breakfast-Table*, 263.
15. See, e.g., Rachel Monroe, "A Medical-History Museum Contends with Its Collection of Human Remains," *The New Yorker*, June 23, 2025; Paul Wolff Mitchell, "Editor's Introduction: The Morton Cranial Collection and Legacies of Scientific Racism in Museums," special issue, *History of Anthropology Review* 45 (2021), https://histanthro.org/news/observations/editors-introduction-morton; Francisco Diaz, "Morton, the Maya, and Me: Reflections from a Yucatec Maya Graduate Student," in "The Morton Cranial Collection and Legacies of Scientific Racism in Museums," ed. Paul Wolff Mitchell, special issue, *History of Anthropology Review* 45 (2021), https://histanthro.org/news/observations/morton-the-maya-and-me; Stephanie Mach, "Affective Responses to Normalized Violence in Museums," in "The Morton Cranial Collection and Legacies of Scientific Racism in Museums," ed. Mitchell, special issue, *History of Anthropology Review* 45 (2021), https://histanthro.org/news/observations/affective-responses; Margaret M. Bruchac, "A Pragmatic Approach to Reconciliation: Thoughts on Transforming Repatriation Practice," in *Pragmatism and the New Museum Anthropology*, ed. Christina J. Hodge and Christina Kreps (Bloomsbury Press, 2024), 120–34; and Tinne Claes and Veronique Deblon, "When Nothing Remains: Anatomical Collections, the Ethics of Stewardship, and the Meanings of Absence," *Journal of the History of Collections* 30, no. 2 (2018): 351–62.
16. Thomas Waddel, "Original Communications: Maternal Impressions," *Detroit Review of Medicine and Pharmacy* 11, no. 11 (1876): 729; Billings, "On Medical Museums," 269.
17. On the history of US medical museums, see Erin McLeary, "Science in a Bottle: The Medical Museum in North America, 1860–1940," PhD diss. (University of Pennsylvania, 2001).
18. On the regulation and management of women's reproduction in institutions of slavery and imperialism, see, e.g., J. Morgan, *Laboring Women*; Cooper Owens, *Medical Bondage*; Theobald, *Reproduction on the Reservation*; and Briggs, *Reproducing Empire.*

19. See, e.g., Hirst, "Teratologic Note," 184; and entries in ledger book, Records of the Mütter Museum, College of Physicians of Philadelphia, Historical Medical Library, Philadelphia, PA.
20. "Medical Items and News," *Medical Record* 19, no. 20 (1881): "Deed of the Wood Museum," 559.
21. Some physicians described plans to give a monstrous specimen as "a present" to an admired professor or medical school. See Samuel Tyler, "Case of Monstrosity," *American Journal of the Medical Sciences* 11, no. 22 (1846): 539; and Garrett, "Singular Case of Monstrosity," 5. For theorization of scientific objects as "gifts" in networks of exchange, see Warwick Anderson, *Collectors of Lost Souls: Turning Kuru Scientists Into Whitemen* (Johns Hopkins University Press, 2008). On specimen collections as a boon to institutional and national status, see Hirst, "Teratologic Note," 184; and Billings, "On Medical Museums," 273.
22. Collections in large cities sometimes included specimens of monstrosity sent in by rural physicians, suggesting how collection activities also engaged practitioners outside of urban centers even in this earlier period. For a notation of one such example, see Jackson, *Descriptive Catalogue of the Anatomical Museum of the Boston Society for Medical Improvement*, 272. On anatomical specimen collections in the antebellum South, see Kenny, "The Development of Medical Museums."
23. Mumford, *Story of the Boston Society for Medical Improvement*, vii; J. Jackson, *Descriptive Catalogue of the Anatomical Museum of the Boston Society for Medical Improvement*, viii.
24. Mumford, *Story of the Boston Society for Medical Improvement*, 8, 6, 7.
25. Series XLI "National Skulls" and Series XLIV "Phrenological Collection," in J. Jackson, *Descriptive Catalogue of the Warren Anatomical Museum*, 699–707, 710–28; J. Jackson, *Descriptive Catalogue of the Monstrosities*. On how physicians invoked imaginaries of racial alterity to characterize monstrosity, see Rich, "Monstrosity in Medical Science."
26. Starr, *The Social Transformation of American Medicine*, 79–144; A. R. Thomas, "Monstrosities," *American Journal of Homeopathic Materia Medica and Record of Medical Science* (1872): 389–94; Purdy, "Case of Monstrosity."
27. D. C. Culver, "Extracts from the Records of the Physicians' Society for Medical Observation," *Southern Medical and Surgical Journal* 8, no. 10 (1852): 603–12; Julius Taylor, "Case of Monstrosity," *Western Lancet* 15, no. 7 (1854): 470–72; J. B. S. Jackson, "Case of Monstrosity: Two Foetuses United," *Boston Society for Medical Improvement* 3 (1859): 147–50; D. Packard, "Anencephalous Monster, with Spina Bifida, and Failure of Development of the Anterior Abdominal Walls," *American Journal of the Medical Sciences* 84 (1861): 437–38; H. D. Holton, "The Connecticut River Valley Medical Association," *American*

Medical Times 4, no. 23 (1862): 325–26; T. C. Duncan, "Cook County (Ill.,) Medical Society: Case of Monstrosity," *Medical Investigator* 4, no. 7 (1867): 76–77.

28. W. T. Wythe, "Proceedings of the San Francisco Medical Society: Acephalous Fetus (Dr. Blach)," *Pacific Medical and Surgical Journal* 7, no. 6 (1873): 288–93; "Medical Items and News," *Medical Record* 19, no. 20 (1881): "Texas State Medical Association," 560; Paul F. Munde, "Transactions of the New York Obstetrical Society," *American Journal of Obstetrics and Diseases of Women and Children* 6, no. 4 (1874): 629.

29. Billings, "On Medical Museums," 268, 272. For examples of how physicians responded to the call, see Museum Records: Accession Records, 1862–present, esp. box 107, Otis Historical Archives, and accessions in Anatomical Collections, National Museum of Health and Medicine, Silver Spring, MD.

30. On changing conceptions of professional identity in the latter third of the nineteenth century, see Warner, *Therapeutic Perspective.*

31. Hirst, "Teratologic Note," 184; Hirst, "Two Recent Additions," 692–93. On imperialism and the medical profession in the nineteenth-century United States, see Christopher Willoughby, "Professors of Racial Medicine: Imperialism and Race in Nineteenth-Century United States Medical Schools," *Medical History* 68, no. 2 (2024): 146–61.

32. John S. Billings, *Medical Museums, with Special Reference to the Army Medical Museum at Washington* (Tuttle, Morehouse & Taylor, 1888), 379 (appendix); Abraham Flexner, *Medical Education in the United States and Canada: A Report to the Carnegie Foundation for the Advancement of Teaching* (Carnegie Foundation for the Advancement of Teaching, 1910), 232.

33. Accessions 93.7531-3 and 93.1853-4, Historical Anatomical Collection and Historical Pathological Collection, Old Red Medical Museum, University of Texas Medical Branch, Galveston; box I, John G. Sinclair Anatomy Papers, 1922–1971, Truman G. Blocker Jr. History of Medicine Collections, Moody Medical Library, University of Texas Medical Branch; Allen J. Smith, "Apparent Fetal Substitution; Medico-Legal Note," *Medical News* 82, no. 11 (1903): 488.

34. Bannan, "Case of Monstrosity"; W. R. Pryor, "Society Meetings: New York Academy of Medicine, Section on Obstetrics and Gynecology," *American Medico-Surgical Bulletin* 10 (1896): 78. On women physicians in the nineteenth-century United States, see Regina Markell Morantz-Sanchez, *Sympathy & Science: Women Physicians in American Medicine*, 2nd ed. (University of North Carolina Press, 2000); and Darlene Clark Hine, "Co-Laborers in the Work of the Lord: Black Women Physicians in the Nineteenth Century," in *Hine Sight: Black Women and the Re-Construction of American History* (Carlson, 1994), 147–62.

35. Thaddeus Taylor, "Report of Medical Societies: Medical Association of Louisiana (Dr. Taylor)," *Journal of the National Medical Association* 1, no. 3 (1909): 175.

On the history of African American physicians, see Gretchen Long, *Doctoring Freedom: The Politics of African American Medical Care in Slavery and Emancipation* (University of North Carolina Press, 2012); Savitt, "The Black Medical Profession," in *Race and Medicine*, 269–338; and Vanessa Northington Gamble, *Making a Place for Ourselves: The Black Hospital Movement, 1920–1945* (Oxford University Press, 1995).

36. John Harley Warner, "Witnessing Dissection: Photography, Medicine, and American Culture," in Warner and James M. Edmonson, *Dissection: Photographs of a Rite of Passage in American Medicine, 1880–1930* (Blast, 2009), 7–29; Ponce, "'They Increase in Beauty and Elegance.'"
37. See, e.g., Horner, *United States Dissector*; and Parsons, *Directions*.
38. Parsons, *Directions*, vi–ii, x. See also Horner, *United States Dissector*, 40.
39. Horner, *United States Dissector*, 26, 38; Parsons, *Directions*, x.
40. Horner, *United States Dissector*, 17–18; Parsons, *Directions*, x.
41. Warner, "Witnessing Dissection," 13.
42. University of Texas, "Catalogue of the Department of Medicine," *Bulletin of the University of Texas* 118, Official Series no. 34 (1909): 30.
43. Hildreth, *Case of Notencephale*, 9; Cunningham, "Case of Monstrosity," 121; J. Jackson, *Descriptive Catalogue of the Anatomical Museum of the Boston Society for Medical Improvement*, 293, 242, 279; Daniel Brown, "A Peculiar Acephalous Monster," *American Journal of Obstetrics and Diseases of Women and Children* 17, no. 10 (1884): 1024; Tuck and Jackson, "Rare Form of Monstrosity," 440; W. T. Lusk, "A Case of Acardia," *Western Lancet* 3, no. 4 (1874): 200.
44. Lichliter, "Anencephalic Monster," 494.
45. J. Jackson, *Descriptive Catalogue of the Warren Anatomical Museum*, 89.
46. Parsons, *Directions*, 119–20; D. Brown, "Peculiar Acephalous Monster," 1021.
47. Meigs, "Case of a Monstrous Birth," 16. See also Francis West, "An Account of an Anencephalous Foetus," *Medical Examiner* 1, no. 4 (1838): 61.
48. Tyler, "Case of Monstrosity," 539; Minot, "Reports of Medical Societies," 161.
49. Henry F. Lewis, "On Iniencephalus," *Journal of the American Medical Association* 28, no. 9 (1897): 388.
50. Thomas Schlich, *The Origins of Organ Transplantation: Surgery and Laboratory Science, 1880–1930* (University of Rochester Press, 2010).
51. Robert Meade Smith and Andrew J. Parker, "Dissection of a Human Otocephalic Cyclops Monstrosity," *American Journal of the Medical Sciences* 84, no. 167 (1882): 138; Billings, "On Medical Museums," 270.
52. Mayer, "Acrania Monsters," 120; H. T. Hanks, "Transactions of the Obstetrical Society of New York: Fetal Monstrosity Without a Trace of Body," *American Journal of Obstetrics* 22, no. 4 (1889): 404; Hirst, "Two Recent Additions," 694.

53. On how aesthetic conventions of anatomical display facilitate "the right to look," see Jane C. Desmond, "Postmortem Exhibitions: Taxidermied Animals and Plastinated Corpses in the Theaters of the Dead," in *Displaying Death and Animating Life: Human–Animal Relations in Art, Science, and Everyday Life* (University of Chicago Press, 2016), 347–77.

54. J. Jackson, *Descriptive Catalogue of the Monstrosities*, 30; J. Jackson, *Descriptive Catalogue of the Anatomical Museum of the Boston Society for Medical Improvement*, 265–66; Wet Specimen Collection in Anatomical Collections, National Museum of Health and Medicine; Historical Anatomical Collection, Old Red Medical Museum.

55. See, e.g., J. Jackson, *Catalogue of the Anatomical Museum of the Boston Society for Medical Improvement*; Garrett, "Singular Case of Monstrosity," 6; J. B. S. Jackson, "Rhinencephalus and Some Allied Forms of Monstrosity," *Boston Medical and Surgical Journal* 98, no. 3 (1878): 67.

56. Parsons, *Directions*, 47.

57. Parsons, *Directions*, 120–23.

58. Freeborn, "Transactions of the New York Obstetrical Society," 255–56.

59. Lichliter, "Anencephalic Monster," 493.

60. Parsons, *Directions*, 51–52; Horner, *United States Dissector*, 38.

61. See, e.g., Hirst and Piersol, *Human Monstrosities*, 2:plates XIX–XX, 3:plate XXIII, 4:plates XXX–XXXIII.

62. Accessions 05786, 05950, and 00825, Warren Anatomical Museum Collection, Countway Library. Other extant preparations include Accessions 1,001,327 and 1,001,019, Anatomical Collections, National Museum of Health and Medicine.

63. Michel Foucault, *The Birth of the Clinic: An Archaeology of Medical Perception* (Pantheon, 1973).

64. Foucault, *Birth of the Clinic*, 165–66. See also Mary Poovey, "Anatomical Realism and Social Investigation in Early Nineteenth-Century Manchester," in *Making a Social Body: British Cultural Formation, 1830–1864* (University of Chicago Press, 1995), 79–80.

65. Claes and Deblon, "When Nothing Remains," 352.

66. Hugh L. Hodge, *The Principles and Practice of Obstetrics* (Henry C. Lea, 1866), xiii–xiv; Oliver Wendell Holmes, "1847 Lecture Before Massachusetts Medical College," in *Medical Essays*, 33; Billings, "On Medical Museums," 269.

67. D. Brown, "Peculiar Acephalous Monster," 1021; University of Texas, "Catalogue of the Department of Medicine," 15–16.

68. Samuel Redman, *Bone Rooms: From Scientific Racism to Human Prehistory in Museums* (Harvard University Press, 2016), 127–28.

69. The history and meanings of "freak shows" have been extensively explored in existing disability studies scholarship. The large literature includes

Garland-Thomson, ed., *Freakery*; Bogdan, *Freak Show*; Durbach, *Spectacle of Deformity*; Marlene Tromp, ed., *Victorian Freaks: The Social Context of Freakery in Britain* (Ohio State University Press, 2008); Samuels, "Examining Millie and Christine McKoy"; and Wu, *Chang and Eng Reconnected*. Though both the popular category of "freak" and the formal medical category of "monstrosity" implicated racialized discourses of deformity, they delimited considerably different populations. Unlike the adults and children who performed in "freak shows," many of whom did *not* meet the formal criteria for teratological monstrosity, most individuals formally classified as teratological monstrosities did not survive past early infancy. However, the two categories notably overlapped for conjoined twins such as Chang and Eng Bunker and Christine and Millie McCoy.

70. Cullen, "A Male Monstrosity," 128; "The Placards and Exhibitions of Freaks and Monstrosities," *Medical News* 59, no. 23 (1891): 665–66.
71. Redman, *Bone Rooms*, 126–57; Durbach, *Spectacle of Deformity*, 23–24. In another example of blurred lines between popular and medical display, some commercial ventures advertised the exhibition of preserved anatomical specimens of "monstrosity" to the public. See Henry Jordan, "Hand-book and Descriptive Catalogue of the Pacific Museum of Anatomy and Natural Science: Now Open at the Eureka Theatre," 1864, and "Jordan & Davieson Grand Anatomical Museum," 1872, Collection of Rare Books and Other Printed Materials, Library Company of Philadelphia.
72. See, e.g., "A Curious Monstrosity," *New York Times*, February 1, 1880; "A Human Monstrosity," *Austin Daily Statesman*, April 4, 1894; "A Monster: A Strange Case Brought Before the Medical Society," *Los Angeles Times*, November 5, 1887; and "This Baby Resembles a Rabbit," *Washington Post*, March 2, 1890.
73. Holmes, "1847 Lecture Before Massachusetts Medical College," in *Medical Essays*, 33; Hodge, *Principles and Practice of Obstetrics*, xiii–xiv; Oliver Wendell Holmes, "Border Lines of Knowledge," in *Medical Essays*, 21–22.
74. For an explicit depiction of the body as text made legible by pathological anatomy, see Holmes, "Border Lines of Knowledge," in *Medical Essays*, 26–27. On representations of the human body "as a text to be read," see Ludmilla Jordanova, "The Art and Science of Seeing in Medicine: Physiognomy 1780–1820," in *Medicine and the Five Senses*, ed. W. F. Bynum and Roy Porter (Cambridge University Press, 1993), 132.
75. Billings, "On Medical Museums," 269.
76. John Metcalf, "A Case of Monstrosity," *Boston Medical and Surgical Journal* 20 (1839): 341; Billings, "On Medical Museums," 269.
77. Park, *Secrets of Women*, 27. See also Kathleen Crowther, *Policing Pregnant Bodies: From Ancient Greece to Post-Roe America* (Johns Hopkins University Press, 2023), 47–86.

78. Hildreth, *Case of Notencephale*, 15; George M. Gould and Walter L. Pyle, *Anomalies and Curiosities of Medicine* (W. B. Saunders, 1896), 1.

79. Shannon Withycombe makes a related point about how late nineteenth-century physicians positioned products of miscarriage as a way to "'see' development." Withycombe, "From Women's Expectations to Scientific Specimens," 250. On twentieth-century prenatal diagnostic technologies, see Rayna Rapp, *Testing Women, Testing the Fetus: The Social Impact of Amniocentesis in America* (Routledge, 1999); and Ilana Löwy, *Tangled Diagnoses: Prenatal Testing, Women, and Risk* (University of Chicago Press, 2016).

80. Warner, *Therapeutic Perspective*, 1. Warner dates a widespread shift in conceptions of professional identity to the latter third of the nineteenth century.

81. Charles D. Meigs, *Obstetrics: The Science and the Art* (Lea & Blanchard, 1849), 25–26. For another midcentury defense of the scientific status of obstetrics by an elite physician, see Hodge, *Principles and Practice of Obstetrics*, viii.

82. Borst, *Catching Babies*, 90–151; and Leavitt, "Growth of Medical Authority."

83. On experimental teratology and embryology in early and mid-nineteenth-century France, see Jane Oppenheimer, "Some Historical Relationships Between Teratology and Experimental Embryology," *Bulletin of the History of Medicine* 42, no. 2 (1968): 145–59. For more on Étienne Geoffroy Saint-Hilaire's early nineteenth-century work in teratology, see Correspondence and Notes, boxes 1–2, Étienne Geoffroy Saint-Hilaire Collection, American Philosophical Society, Philadelphia, PA. On obstetric practitioners' engagement with the science of teratology in Britain and in Mexico, see Al-Gailani, "Teratology and the Clinic"; and Jaffary, "The Monstrous Nation."

84. See, e.g., J. Jackson, "Rhinencephalus"; Minot, *Extracts*, 77; H. T. Hanks, "Specimen of Human Monstrosity Presented to the Society by Dr. H. J. Boldt," *American Journal of Obstetrics* 22, no. 12 (1889): 1292–97; Hirst and Piersol, *Human Monstrosities*, 1:11–18; and Fisher, *Diploteratology*.

85. D. Brown, "Peculiar Acephalous Monster," 1021.

86. Hirst, "Two Recent Additions," 693.

87. Metcalf, "Case of Monstrosity," 341. See also W. W., "Monstrosities"; Hildreth, *Case of Notencephale*; and Nicoll and Arnold, "Account of an Anencephalus" (1837).

88. Terry, "Remarks Upon Some Recently Reported Cases of Monstrosity," 369; Ramsbotham, *Principles and Practice of Obstetric Medicine*, 443–44; Purple, "A Literary, Historical, and Practical Sketch of Acrania," 40; Hirst and Piersol, *Human Monstrosities*, 1:i.

89. West, "An Account of an Anencephalous Foetus," 61; E. W. Taylor, "The Spinal Cord in a Case of Anencephalus," *Journal of the Boston Society of Medical Sciences* 2, no. 4 (1897): 32.

90. Dana, "Report of a Case of Anencephaly," 22.
91. Dana, "Report of a Case of Anencephaly," 23.
92. "Microscopy," *American Naturalist* 19, no. 8 (1885): 828.
93. "Microscopy," 828–29.
94. Dana, "Report of a Case of Anencephaly," 21–22, 31, 26.
95. See, e.g., both histological slides and gross anatomical specimens in Anatomical Collections, National Museum of Health and Medicine.
96. One case report urged the necessity of mastering "pathological anatomy, which alone can enable [physicians] to detect the various derangements of any, or all of the parts of the system; to trace their origin and explain the processes by which such monstrosities are produced." C. M. E., "Monstrosity," *Chicago Medical Examiner* 12, no. 1 (1871): 16–17.
97. Parsons, *Directions*, 120; J. Jackson, *Descriptive Catalogue of the Warren Anatomical Museum*, 89.
98. On ways of knowing the body in the medieval and early modern periods, see Park, *Secrets of Women*; Duden, *Woman Beneath the Skin*; and Gianna Pomata, *Contracting a Cure: Patients, Healers, and the Law in Early Modern Bologna* (Johns Hopkins University Press, 1998), 120–39.
99. Cryle and Stephens, *Normality*, 142–79.
100. Holmes, "Scholastic and Bedside Teaching," in *Medical Essays*, 279–80.

4. MONSTROUS IMAGES: MEDICAL ILLUSTRATION AND PHOTOGRAPHY

1. H. Lewis, "On Iniencephalus," 388.
2. West, "An Account of an Anencephalous Foetus."
3. West, "An Account of an Anencephalous Foetus," 61, 60.
4. West, "An Account of an Anencephalous Foetus," 61.
5. Hildreth, *Case of Notencephale*, frontispiece.
6. J. Taylor, "Case of Monstrosity," 471.
7. P. H. Thompson, "Three Monstrosities," *Atlanta Medical and Surgical Journal* 2, no. 10 (1885): 593.
8. Hirst and Piersol, *Human Monstrosities*, 2:plate XIX.
9. J. Jackson, "Case of Monstrosity, in Which the Brain, Heart . . . Were Wanting," 362; J. Taylor, "Case of Monstrosity," 471.
10. Meigs, "Case of a Monstrous Birth," 13; J. Jackson, *Descriptive Catalogue of the Anatomical Museum of the Boston Society for Medical Improvement*, plate II (appendix).
11. J. Jackson, *Descriptive Catalogue of the Anatomical Museum of the Boston Society for Medical Improvement*, plate VI (appendix); A. Charpentier and

E. H. Grandin, trans., "Exencephalic Foetus," in *Cyclopaedia of Obstetrics and Gynecology*, vol. 3 (W. Wood, 1887), 295; Hirst and Piersol, *Human Monstrosities*, 2:99; Saint-Hilaire, *Histoire générale et particulière des anomalies*, 2:313.

12. Martin Kemp, "Style and Non-Style in Anatomical Illustration: From Renaissance Humanism to Henry Gray," *Journal of Anatomy* 216, no. 2 (2010): 192–208; Lorraine Daston and Peter Galison, *Objectivity* (Zone, 2007), 69–104.
13. See, e.g., "Reports of Societies: American Medical Institute," *Medical Investigator* 4, no. 11 (1867): 125; Terry, "Remarks Upon Some Recently Reported Cases of Monstrosity"; Harrel, "Acephalous Monstrosity"; and Charles Jewett, "Transactions of the New York Obstetrical Society: Dr. Coe," *American Gynaecological and Obstetric Journal* 4 (1894): 431.
14. Martin Kemp, "A Perfect and Faithful Record: Mind and Body in Medical Photography Before 1900," in *Beauty of Another Order: Photography in Science*, ed. Ann Thomas (Yale University Press, 1997), 120; Chris Amirault, "Posing the Subject of Early Medical Photography," *Discourse: Journal for Theoretical Studies in Media and Culture* 16, no. 2 (1993): 60.
15. Kemp, "Perfect and Faithful Record," 120–22.
16. Amirault, "Posing the Subject," 55. On historical clinical photography as one of the "constitutive elements of biomedical knowledge production," see Imada, *Archive of Skin*, 14.
17. Frank Spencer, "Some Notes on Attempt to Apply Photography to Anthropometry During the Second Half of the Nineteenth Century," in *Anthropology and Photography, 1860–1920*, ed. Elizabeth Edwards (Yale University Press, 1992), 99–107; Elizabeth Edwards, "Photographic 'Types': The Pursuit of Method," *Visual Anthropology* 3, nos. 2–3 (1990): 235–58.
18. For a deeply thoughtful discussion of one historian's decision to include historical clinical photographs in her book, see Imada, *Archive of Skin*, vii–ix, 29–32.
19. See, e.g., Gould Smith, "A Few Cases from My Experience in Obstetrics"; and J. Johnson, "Correspondence: A Double Monstrosity," 263.
20. Kenny, "The Development of Medical Museums"; D. Berry, *Price for Their Pound of Flesh*; Susan Lawrence and Susan E. Lederer, "Medical Specimens and the Erasure of Racial Violence: The Case of Harriet Cole," *Medical Humanities* 49, no. 3 (2023): 457–67; Lindquist, "Stealing from the Dead"; Engel, "A 'Most Remarkable Trait.'"
21. West, "An Account of an Anencephalous Foetus," 60–61.
22. West, "An Account of an Anencephalous Foetus," 60. On the "scale of being," see Arthur O. Lovejoy, *The Great Chain of Being: A Study of the History of an Idea* (1936; Harvard University Press, 2001).

23. Z. Jackson, *Becoming Human*, 49–50, emphasis in original.
24. D. S. Conant, "The Science, Causes, and Anatomical Peculiarities of Human Monstrosities," *Transactions of the New York Academy of Medicine* 2 (1862): 278.
25. P. Thompson, "Three Monstrosities," 593.
26. Hirst and Piersol, *Human Monstrosities*, 2:plate XIX.
27. Spencer, "Some Notes," 103. On the study and significance of skulls in nineteenth-century racial sciences, see Stepan, *Idea of Race in Science*, 20–46, 83–110; Fabian, *Skull Collectors*; Stephen Jay Gould, *The Mismeasure of Man* (Norton, 1996), esp. 62–141; and John S. Haller, *Outcasts from Evolution: Scientific Attitudes of Racial Inferiority, 1859–1900* (University of Illinois Press, 1971), 3–39.
28. Spencer, "Some Notes," 103, 103–6; J. Jackson, "National Skulls," in *Descriptive Catalogue of the Anatomical Museum of the Boston Society for Medical Improvement*, 39–76; Elise Juzda, "Skulls, Science, and the Spoils of War: Craniological Studies at the United States Army Medical Museum, 1868–1900," *Studies in History and Philosophy of Science Part C: Studies in History and Philosophy of Biological and Biomedical Sciences* 40, no. 3 (2009): 156–67; Willoughby, "Professors of Racial Medicine."
29. Abraham Jacobi, "On the Etiological and Prognostic Importance of the Premature Closure of the Fontanels and Sutures of the Infantile Cranium," in *Contributions to Midwifery and Diseases of Women and Children, with a Report on the Progress of Obstetrics*, ed. E. Noeggerath and A. Jacobi (Bailiere Brothers, 1859), 78; Adolf Meyer, "A Review of the Signs of Degeneration and of Methods of Registration," *American Journal of Insanity* 52, no. 3 (1896): 344–63.
30. L. Manouvrier and George Grant MacCurdy, "On *Pithecanthropus Erectus*," *American Journal of Science* 4, no. 21 (1897): 216, 233.
31. L. E. Russell, "Obstetrical Problems," *Western Medical Reformer* 59 (1899): 20.
32. Nicoll and Arnold, "Account of an Anencephalus" (1837), 14.
33. P. Thompson, "Three Monstrosities," 593.
34. J. G. Stokes, "Original Communications: Description of a Double Monster," *Medical Examiner* 15, no. 18 (1874): 435.
35. J. Taylor, "Case of Monstrosity," 470.
36. J. Edwards, "Case of Acephalous Monster," 228.
37. Crossen, "Transactions," 215.
38. Stahl, "Maternal Impressions," 502–3.
39. Lorraine Daston, "Type Specimens and Scientific Memory," *Critical Inquiry* 31, no. 1 (2004): 153–82.
40. Hirst and Piersol, *Human Monstrosities*, 1:11.
41. Daston, "Type Specimens."

42. Fisher, *Diploteratology*, 4; Hirst and Piersol, *Human Monstrosities*, 2:plate XVII, 2:plate X.
43. Hirst and Piersol, *Human Monstrosities*, 2:plate XIX.
44. See, e.g., Lichliter, "Anencephalic Monster," 493; B. P. Goode, "Anencephalic Foetus," *Cincinnati Lancet and Clinic* 6, no. 25 (1881): 566–67; Mayer, "Acrania Monsters," 118; Koogler, "Report of Three Human Monstrosities," 129; Edward Winthrop Penney, "A Case of Triplets, Hydramnion, and Monstrosity," *American Journal of Obstetrics* 22, no. 11 (1889): 1151–57; W. W. Jaggard, "Transactions of the Gynecological Society of Chicago: A Case of Fetal Aplasia," *American Journal of Obstetrics* 22, no. 11 (1889): 1209–22.
45. See, e.g., Harrel, "Acephalous Monstrosity," 103; Brettauer, "Transactions," 231; Ballard, "Case of Exencephalia," 744; Burton, "Iniencephalic Monster," 210–12; Russell, "Obstetrical Problems," 21.
46. On photography as a way to "present the object just as it was seen" within nineteenth-century aspirations to "mechanical objectivity," see Daston and Galison, *Objectivity*, 45.
47. Spencer, "Some Notes," 102; Jeff Rosen, "Of Monsters and Fossils: The Making of Racial Difference in Malvina Hoffman's Hall of the Races of Mankind," *History and Anthropology* 12, no. 2 (2001): 122.
48. Spencer, "Some Notes"; Elizabeth Edwards, "Photography and Anthropological Intention in Nineteenth Century Britain," *Revista de dialectología y tradiciones populares* 53, no. 2 (1998): 36; E. Edwards, "Photographic 'Types.'"
49. Lowman, "Résumé on Maternal Impressions," 177; "Notes and Comments," *Atlanta Medical and Surgical Journal* 1, no. 2 (1884): "Poisonous Snakes and Their Venom," 123.
50. Bannan, "Case of Monstrosity," 788; Robert P. Harris, "The Practice of Obstetrics Among the Chinese," *American Journal of Obstetrics and Diseases of Women and Children* 14, no. 3 (1881): 575; "Medical Items," *Medical Record* 30, no. 16 (1886): "Differences in the Blood of the Human Races," 445; L. McLane Tiffany, "Surgical Disease of the White and Colored Races Compared," *Boston Medical and Surgical Journal* 116 (1887): 524–25; Francis L. Galt, "Medical Notes on a Trip Through the Pampa del Sacramento, Peru," *American Journal of the Medical Sciences* 134 (1874): 400; Eugene Corson, "Some Clinical Jottings on Five Hundred Cases of Labor," *American Journal of Obstetrics and Diseases of Women and Children* 35, no. 2 (1897): 175–76; J. C. McCassey, "Criminals and Defectives: How Best to Reduce Their Number," *Medical News* 79 (1901): 139; Manouvrier and MacCurdy, "On *Pithecanthropus Erectus*," 216, 233.
51. Z. Jackson, *Becoming Human*, 49–50.

5. MONSTROUS LOGICS: CONCEPTS OF RACE, SEX, AND DISABILITY

1. Aims McGuinness, *Path of Empire: Panama and the California Gold Rush* (Cornell University Press, 2008), 10.
2. Joan Flores-Villalobos, *The Silver Women: How Black Women's Labor Made the Panama Canal* (University of Pennsylvania Press, 2023), 9–10.
3. Badger, "Rare Case of Monstrosity," 166, emphasis in original.
4. Terry, "Remarks Upon Some Recently Reported Cases of Monstrosity," 372.
5. Willoughby, *Masters of Health*, esp. 1–46; Dain, *Hideous Monster of the Mind*, 197–226.
6. Fisher, *Diploteratology*, 12.
7. Pedro Velasquez, John Stephens, and Barnum's American Museum, *Life of the Living Aztec Children* (Wynkoop, Hallenbeck & Thomas, 1860).
8. Peck, "Bureau of Obstetrics," 120.
9. Durbach, *Spectacle of Deformity*, 115. See also Sadiah Qureshi, *Peoples on Parade: Exhibitions, Empire, and Anthropology in Nineteenth Century Britain* (University of Chicago Press, 2011).
10. Bogdan, *Freak Show*, 127; Henry Ashby and George Wright, *The Diseases of Children: Surgical and Medical* (Longman, Greens, 1889), 425.
11. Peck, "Bureau of Obstetrics," 118–19, emphasis in original.
12. Peck, "Bureau of Obstetrics," 119–21.
13. Hanks, "Transactions," 404–5.
14. Hanks, "Transactions," 403–4; Hanks, "Specimen of Human Monstrosity," 1296, 1292.
15. Hanks, "Specimen of Human Monstrosity," 1296, 1294; Hanks, "Transactions," 404–5.
16. Cooper Owens, *Medical Bondage*; Hogarth, *Medicalizing Blackness*. See also D. Roberts, *Fatal Invention*, 26–36; and Schwalm, *Medicine, Science, and Making Race*.
17. Cooper Owens, *Medical Bondage*, 8, quoting W. Johnson, *Soul by Soul*.
18. D. Roberts, *Fatal Invention*, 4; Stepan, "Race, Gender, Science, and Citizenship," 29; Hammonds, "Straw Men and Their Followers."
19. Dain, *Hideous Monster of the Mind*, 197–226; Jennifer Morgan, "Partus sequitur ventrem: Law, Race, and Reproduction in Colonial Slavery," *Small Axe: A Caribbean Journal of Criticism* 22, no. 1 (2018): 1–17; D. Roberts, *Fatal Invention*, 26–36; Smedley, *Race in North America*, esp. 213–50.
20. On the "protean character" and "mercurial nature" of race, see Hammonds and Herzig, *The Nature of Difference*, xiii–xiv; and Martha Hodes, "The Mercurial Nature and Abiding Power of Race: A Transnational Family Story," *American*

Historical Review 108 (2003): 84–118. On the legal codification of racial discrimination and the legal construction of race, see Browne-Marshall, *Race, Law, and American Society*; and Haney-López, *White by Law.* On formations and doctrines of race in US history more generally, see Omi and Winant, *Racial Formation in the United States*; and Fields and Fields, *Racecraft*.

21. Evelyn Brooks Higginbotham, "African-American Women's History and the Metalanguage of Race," *Signs* 17 (1992): 252.

22. Thomas Laqueur, *Making Sex: Body and Gender from the Greeks to Freud* (Harvard University Press, 1992).

23. Velocci, *Sex Isn't Real*; Bederman, *Manliness and Civilization*; Welter, "Cult of True Womanhood"; Carby, *Reconstructing Womanhood.*

24. For an example of "disability" used to denote incapacity for labor, see "Report of the Surgeon General" (1885), 782.

25. Garland-Thomson, *Extraordinary Bodies*, 6; Schalk, *Bodyminds Reimagined*, 3; Kudlick, "Disability History."

26. Walter Atlee, "Account of a Monster of the Genus *Peracephalus*," *American Journal of the Medical Sciences* 70 (1858): 370; H. Lewis, "Iniencephalus," 11; Fisher, *Diploteratology*, 17.

27. Jeffries Wyman, "Description of an Anencephalous Foetus with Unusual Malformation," *Boston Medical and Surgical Journal* 71, no. 3 (1864): 49–52; A. Moore, "Anencephalic Monster" (1867), 281–82.

28. Jeffries Wyman was a colleague of Louis Agassiz at Harvard and engaged with the work of Samuel Morton in measuring racial crania. See Jeffries Wyman, "On the Measurement of Crania," *Anthropological Review* 6, no. 23 (1868): 345–49. A. A. Moore's colleague in the South Carolina Medical Association, Robert Gibbes, assisted Agassiz in attempts to offer proof of polygenesis and was a close associate of Josiah Nott. See Kenny, "Development of Medical Museums," 52.

29. H. Lewis, "Iniencephalus," 11; Tingley, "Observations," 219; Fisher, *Diploteratology*, 16.

30. Aristotle, *Generation of Animals*, 401; J. Morgan, "Partus sequitur ventrem."

31. Oslin, "A Monstrosity," 197; J. Johnson, "Correspondence: Double Monstrosity," 263; Cunningham, "Case of Monstrosity," 120; Cohen and Durr, "Case of Monstrosity," 68; W. W., "Monstrosities," 421; J. E. Benton, "Monstrosity or Double Fetus," *Journal of the American Medical Association* 33, no. 3 (1899): 131; C. S. Hoffman, "A Peculiar Monstrosity," *American Journal of Obstetrics and Diseases of Women and Children* 29, no. 3 (1894): 367–68.

32. J. W. Palmer, "Hermaphroditism, or Monstrosity," *Boston Medical and Surgical Journal* (1836): 377–78. On the taxonomic separation of monstrosity and hermaphroditism in later nineteenth-century work, see Hirst and Piersol, *Human Monstrosities*, 1:75.

33. For examples of reference works and museum catalogs that cited Saint-Hilaire, see "Anencephalus," in *The American Cyclopedia of Practical Medicine and Surgery Literature; a Digest of Medical Literature*, ed. Isaac Hays (Carey, Lea, and Blanchard, 1834), 480–92; Hirst and Piersol, *Human Monstrosities*, 1:11–12; and Jackson, *Descriptive Catalogue of the Anatomical Museum of the Boston Society for Medical Improvement*, vii. For examples of case reports that cited Saint-Hilaire, see Hildreth, *Case of Notencephale*; Purple, "A Literary, Historical, and Practical Sketch of Acrania"; Johnston, "Description of a Pseudencephalic Monster," 96; L. E. Neal, "Gynaecological and Obstetrical Society of Baltimore: Foetal Monstrosity, Placenta Praevia. Discussion," *Medical and Surgical Reporter of Philadelphia* 56, no. 15 (1887): 459–60; H. Lewis, "On Iniencephalus," 388; J. Jackson, "Rhinencephalus"; Dana, "Report of a Case of Anencephaly"; and T. M. Drysdale, "Transactions of the Obstetrical Society of Philadelphia," *American Journal of Obstetrics* 21, no. 6 (1888): 622–35.
34. Fisher, *Diploteratology*, 3–4.
35. "Craniopagus," Historical Anatomical Collection and Historical Pathology Collection, Old Red Medical Museum; Henry O. Marcy and R. H. Fitz, "A Case of Double Monstrosity—Union Upon the Anterior Median Line from Clavicle to Umbilicus," *Boston Medical and Surgical Journal* 8, no. 2 (1871): 17–20.
36. "Book Reviews: *Human Monstrosities*," *Journal of the American Medical Association* 20, no. 18 (1893): 512; Hirst and Piersol, *Human Monstrosities*, 1:11.
37. This chart was later reprinted under the entry for "Monstrosity" in a prominent US medical dictionary. See George Gould, *An Illustrated Dictionary of Medicine, Biology, and Allied Sciences*, 4th ed. (P. Blakiston's Son, 1899), s.v. "monstrosity," 779–80.
38. Hirst and Piersol, *Human Monstrosities*, 1:11–2.
39. In medical museum collections, "monstrosities" were sometimes classified as specimens of "healthy anatomy," sometimes as specimens of "morbid anatomy" or "pathology," and sometimes as both. For contrasting examples, see J. Jackson, *Descriptive Catalogue of the Anatomical Museum of the Boston Society for Medical Improvement*; J. Jackson, *Descriptive Catalogue of the Warren Anatomical Museum*; and Historical Anatomical Collection and Historical Pathological Collection, Old Red Medical Museum.
40. L. N. Beardsley, "An Acephalous Foetus," *Boston Medical and Surgical Journal* 59, no. 2 (1858): 39. See also Cullen, "A Male Monstrosity"; M. Baxter, "Acephalous Monstrosity," *Nashville Journal of Medicine and Surgery* 27, no. 1 (1881): 15; and A. Moore, "Anencephalic Monster" (1867).
41. W. W., "Monstrosities," 415.
42. Hirst and Piersol, *Human Monstrosities*, 1:11.

43. A. Taylor, *A Manual of Medical Jurisprudence*, 396; Purple, "A Literary, Historical, and Practical Sketch of Acrania," 56–58.

44. On eighteenth- and early nineteenth-century theories of development and the intellectual genesis of teratology, see S. Ray, "From Monsters to Malformations"; and Shirley Roe, *Matter, Life, and Generation: Eighteenth-Century Embryology and the Haller–Wolff Debate* (Cambridge University Press, 1981).

45. Roe, *Matter, Life, and Generation.*

46. Purple, "A Literary, Historical, and Practical Sketch of Acrania," 53, quoting Saint-Hilaire.

47. E. Richards, "Political Anatomy of Monsters," 380; Ballantyne, *Manual of Antenatal Pathology*, 334.

48. "Anencephalus," in *American Cyclopedia of Practical Medicine*, ed. Hays, 491.

49. Purple, "A Literary, Historical, and Practical Sketch of Acrania," 54.

50. Hirst and Piersol, *Human Monstrosities*, 1:38.

51. D. Hayes Agnew, "Regional Anatomy in Its Relation to Medicine and Surgery," *Medical and Surgical Reporter* 2, no. 4 (1859): 71, emphasis in original.

52. John North, "A Lecture on Monstrosities," *American Medical Intelligencer* 4, no. 9 (1840): 133; Waddel, "Original Communications," 730; Lowman, "Résumé on Maternal Impressions," 177.

53. "Anencephalus," in *American Cyclopedia of Practical Medicine*, ed. Hays, 483–84, 491. For more on the concept of temporal deviance in nineteenth-century sciences of development, see Caroline Arni, "Traversing Birth: Continuity and Contingency in Research on Development in Nineteenth-Century Life and Human Sciences," *History and Philosophy of the Life Sciences* 37, no. 1 (2015): 52, 60, 64.

54. Hodge, *Principles and Practice of Obstetrics*, 48.

55. J. Jackson, *Descriptive Catalogue of the Anatomical Museum of the Boston Society for Medical Improvement*, 248; Purple, "A Literary, Historical, and Practical Sketch of Acrania," 43, 40.

56. Lovejoy, *The Great Chain of Being.*

57. Emmanuel Chukwudi Eze, introduction to *Race and the Enlightenment: A Reader*, ed. Eze (Blackwell, 1997), 5–6; Georges-Louis Leclerc, Comte de Buffon, "The Geographical and Cultural Distribution of Mankind," from *A Natural History, General and Particular* (trans. 1785; orig. French pub. 1748–1804), in *Race and the Enlightenment*, ed. Eze, 15–28.

58. Louis Agassiz, *Twelve Lectures on Comparative Embryology* (Henry Flanders, 1849), 1, 7.

59. Atlee, "Account of a Monster," 372. See similar discussions in W. W., "Monstrosities," 417–18; and Tingley, "Observations."

60. Charles Darwin's *Origin of Species* was published in 1859, and *Descent of Man and Selection in Relation to Sex* was published in 1871.

61. Ernst Haeckel, *Generelle Morphologie der Organismen. Allgemeine Grundzüge der Organischen Formen-Wissenschaft, mechanisch begründet durch die von Charles Darwin reformirte Descendenztheorie* (G. Reimer, 1866). In an 1879 work for a popular American audience, Haeckel explained that "the series of forms through which the Individual Organism passes during its progress from the egg cell to its fully developed state" composed a "brief, compressed reproduction of the long series of forms through which the animal ancestors of that organism have passed from the earliest periods . . . down to the present time." Ernst Haeckel, *The Evolution of Man: A Popular Exposition of the Principal Points of Human Ontogeny and Phylogeny*, trans. from German (D. Appleton, 1879), 6–7. See also Nick Hopwood, *Haeckel's Embryos: Images, Evolution, and Fraud* (University of Chicago Press, 2015).
62. Thomas, "Monstrosities," 393, emphasis in original; Stanford E. Chaillé, "Evolution and Human Anatomy," *Medical Record* 15, no. 8 (1879): 172.
63. On discourses that positioned binary sex as a marker of evolutionary development, see Bederman, *Manliness and Civilization*, 25–8, 121–69; and Velocci, *Sex Isn't Real*.
64. Laqueur, *Making Sex*.
65. On the coexistence of multiple and contradictory models of sex difference in the nineteenth and twentieth centuries, see Velocci, *Sex Isn't Real*. On the coexistence of multiple and contradictory models of sex difference in the medieval period, see Joan Cadden, *Meanings of Sex Difference in the Middle Ages: Medicine, Science, and Culture* (Cambridge University Press, 1993).
66. Nicoll and Arnold, "Account of an Anencephalus" (1837), 18, emphasis in original.
67. W. W., "Monstrosities," 417–18, emphasis added.
68. Tingley, "Observations," 228.
69. W. W., "Monstrosities," 417–18; Hoffman, "A Peculiar Monstrosity," 367–68.
70. Velocci, *Sex Isn't Real*. On linkages of race and sex in nineteenth-century science, also see Myrna Perez Sheldon, "Sexual Selection as Race Making," *British Journal for the History of Science* 6 (2021): 9–23; and Stepan, "Race and Gender."
71. Jacobson, *Barbarian Virtues*, 139–41; Stocking, *Victorian Anthropology*.
72. See, e.g., Jacobson, *Barbarian Virtues*, 139–72.
73. Daniel Garrison Brinton, *Races and Peoples: Lectures on the Science of Ethnography* (N. D. C. Hodges, 1890), 41–48. On teratological monstrosity as deviation from "type," see H. Lewis, "On Iniencephalus"; North, "A Lecture on Monstrosities," 130; and "Monster/Monstrosity," in *Globe Encyclopaedia*, ed. Ross, 305.
74. Brinton, *Races and Peoples*, 47.
75. J. Jackson, *Descriptive Catalogue of the Warren Anatomical Museum*, 101–2.

76. Gould and Pyle, *Anomalies and Curiosities*, 248. On the collection and pathologization of Native American skulls by Euro-American medical and scientific professionals in this period, see Engel, "'A Most Remarkable Trait.'"
77. Montgomery, "Cases of Monstrosity."
78. Stevenson, "Case of Monstrosity," 223–24.
79. Lueck, "Acephalic Babe," 150.
80. Henry Fairfield Osborn, *Present Problems in Evolution and Heredity*, Cartwright Lectures (Columbia College, 1892), 314, 320.
81. Baynton, "Disability and the Justification of Inequality," 34. On the nexus of race, gender, and disability, see Schalk and Kim, "Integrating Race"; Schalk, *Bodyminds Reimagined*; Samuels, *Fantasies of Identification*; Erevelles, *Difference and Disability*; Khater, "No Use to the State"; and Livingston, "Comment."
82. Brinton, *Races and Peoples*, 47; "Anencephalus," in *American Cyclopaedia of Practical Medicine*, ed. Hays, 491.
83. E. Richards, "Political Anatomy of Monsters," 381, 394; Toby A. Appel, *The Cuvier–Geoffroy Debate: French Biology in the Decades Before Darwin* (Oxford University Press, 1987), 125–36; Michael R. Dietrich, "From Hopeful Monsters to Homeotic Effects: Richard Goldschmidt's Integration of Development, Evolution, and Genetics," *American Zoologist* 40, no. 5 (2000): 738–47. On alterations of development as "the motor of evolutionary innovation," see Scott F. Gilbert, "The Generation of Novelty: The Province of Developmental Biology," *Biological Theory* 1, no. 2 (2006): 209–12.
84. See Terence Keel, "Impure Thoughts: Johann Blumenbach and the Birth of Racial Science," in *Divine Variations: How Christian Thought Became Racial Science* (Stanford University Press, 2018), 23–54; Eze, introduction to *Race and the Enlightenment*, ed. Eze, 5–6; Buffon, "The Geographical and Cultural Distribution of Mankind"; Justin Smith-Ruiu, "Diversity as Degeneration," in *Nature, Human Nature, and Human Difference: Race in Early Modern Philosophy* (Princeton University Press, 2015), 114–39; and Nancy Stepan, "Biology and Degeneration: Races and Proper Places," in *Degeneration: The Dark Side of Progress*, ed. J. Edward Chamberlin and Sander L. Gilman (Columbia University Press, 1985), 97–120.
85. Atlee, "Account of a Monster," 372–73; Tingley, "Observations."
86. This discourse was particularly pervasive in countries such as France, Germany, and Great Britain as well as in the United States. See Stephan Karschay, *Degeneration, Normativity, and the Gothic at the Fin de Siècle* (Palgrave Macmillan, 2015); and R. B. Kershner, "Degeneration: The Explanatory Nightmare," *Georgia Review* 40, no. 2 (1986): 416–44. On engagement with "European notions of racial degeneracy" in late nineteenth-century Brazil, see Cassia Roth,

"The Degenerating Sex: Female Sterilisation, Medical Authority and Racial Purity in Catholic Brazil," *Medical History* 64, no. 2 (2020): 175.

87. Meyer, "Review of Signs of Degeneration and of Methods of Registration," 345.
88. Bederman, *Manliness and Civilization*, 90, 77–120.
89. Bederman, *Manliness and Civilization*; Jacobson, *Barbarian Virtues*.
90. Douglas Baynton, *Defectives in the Land: Disability and Immigration in the Age of Eugenics* (University of Chicago Press, 2016).
91. Anderson, *Colonial Pathologies*, 44.
92. On obstetrics and "racial degeneration," see Corson, "Some Clinical Jottings," 175. On characters of monstrosities as evolutionary "reversions," see Chaillé, "Evolution and Human Anatomy," 172; and Hirst and Piersol, *Human Monstrosities*, 1:20.
93. J. Taylor, "Case of Monstrosity," 470; Snively, "Remarkable Case of Monstrosity," 383.
94. On Black women's reproduction and the racial logics of slavery, see J. Morgan, "Partus sequitur ventrem."
95. Sweet, "Interesting Obstetric Case," 439; A. Moore, "Anencephalic Monster" (1867), 281; Terry, "Remarks Upon Some Recently Reported Cases of Monstrosity"; Crossen, "Transactions," 214–15. On the association of monstrosity with "illegitimate conceptions," see "Strange Case Brought Before the Medical Society," *Los Angeles Times*, November 5, 1887.
96. Manlove, "Remarks on a Case of an Acephalous Monster," 401; A. Woodward, "A Case of Melancholia," 319. See also, e.g., Brouillette "Anencephalous Foetus," 238; F. Smith, "Case of Monstrosity," 154; Keyes, "Two Cases of Monstrosity," 501; H. Clippinger, "An Anencephalus Monster," *Medical and Surgical Reporter* 40, no. 7 (1879): 153; Baxter, "Acephalous Monstrosity," 15; and L. Woodruff, "Anencephalic Monsters," *Cincinnati Lancet and Clinic* 37, no. 24 (1896): 622–23.
97. "Anencephalus," in *American Cyclopaedia of Practical Medicine*, ed. Hays, 483.
98. On concepts of immutable biological difference in later nineteenth-century racial science, see Haller, *Outcasts from Evolution*; Jacobson, *Barbarian Virtues*, 139–72; and Rich, "Curse of Civilised Woman," 64–66.
99. John North, "A Lecture on Monstrosities: Part II," *American Medical Intelligencer* 4, no. 10 (1840): 150.
100. Tiffany, "Surgical Disease of the White and Colored Races Compared," 524.
101. Galt, "Medical Notes," 400. Here, claims about low rates of monstrosity converged with a broader claim that vigorous "primitive" women were not subject to the same difficulties in birth as more "civilized" white women. See Rich, "Curse of Civilised Woman."

102. For examples of eugenicists' discourse on degeneracy, see John Harvey Kellogg, *Tendencies Toward Race Degeneracy* (n.p., 2012), reprinted from Senate Document no. 648, *New York Medical Journal* (1911), and digitized by the HathiTrust from a copy held by the University of Michigan, https://catalog.hathitrust.org/Record/005034851; Madison Grant, *The Passing of the Great Race; or, The Racial Basis of European History* (Scribner, 1916); and Edwin Augustus Down, *The Sterilization of Degenerates* (n.p., 1910).

103. Jennifer L. Morgan, *Reckoning with Slavery: Gender, Kinship, and Capitalism in the Early Black Atlantic* (Duke University Press, 2021), 251.

104. On these varied historical concepts of race, see, e.g., Stepan, *Idea of Race in Science*; Dain, *Hideous Monster of the Mind*; Stocking, *Victorian Anthropology*; George Fredrickson, *The Black Image in the White Mind: The Debate on Afro-American Character and Destiny, 1817–1914* (Wesleyan University Press, 1987); and Haller, *Outcasts from Evolution.*

105. George W. Stocking, "The Turn-of-the Century Concept of Race," *Modernism/Modernity* 1, no. 1 (1994): 12.

106. Stocking, "Turn-of-the Century Concept of Race," 12.

6. MONSTROUS LEGACIES: EUGENIC AFTERLIVES OF MONSTROSITY

1. J. L. to Charles Davenport, n.d. [1924], A:221, box I-33, ERO Trait Files, Records of the Eugenics Record Office (ERO), American Philosophical Society.
2. Apple, *Perfect Motherhood.*
3. Davenport, *Heredity in Relation to Eugenics*, 1.
4. J. L. to Davenport, n.d. [1924], Records of the ERO.
5. J. L. to Davenport, n.d. [1924], Records of the ERO.
6. J. L. to Davenport, n.d. [1924], Records of the ERO.
7. Kline, *Building a Better Race*, 1–31.
8. J. L. to Davenport, n.d. [1924], Records of the ERO.
9. J. L. to Davenport, n.d. [1924], Records of the ERO.
10. For more on the ERO researchers' mission and beliefs, see H. H. Laughlin, "History of the Eugenics Record Office" (1940), box 21, Carnegie Institution of Washington Eugenics Record Office (ERO) Collection, Cold Spring Harbor Laboratory and Archives, Cold Spring Harbor, NY; and Davenport, *Heredity in Relation to Eugenics.*
11. Davenport, *Heredity in Relation to Eugenics*, v.
12. H. H. Laughlin, "The Biological Aspects of Immigration," box 21, Carnegie Institution ERO Collection.

13. Herbert Eugene Walter, *Genetics: An Introduction to the Study of Heredity* (Macmillan, 1913), 248. An ERO pamphlet produced for a popular audience explained, quoting E. A. Ross, that "a moral obligation rests upon the ill-constituted not to reproduce, and upon the superior to rear a real family instead of just one or two." *Of Minds and Bodies* (pamphlet), box 13, Carnegie Institution ERO Collection.
14. Charles Davenport to J. L., September 4, 1924, A:221, box I-33, ERO Trait Files, Records of the ERO.
15. Kline, *Building a Better Race*, 64.
16. George Ritter Smith, "Report of a Case of Monstra per Defectum," *American Journal of Obstetrics and Diseases of Women and Children* 69, no. 4 (1914): 664–70.
17. Leavitt, *Brought to Bed*, 142–70.
18. G. R. Smith, "Report of a Case of Monstra per Defectum," 665.
19. G. R. Smith, "Report of a Case of Monstra per Defectum," 665–66.
20. By the 1920s, the majority of US-born white women gave birth in hospitals; in most Black and recent immigrant communities, midwife-assisted home births continued to predominate until the mid–twentieth century. See Leavitt, *Brought to Bed*, 171–95; G. Fraser, *African American Midwifery in the South*; and Borst, *Catching Babies*, 1–12.
21. G. R. Smith, "Report of a Case of Monstra per Defectum," 667.
22. G. R. Smith, "Report of a Case of Monstra per Defectum," 664–65.
23. For discussion of the teratological experiments of European scientists such as Camille Dareste in nineteenth-century US journals, see "Medical Items and News," *Medical Record* 4 (1869): "Heat as Affecting the Production of Monstrosity," 308; "Teratology," *American Naturalist* 3, no. 3 (1869): 152–54; and Lowman, "Résumé on Maternal Impressions," 177.
24. Oppenheimer, "Some Historical Relationships Between Teratology and Experimental Embryology"; Jane Maienschein, "Shifting Assumptions in American Biology: Embryology, 1890–1910," *Journal of the History of Biology* 14, no. 1 (1981): 98.
25. Franklin Paine Mall and Arthur William Meyer, *Studies on Abortuses: A Survey of Pathologic Ova in the Carnegie Embryological Collection* (Carnegie Institution of Washington, 1921), 34. For more on Mall's work in teratology, see "Mall, Franklin Paine 1893–1934" (folder), Minot Collection, and Franklin P. Mall (box), Carnegie Reprint Collection, both in Human Developmental Anatomy Collections, National Museum of Health and Medicine.
26. Franklin Paine Mall, "A Study of the Causes Underlying the Origin of Human Monsters: Third Contribution to the Study of the Pathology of Human Embryos," *Journal of Morphology* 19, no. 1 (1908): 4. On the emergence and

growth of "academic biology" in US universities and research institutions, see Philip Pauly, *Biologists and the Promise of American Life: From Meriwether Lewis to Alfred Kinsey* (Princeton University Press, 2000), 126–64.

27. Mall and Meyer, *Studies on Abortuses*, 6, 193, 18. For more on the embryo-collecting project, see Lynn Morgan, *Icons of Life: A Cultural History of Human Embryos* (University of California Press, 2009).
28. Mall and Meyer, *Studies on Abortuses*, 18–19.
29. Reagan, *Dangerous Pregnancies*; Heather Dron, "Teratology Transformed: Uncertainty, Knowledge, and Conflict Over Birth Defects in Midcentury America," PhD diss. (University of California, San Francisco, 2016); Josef Warkany, "The Medical Profession and Congenital Malformations," *Teratology* 20, no. 2 (1979): 201–4. By the late twentieth century, a widespread "maxim" held that experts prior to the 1960s had uniformly believed an impermeable "placental barrier" protected developing fetuses from exposure to external environmental agents. On the origins and implications of this "maxim," see Aryn Martin and Kelly Holloway, "'Something There Is That Doesn't Love a Wall': Histories of the Placental Barrier," *Studies in History and Philosophy of Science Part C: Studies in History and Philosophy of Biological and Biomedical Sciences* 47, Part B (2014): 300–310.
30. Charles R. Stockard, "The Artificial Production of One-Eyed Monsters and Other Defects, Which Occur in Nature, by the Use of Chemicals," *Anatomical Record* 3, no. 4 (1909): 167–73; Stockard, "The Influence of Alcohol and Other Anæsthetics on Embryonic Development," *American Journal of Anatomy* 10, no. 1 (1909): 369–92; Stockard, "An Experimental Study of Racial Degeneration in Mammals Treated with Alcohol," *Archives of Internal Medicine* 10, no. 4 (1912): 369–98. See also Philip Pauly, "How Did the Effects of Alcohol on Reproduction Become Scientifically Uninteresting?," *Journal of the History of Biology* 29, no. 1 (1996): 1–28.
31. Michael F. Guyer and Elizabeth A. Smith, "Studies on Cytolysins. I. Some Prenatal Effects of Lens Antibodies," *Journal of Experimental Zoology* 26, no. 1 (1918): 65–82; Halsey J. Bagg, "Disturbances in Mammalian Development Produced by Radium Emanation," *American Journal of Anatomy* 30, no. 1 (1922): 134–61. See also J. F. McClendon, "An Attempt Toward the Physical Chemistry of the Production of One-Eyed Monstrosities," *American Journal of Physiology* 29, no. 3 (1912): 289–97; and E. I. Werber, "Experimental Studies Aiming at the Control of Defective and Monstrous Development. A Survey of Recorded Monstrosities with Special Attention to the Ophthalmic Defects," *Anatomical Record* 9, no. 7 (1915): 529–62.
32. Schumann, "Observations Upon the Formation of Terata," 1161; J. Torbert, "An Unusual Monstrosity," *Boston Medical and Surgical Journal* 165, no. 7 (1911):

251; and H. K. Thompson, "Anencephalic Monster; One of Twins," *Boston Medical and Surgical Journal* 193, no. 27 (1925): 1241. On recognition of radiation as a teratogenic agent in the research literature of this period, see Bagg, "Disturbances in Mammalian Development"; and Douglas P. Murphy, "Outcome of 625 Pregnancies in Women Subjected to Pelvic Radium or Roentgen Irradiation," *American Journal of Obstetrics and Gynecology* 18 (1929): 79.

33. Mall, "A Study of the Causes Underlying the Origin of Human Monsters," 5, 15.
34. C. L. H. to US Children's Bureau, September 1, 1916, 4-1-1: Heredity vs. Environment, box 24, Records of the Children's Bureau (Record Group 102), Central File (1914–1940), National Archives, College Park, MD.
35. Julia Lathrop to F. B. H., April 10, 1913, 4-1-1: Heredity vs. Environment, box 24, Records of the Children's Bureau.
36. Charles E. Rosenberg, "The Bitter Fruit: Heredity, Disease, and Social Thought in Nineteenth-Century America," *Perspectives in American History* 8 (1974): 189–95; Jane Maienschein, "Heredity/Development in the United States, Circa 1900," *History and Philosophy of Life Sciences* 9 (1987): 79–83.
37. Garland, "Acephalous Monster," 212.
38. F. B. Churchill, *August Weismann: Development, Heredity, and Evolution* (Harvard University Press, 2015).
39. Stahl, "Maternal Impressions," 505.
40. See, e.g., H. B. to Children's Bureau, February 28, 1916, 4-2-0-3: Inability to Provide Adequate Maternal Care, box 25, Records of the Children's Bureau; E. R. to Children's Bureau, March 17, 1916, 4-2-1-5: Prenatal Influences, box 25, Records of the Children's Bureau; and M. C. to ERO, March 12, 1938, box 6, Carnegie Institution ERO Collection. See also Michele Mitchell, *Righteous Propagation: African Americans and the Politics of Racial Destiny After Reconstruction* (University of North Carolina Press, 2004), 86–87.
41. Mall, "A Study of the Causes Underlying the Origin of Human Monsters"; John Wilfrid Jenkinson, *Experimental Embryology* (Clarendon Press, 1909), 78–157; G. R. Smith, "Report of a Case of Monstra per Defectum," 666; Stockard, "Influence of Alcohol."
42. Correspondence in 4-1-1: Heredity vs. Environment, box 24; 4-2-1-5: Prenatal Influences, box 25; 4-2-0-3: Inability to Provide Adequate Maternity Care, box 25; 4-2-1-2: Personal Hygiene During Pregnancy, box 25; 4-2-1-3: Exertion During Pregnancy, box 25; and 4-2-1-4: Complications of Pregnancy, box 25, all in Records of the Children's Bureau.
43. H. R. to Children's Bureau, June 14, 1920, and H. B. to Children's Bureau, February 28, 1916, both in 4-2-0-3: Inability to Provide Adequate Maternal Care, box 25, Records of the Children's Bureau.

44. Sadie Black Hamilton, "Child Welfare Department," *National Notes* (1924): 7; "How These Problems Should be Treated by Colored Club Women," *National Notes* (1931): 9; "Tuskegee Institute Health Center Report Shows Improved Health Conditions in Macon County: Mother's Club Effective," *National Notes* (1928): 10. See also M. Mitchell, *Righteous Propagation*, 76–107.
45. Charles R. Stockard, "Is the Control of Embryonic Development a Practical Problem?," *Proceedings of the American Philosophical Society* 51 (1912): 199.
46. Davenport, *Heredity in Relation to Eugenics*, 1; Laughlin, "History of the Eugenics Record Office," 95, box 21, Carnegie Institution ERO Collection.
47. Stern, *Eugenic Nation*; Wendy Kline, "Eugenics in the United States," in *The Oxford Handbook of the History of Eugenics*, ed. Alison Bashford and Philippa Levine (Oxford University Press, 2010), 511–22; Kline, *Building a Better Race*. For examples of early twentieth-century support for eugenics among "seemingly unlikely populations," see M. Mitchell, *Righteous Propagation*, 86–87; Ayah Nuriddin, "Engineering Uplift: Black Eugenics as Black Liberation," in *Nature Remade: Engineering Life, Envisioning Worlds*, ed. Luis A. Campos et al. (University of Chicago Press, 2021), 186–202; and Max Reichler, *Jewish Eugenics: A Paper Read Before the New York Board of Jewish Ministers* (Bloch, 1916).
48. Irving Fisher to Charles Davenport, March 2, 1912, Irving Fisher—Correspondence, folder 1, Charles Benedict Davenport Papers, American Philosophical Society.
49. Davenport, *Heredity in Relation to Eugenics*, iv. Davenport argued that "the great differential factor is not conditions of life but differences of chromosomes and their content" (iv). See also Charles Benedict Davenport, "Lecture: Modification of the Germ Plasm" (1923), Series B:D27, Davenport Papers.
50. On the ERO's involvement in sterilization programs, see Harry Hamilton Laughlin, *Eugenical Sterilization: Historical, Legal, and Statistical Review of Eugenical Sterilization in the United States* (American Eugenics Society, 1926); Laughlin, *Eugenical Sterilization in the United States* (Psychopathic Laboratory of the Municipal Court of Chicago, 1922); and Laughlin, "History of the Eugenics Record Office," 125–28, box 21, Carnegie Institution ERO Collection. On the ERO's involvement in immigration policy, see Harry Laughlin, "The Biological Aspects of Immigration," box 21, and Laughlin, "A Report of the Special Committee on Immigration and Naturalization, Submitting a Research," box 1, Carnegie Institution ERO Collection.
51. See, e.g., Jamie Marsella, "'Better Babies, Better Mothers, Better City': Eugenic Maternalism, the Babies Welfare Association, and the Urban Better Baby Contest," *Bulletin of the History of Medicine* 98, no. 3 (2024): 370–93; and Nuriddin, "Engineering Uplift." For one early twentieth-century physician's critique of sterilization laws and interpretation of "the germ plasm and the environment"

as "not opposing but complementary forces," see "Conference on Medicine and Eugenics," American Eugenics Society Records, American Philosophical Society. On how Latin American eugenics movements incorporated environmental reform as a eugenic intervention, see Nancy Leys Stepan, *"The Hour of Eugenics": Race, Gender, and Nation in Latin America* (Cornell University Press, 1996).

52. Edwin Conklin, director of the American Eugenics Society from 1923 to 1930, explained that the eugenics movement was distinguished by its focus on "the improvement of heredity," which contrasted with movements "aimed at the improvement of the environment." Conklin, "The Purposive Improvement of the Human Race," in *Human Biology and Racial Welfare*, ed. Edmund V. Cowdry (P. B. Hoeber, 1930), 568.
53. Charles Benedict Davenport, "Marriage Laws and Customs," in *Problems in Eugenics: Papers Communicated in 1st International Eugenics Conference* (Eugenics Education Society, 1912), 154–55; Charles Benedict Davenport, *How We Came by Our Bodies* (H. Holt, 1936), 9; Charles Benedict Davenport, "From Generation to Generation," n.p., Davenport Papers.
54. Irving Fisher to Charles Davenport, November 30, 1923, and Charles Davenport to Irving Fisher, December 6, 1923, Irving Fisher—Correspondence, folder 5, Davenport Papers.
55. Florence Rena Sabin, *Franklin Paine Mall: The Story of a Mind* (Johns Hopkins Press, 1934), 111.
56. Scott F. Gilbert and David Epel, *Ecological Developmental Biology: The Environmental Regulation of Development, Health, and Evolution*, 2nd ed. (Oxford University Press, 2015), 7; Warkany, "The Medical Profession and Congenital Malformations," 201–2. On how the historical selection of model organisms constrained researchers' ability to study environmental influences on development, see Jessica A. Bolker, "Model Species in Evo-Devo: A Philosophical Perspective," *Evolution & Development* 16, no. 1 (2014): 49–56.
57. *Eugenics Record Office Bulletin* 1 (1911), box 9, Carnegie Institution ERO Collection.
58. Davenport correspondence, 1915, A-015—Abnormal Development, Trait Files: box I-4, Records of the ERO.
59. Robert Dickinson to Charles Davenport, September 16, 1915; Joshua Ronsheim to Davenport, September 18, 1915; Herbert Allen to Davenport, September 22, 1915; and Julia Lathrop to ERO, February 17, 1916, all in A-015—Abnormal Development, Trait Files: box I-4, Records of the ERO.
60. Elizabeth Muncey, "Lying In Hospital: Anencephalic Baby," July 17, 1917, A:312—Anencephal, Trait Files: box I-34, Records of the ERO.
61. Davenport, *Heredity in Relation to Eugenics*, 256, 4.

62. Foucault, *Abnormal*, 56. Foucault writes that "the species of great exceptional monstrosity end up divided up into this host of little abnormalities" in the modern age (110).

63. Hirst and Piersol, *Human Monstrosities*, 1:11. For an example of early twentieth-century eugenic interest in traits previously identified by Hirst and Piersol as "hemiterata," see "Hill Folk: Report on Rural Community of Hereditary Defectives," which lists conditions including "hare-lip," "cleft palate," "club foot," and "a congenital union of the second and third digits on both hands and feet" as proofs of hereditary degeneracy. ERO Family Studies Reports, box 24, Carnegie Institution ERO Collection.

64. Hirst and Piersol, *Human Monstrosities*, 1:65, 11.

65. Cryle and Stephens, *Normality*, 294–332. As one example of how categories of "normality" and "abnormality" circulated in medical obstetric practice, late nineteenth- and early twentieth-century New York maternity hospitals began to include a section documenting newborn "abnormalities" on their standardized patient forms. See Sloane Maternity Hospital Obstetric Records, 1892–1896; Blackwell's Island Maternity Hospital Records, 1894–1900; and Mothers' and Babies' Hospital Records, 1899–1900, all in Archives and Manuscript Collections, New York Academy of Medicine, New York.

66. Charles H. Mead, "A Quantitative Study in Human Teratology," *Human Biology* 2, no. 1 (1930): 1 (quote); 10, 12, 16, 22–23 (figures).

67. Kansas Free Fair, 1924–1928, Fitter Families Studies: box VI-4, Records of the ERO.

68. Kansas Free Fair, 1924–1929, Fitter Families Studies: box VI-4, Records of the ERO.

69. Stahl, "Maternal Impressions," 505.

70. See, e.g., Henry Goddard, *The Kallikak Family: A Study in the Heredity of Feeble-Mindedness* (Macmillan, 1912).

71. Michael Rembis, *Defining Deviance: Sex, Science, and Delinquent Girls: 1890–1960* (University of Illinois Press, 2013).

72. Davenport, *Heredity in Relation to Eugenics*, 4.

73. See, e.g., Susan Schweik, "Archaeology of the 'Feebleminded': In the Archives with Lee Swearengin," *Osiris* 39 (2024): 135–49; Jess Whatcott, *A Menace to the Future: A Disability and Queer History of Carceral Eugenics* (Duke University Press, 2024); Natalie Lira, *Laboratory of Deficiency: Sterilization and Confinement in California, 1910s–1950s* (University of California Press, 2021); Molly Ladd-Taylor, *Fixing the Poor: Eugenical Sterilization and Child Welfare in the Twentieth Century* (Johns Hopkins University Press, 2017); Miroslava Chávez-García, *States of Delinquency: Race and Science in the Making of California's*

Juvenile Justice System (University of California Press, 2012); Rembis, *Defining Deviance*; and Stern, *Eugenic Nation*, 82–114.

74. Meyer, "A Review of the Signs of Degeneration," 348.

75. Pedigree chart, "The Hovel Type of Source of Defectives," ERO Family Studies, box 23, Carnegie Institution ERO Collection, reprinted in Charles Benedict Davenport and David Weeks, "A First Study of Inheritance of Epilepsy," *Journal of Nervous and Mental Disease* 38, no. 11 (1911): 646. See also "Exhibit D-3," *Proceedings of 1st International Eugenics Conference: Index of Exhibits* (1912): 49, Carnegie Institution ERO Collection.

76. Davenport and Weeks, "First Study of Inheritance of Epilepsy," 646.

77. F. Mott, "Heredity in Relation to Mental Disease," *British Medical Journal* 2 (1925): 727, excerpt in A-0 #7—Heredity and Eugenics, Trait Files: box I-1, Records of the ERO.

78. Davenport, *How We Came by Our Bodies*, 299.

79. Daniel Kevles, *In the Name of Eugenics: Genetics and the Uses of Human Heredity* (University of California Press, 1985); Garland Allen, "The Eugenics Record Office at Cold Spring Harbor, 1910–1940: An Essay in Institutional History," *Osiris* 2, no. 1 (1986): 225–64; Charles Rosenberg, "Charles Benedict Davenport and the Irony of American Eugenics," in *No Other Gods: Science and American Social Thought*, rev. and exp. ed. (John Hopkins University Press, 1997), 89–97; Diane B. Paul, "Reflections on the Historiography of American Eugenics: Trends, Fractures, Tensions," *Journal of the History of Biology* 49, no. 4 (2016): 641–58.

80. E. R. Downing, "Inheritance of Human Characters, Physical and Mental," in Horatio Hackett Newman, *Readings in Evolution, Genetics, and Eugenics* (University of Chicago Press, 1921), 462. For one influential example, see Goddard, *Kallikak Family*.

81. Davenport, "Generation to Generation," n.p., Davenport Papers; Charles Benedict Davenport, "How Far and in What Way Is It True That a Child Is Bound by Heredity?" (1909), Lecture Series, Davenport Papers.

82. Goddard, *Kallikak Family*, 57; William E. Castle, *Genetics and Eugenics: A Text-Book for Students of Biology and a Reference Book for Animal and Plant Breeders* (Harvard University Press, 1916), 254; Henry Goddard, "The Height and Weight of Feeble-Minded Children in American Institutions," *Journal of Nervous and Mental Disease* 39, no. 4 (1912): 234.

83. For examples of scholarship that portrays this shift, see, e.g., Kathryn Brammall, "Monstrous Metamorphosis: Nature, Morality, and the Rhetoric of Monstrosity in Tudor England," *Sixteenth Century Journal* 27, no. 1 (1996): 3–21; and Canguilhem, "Monstrosity and the Monstrous," 143.

84. Foucault, *Abnormal*, 74–75.

85. Early twentieth-century embryologists also explicitly conflated "arrests of ontogeny" and "racial degeneration"; see, e.g., Charles R. Stockard, "The Artificial Production of Structural Arrests and Racial Degeneration," *Proceedings of Meetings of the New York Pathological Society* 13 (1913): 83–88.
86. Atlee, "Account of a Monster," 372.
87. Davenport, *Heredity in Relation to Eugenics*, 262–63; Davenport, *How We Came by Our Bodies*, 382.
88. Charles Benedict Davenport and Morris Steggerda, *Race Crossing in Jamaica*, Publication no. 395 (Carnegie Institution of Washington, 1929), 192.
89. "Mongoloids," *Eugenical News* 9 (1924): 90, Eugenical News Print Collection, Cold Spring Harbor Laboratory and Archives.
90. On race, disability, and the history of Down syndrome, see Mel Y. Chen, "'The Stuff of Slow Constitution': Reading Down Syndrome for Race, Disability, and the Timing That Makes Them So," *Somatechnics* 6, no. 2 (2016): 235–48.
91. Newman quoted in "Hybrid Vigor and Hybrid Weakness," *Eugenical News* 9 (1924): 81, Eugenical News Print Collection.
92. Walter, *Genetics*, 248.
93. For more on popular engagement with eugenics in relation to pregnancy, childbirth, and motherhood, see, e.g., Kline, *Building a Better Race*, 1–31; Marsella, "'Better Babies, Better Mothers, Better City'"; and Martin S. Pernick, *The Black Stork: Eugenics and the Death of "Defective" Babies in American Medicine and Motion Pictures Since 1915* (Oxford University Press, 1996).
94. Apple, *Perfect Motherhood*; Reagan, *Dangerous Pregnancies*, 1–21.
95. See, e.g., "Clinical Inquiries in Human Heredity," box 6, Carnegie Institution ERO Collection.
96. Noliwe Rooks, *Ladies' Pages: African American Women's Magazines and the Culture That Made Them* (Rutgers University Press, 2004).
97. J. L. to Davenport, n.d. [1924], Records of the ERO.
98. E. R. to Children's Bureau, March 17, 1916, and L. M. to Dr. Meigs, March 15, 1920, Folder 4-2-1-2: Personal Hygiene During Pregnancy, box 25, Records of the Children's Bureau.
99. Quoted in M. Mitchell, *Righteous Propagation*, 77, 87.
100. R. B. to Eugenics Laboratory, April 19, 1938; E. G. to New York Academy of Medicine, January 3, 1938; and R. G. to Rockefeller Institute for Medical Research, May 11, 1937, all in box 6, Carnegie Institution ERO Collection.
101. Hirst and Piersol, *Human Monstrosities*, 1:13.
102. E. G. to New York Academy of Medicine, January 3, 1938, Carnegie Institution ERO Collection.

103. A. L. to Dr. H. H. Lauglin, October 28, 1937; G. N. to ERO, December 3, 1937; and R. G. to Rockefeller Institute for Medical Research, May 11, 1937, all in box 6, Carnegie Institution ERO Collection.
104. M. H. to ERO, May 16, 1938, box 6, Carnegie Institution ERO Collection.
105. M. C. to ERO, March 12, 1938, Carnegie Institution ERO Collection.
106. M. C. to ERO, March 12, 1938, Carnegie Institution ERO Collection.
107. M. C. to ERO, March 12, 1938, Carnegie Institution ERO Collection.
108. M. C. to ERO, March 12, 1938, Carnegie Institution ERO Collection.
109. M. C. to ERO, March 12, 1938, Carnegie Institution ERO Collection.
110. M. C. to ERO, March 12, 1938, Carnegie Institution ERO Collection.
111. M. C. to ERO, March 12, 1938, Carnegie Institution ERO Collection.
112. Canguilhem, "Monstrosity and the Monstrous," 143.

EPILOGUE

1. Thelander, "Use of the Term 'Monster.'"
2. See, e.g., Hugh Newbill, "Sirenomelian Monster (Sympus): An Anatomic Presentation," *American Journal of Diseases of Children* 62, no. 6 (1941): 1233–41; Natalie Feuerlicht, "Recurrent Anencephaly," *Journal of the American Medical Association* 143, no. 1 (1950): 23; and Raymond S. Rosedale, "Polygnathus Epignathus: A Case Report," *Archives of Otolaryngology* 74, no. 5 (1961): 529–31.
3. Gilbert and Epel, *Ecological Developmental Biology*, 7; Warkany, "Medical Profession"; Dron, "Teratology Transformed."
4. On the rubella epidemic and emerging awareness of teratogens in the 1960s, see Reagan, *Dangerous Pregnancies*.
5. David W. Smith, "Dysmorphology (Teratology)," *Journal of Pediatrics* 69, no. 6 (1966): 1150–69.
6. Lindsey Patterson, "The Disability Rights Movement in the United States," in *The Oxford Handbook of Disability History*, ed. Michael Rembis et al. (Oxford University Press, 2018), 439–57; Richard K. Scotch, "'Nothing About Us Without Us': Disability Rights in America," *OAH Magazine of History* 23, no. 3 (2009): 17–22.
7. Robert Bogdan et al., "The Disabled: Media's Monster," *Social Policy* 13, no. 2 (1982): 35; Paul Longmore, "A Note on Language and the Social Identity of Disabled People," *American Behavioral Scientist* 28, no. 3 (1985): 419–21.
8. Ramsbotham, *Principles and Practice of Obstetric Medicine*, 511; Thelander, "Use of the Term 'Monster,'" 621.
9. Longmore, "Note on Language," 421–22.
10. Simpson et al., "The Intrauterine Treatment of Fetal Cardiac Failure in a Twin Pregnancy."

11. Jamelle Bouie, "Michael Brown Wasn't a Superhuman Demon, but Darren Wilson's Racial Prejudice Told Him Otherwise," *Slate*, November 26, 2014, https://slate.com/news-and-politics/2014/11/darren-wilsons-racial-portrayal-of-michael-brown-as-a-superhuman-demon-the-ferguson-police-officers-account-is-a-common-projection-of-racial-fears.html.
12. Lorenah Vásquez et al., "Beyond Policing Bodies: A Broader Conception of Fairness in Women's Sports," *American Journal of Bioethics* 24, no. 11 (2024): 29–30; Paul Longmore, "Screening Stereotypes: Images of Disabled People in Television and Motion Picture," in *Why I Burned My Book and Other Essays on Disability* (Temple University Press, 2003), 131–46.
13. Centers for Disease Control and Prevention, "Updated Estimates of Neural Tube Defects."
14. These cases concerned infants identified as "Baby K" and "Baby Theresa." See Mark A. Bonanno, "The Case of Baby K: Exploring the Concept of Medical Futility," *Annals of Health Law* 4 (1995): 151–72; and Robert M. Veatch, "Abandon the Dead Donor Rule or Change the Definition of Death?," *Kennedy Institute of Ethics Journal* 14, no. 3 (2004): 261–76.
15. Quoted in Selena Simmons-Duffin, "Good Friday Funeral in Texas: Baby Halo's Parents Had Few Choices in Post-Roe Texas," NPR, April 6, 2023, https://www.npr.org/sections/health-shots/2023/04/06/1168399423/a-good-friday-funeral-in-texas-baby-halos-parents-had-few-choices-in-post-roe-te. Casiano chose to "tell her story publicly in the hope that others would not have to go through the same experience." Center for Reproductive Rights, "The Plaintiffs and Their Stories: *Zurawski v. State of Texas*," November 14, 2023, https://reproductiverights.org/zurawski-v-texas-plaintiffs-stories-remarks.
16. On the 2024 ruling, see Center for Reproductive Rights, "Texas Supreme Court Refuses to Clarify Abortion Ban Exceptions," May 31, 2024, https://reproductiverights.org/texas-supreme-court-refuses-to-clarify-abortion-ban-exceptions. Physicians charged with violating the ban face up to ninety-nine years in prison, at least $100,000 in fines, and the revocation of their medical license, all of which strongly deter providers from taking the risk of providing care. On the subsequent surge in rates of life-threatening complications and mortality associated with pregnancy and birth in Texas, especially in cases of miscarriage, see Lizzie Presser, Andrea Suozzo, Sophie Chou, and Kavitha Surana, "Texas Banned Abortion. Then Sepsis Rates Soared," ProPublica, February 20, 2025, https://www.propublica.org/article/texas-abortion-ban-sepsis-maternal-mortality-analysis; and other investigative reports from ProPublica Series, *Life of the Mother: How Abortion Bans Lead to Preventable Death*, https://www.propublica.org/series/life-of-the-mother.

17. American Medical Association, "*Dobbs* Ruling Is an Assault on Reproductive Health, Safe Medical Practice," June 24, 2022, https://www.ama-assn.org/about/leadership/dobbs-ruling-assault-reproductive-health-safe-medical-practice. The statement also warns that the decision will exacerbate health inequities by disproportionately burdening those from economically, racially, and regionally marginalized communities.
18. For more on these continuities across time, see Crowther, *Policing Pregnant Bodies*.
19. Thelander, "Use of the Term 'Monster,'" 261.
20. Darshali A. Vyas et al., "Hidden in Plain Sight: Reconsidering the Use of Race Correction in Clinical Algorithms," *New England Journal of Medicine* 383, no. 9 (2020): 874–82.
21. Anil Oza, "Trump's Talk of 'Bad Genes' Is Rooted in Eugenics. Experts Explain Why It's Making a Comeback," *STAT News*, October 28, 2024, https://www.statnews.com/2024/10/28/eugenics-in-political-rhetoric-open-science-movement-expert-analysis/; Tonya Mosley, "What's Behind the 'Pronatalist' Movement to Boost the Birth Rate?," *Fresh Air*, NPR, April 30, 2025.
22. Executive Order No. 14168, 90 *Federal Register* 8615 (January 30, 2025); Charles Benedict Davenport, "Generation to Generation," Davenport Papers. Executive Order No. 14168, which claims to "restore biological truth to the federal government," describes sex as "an individual's immutable biological classification as either male or female" and specifies that "it is the policy of the United States to recognize two sexes, male and female." Notably, this would appear to prohibit recognition of many of the infants described in this book, whose biological sex (as discussed in chapter 5) often fell outside of a male/female binary. Belying its own premise that binary sex distinction is a matter of clearcut "biological truth," the order struggles to offer a cogent definition of the "two sexes": It defines a female as "a person belonging, at conception, to the sex that produces the large reproductive cell" and a male as "a person belonging, at conception, to the sex that produces the small reproductive cell"—but conspicuously leaves unanswered the question of how said belonging is determined, given that zygotes "at conception" do not produce reproductive cells of any size.
23. Zachary Small, "Taking Aim at Smithsonian, Trump Wades Into Race and Biology," *New York Times*, March 31, 2025.
24. American Historical Association, "Joint Statement on Legislative Efforts to Restrict Education About Racism in American History," July 16, 2021, https://www.historians.org/news/joint-statement-on-legislative-efforts-to-restrict-education-about-racism-in-american-history/.

Bibliography

ARCHIVAL SOURCES

American Philosophical Society. Philadelphia, PA.

American Eugenics Society Records.
Charles Benedict Davenport Papers.
Étienne Geoffroy Saint-Hilaire Collection.
Records of the Eugenics Record Office (ERO).

Barbara Bates Center for History of Nursing. Philadelphia, PA.

Woman's Hospital of Philadelphia Records.

Cold Spring Harbor Laboratory Library and Archives. Cold Spring Harbor, NY.

Carnegie Institution of Washington Eugenics Record Office (ERO) Collection.
Eugenical News Print Collection.

College of Physicians of Philadelphia, Historical Medical Library. Philadelphia, PA.

Records of the Mütter Museum.

Countway Library, Center for the History of Medicine, Harvard Medical School. Boston.

John Barnard Swett (J. B. S.) Jackson Papers.
Warren Anatomical Museum Collection.

Library Company of Philadelphia.

Collection of Rare Books and Other Printed Materials.

Moody Medical Library, Truman G. Blocker Jr. History of Medicine Collections, University of Texas Medical Branch. Galveston.

John G. Sinclair Anatomy Papers.

National Archives. College Park, MD.

Records of the Children's Bureau (Record Group 102).

National Museum of Health and Medicine. Silver Spring, MD.

Anatomical Collections.
Human Developmental Anatomy Collections.
Otis Historical Archives.

New York Academy of Medicine, Archives and Manuscript Collections. New York.

Blackwell's Island Maternity Hospital Records.
Mothers' and Babies' Hospital Records.
Sloane Maternity Hospital Obstetric Records.

Old Red Medical Museum, University of Texas Medical Branch. Galveston.

Historical Anatomical Collection.
Historical Pathological Collection.

PUBLISHED PRIMARY SOURCES

Agassiz, Louis. *Twelve Lectures on Comparative Embryology*. Henry Flanders, 1849.

Agnew, D. Hayes. "Regional Anatomy in Its Relation to Medicine and Surgery." *Medical and Surgical Reporter* 2, no. 4 (1859): 71–76.

A. J. E. "Acephalous Foetus—Imperfect Spinal Column." *Boston Medical and Surgical Journal* 24, no. 8 (1841): 123–24.

Aristotle. *Generation of Animals, with an English Translation by A. L. Peck*. Harvard University Press, 1902.

Ashby, Henry, and George Wright. *The Diseases of Children: Surgical and Medical*. Longman, Greens, 1889.

Atlee, Walter. "Account of a Monster of the Genus *Peracephalus*." *American Journal of the Medical Sciences* 70 (1858): 370–73.

Badger, George. "A Rare Case of Monstrosity." *Medical Record* (1869): 166.

Baer, O. P. "First Causes of Structure and Character of the Embryo in Utero." *United States Medical Investigator* 7 (1878): 151–58.

Bagg, Halsey J. "Disturbances in Mammalian Development Produced by Radium Emanation." *American Journal of Anatomy* 30, no. 1 (1922): 134–61.

Ballantyne, John W. *Manual of Antenatal Pathology and Hygiene: The Embryo*. Wood, 1905.

Ballard, C. N. "A Case of Exencephalia." *American Gynaecological and Obstetrical Journal* 9, no. 6 (1896): 744–49.

Bannan, Theresa. "A Case of Monstrosity." *Medical Record* 45, no. 25 (1894): 788–89.

Barry, John. "Cases of Monstrosities, with Special Reference to the Theory of Maternal Impressions." *Medical Record* 46, no. 26 (1894): 811–13.

Battson, O. A. "Communications." *Medical and Surgical Reporter* 24 (1871): 47–51.

Baxter, M. "Acephalous Monstrosity." *Nashville Journal of Medicine and Surgery* 27, no. 1 (1881): 15.

Beardsley, L. N. "An Acephalous Foetus." *Boston Medical and Surgical Journal* 59, no. 2 (1858): 39.

Benton, J. E. "Monstrosity or Double Fetus." *Journal of the American Medical Association* 33, no. 3 (1899): 131.

Billings, John S. *Medical Museums, with Special Reference to the Army Medical Museum at Washington*. Tuttle, Morehouse & Taylor, 1888.

Billings, John S. "On Medical Museums, with Special Reference to the Army Medical Museum at Washington." *Boston Medical and Surgical Journal* 119, no. 12 (1888): 265–73.

Birdsell, S. "A Monstrosity." *New Jersey Medical Reporter and Transactions of the New Jersey Medical Society* 4, no. 7 (1851): 312.

Boerstler, G. P. "Monstrosity." *Nashville Journal of Medicine and Surgery* 9 (1855): 121–22.

"Book Reviews: *Human Monstrosities*." *Journal of the American Medical Association* 20, no. 18 (1893): 512.

Bowerman, Albert. "Anencephalous Monsters." *Medical Record* 48, no. 9 (1895): 309–10.

Boylston, Ward Nicholas. "Case of Monstrosity." *Boston Medical and Surgical Journal* 16, no. 24 (1837): 382–83.

Breed, J. E. "Case of Monstrosity: Deficiency of Posterior Parts of Cranium and Spinal Column—Deformity of Genital Organs, &c." *American Journal of the Medical Sciences* 11 (1849): 408–10.

Brettauer, Joseph. "Transactions of the New York Obstetrical Society: Acrania with Anencephalia." *American Journal of Obstetrics and Diseases of Women and Children* 31, no. 2 (1895): 231–32.

"Brief of Current Literature: Obstetrics." *American Journal of Obstetrics and Diseases of Women and Children* 37, no. 4 (1898): 551.

Brinton, Daniel Garrison. *Races and Peoples: Lectures on the Science of Ethnography*. N. D. C. Hodges, 1890.

Brouillette, P. "An Anencephalous Foetus." *The Clinic* 6, no. 20 (1874): 238.

Brown, Daniel. "A Peculiar Acephalous Monster." *American Journal of Obstetrics and Diseases of Women and Children* 17, no. 10 (1884): 1021.

Buck, H. B. "Report on Obstetrics." *Chicago Medical Examiner* 10 (1869): 457–69.

Buffon, Georges-Louis Leclerc, Comte de. "The Geographical and Cultural Distribution of Mankind." From *A Natural History, General and Particular* (trans. 1785; orig. French pub. 1748–1804). Reprinted in *Race and the Enlightenment: A Reader*, ed. Emmanuel Chukwudi Eze, 15–28. Blackwell, 1997.

Bulkley, L. Duncan. "Society Proceedings: Northwestern Medical and Surgical Society of New York." *Medical News* 73, no. 5 (1898): 155–59.

Burton, T. W. "An Iniencephalic Monster." *Western Medical Reformer* 57, no. 4 (1897): 209–13.

Caldwell, J. "A Monstrosity." *Medical and Surgical Reporter* 29, no. 5 (1873): 87–88.

Carpenter, J. G. "Report of a Case of Monstra Deficientia to the Central Kentucky Medical Association." *Missouri Medical and Surgical Journal* 37, no. 3 (1879): 281–82.

Castle, William E. *Genetics and Eugenics: A Text-Book for Students of Biology and a Reference Book for Animal and Plant Breeders*. Harvard University Press, 1916.

Chaillé, Stanford E. "Evolution and Human Anatomy." *Medical Record* 15, no. 8 (1879): 169–74.

Charpentier, A., and E. H. Grandin, trans. *Cyclopaedia of Obstetrics and Gynecology*. Vol. 3. W. Wood, 1887.

Clippinger, H. "An Anencephalus Monster." *Medical and Surgical Reporter* 40, no. 7 (1879): 152–53.

C. M. E. "Monstrosity." *Chicago Medical Examiner* 12, no. 1 (1871): 16–17.

Cohen and Durr, Drs. "Case of Monstrosity." *Charleston Medical Journal and Review* 7 (1852): 67–8.

Conant, D. S. "The Science, Causes, and Anatomical Peculiarities of Human Monstrosities." *Transactions of the New York Academy of Medicine* 2 (1862): 269–98.

Conger, Horace O., and Caroline P. Crane. *Obstetrics and Womanly Beauty: A Treatise on the Physical Life of Woman, Embracing Full Information on All Important Matters for Both Mothers and Maidens.* American Publishing House, 1900.

Conklin, Edwin. "The Purposive Improvement of the Human Race." In *Human Biology and Racial Welfare*, ed. Edmund V. Cowdry, 566–88. P. B. Hoeber, 1930.

Cook, E. G. *Mothers and Daughters: A Manual of Hygiene for Women and the Household.* New York Arcade, Fowler & Wells, 1884.

Corson, Eugene. "Some Clinical Jottings on Five Hundred Cases of Labor." *American Journal of Obstetrics and Diseases of Women and Children* 35, no. 2 (1897): 175–76.

Courtright, George. "Gynecology: Monstrosities vs. Maternal Impressions." *Transactions of the Ohio State Medical Society* (1898): 319–22.

Cowdry, E. V. *Human Biology and Racial Welfare.* P. B. Hoeber, 1930.

Crossen, H. S. "Transactions of the St. Louis Obstetrical and Gynecological Society: Anencephalus." *American Journal of Obstetrics and Diseases of Women and Children* 39, no. 2 (1899): 214–15.

Cullen, Thomas. "A Male Monstrosity." *Transactions of the New Jersey Medical Society* (1875): 125–29.

Culver, D. C. "Extracts from the Records of the Physicians' Society for Medical Observation." *Southern Medical and Surgical Journal* 8, no. 10 (1852): 603–12.

Cunningham, S. B. "A Case of Monstrosity." *Southern Medical and Surgical Journal* 1, no. 3 (1845): 120–22.

Dana, Charles L. "Report of a Case of Anencephaly, with a Microscopical Study Bearing on Its Relation to the Sensory and Motor Tracts." *Journal of Nervous and Mental Disease* 13, no. 1 (1888): 21–32.

Davenport, Charles Benedict. *Heredity in Relation to Eugenics.* H. Holt, 1911.

Davenport, Charles Benedict. *How We Came by Our Bodies.* H. Holt, 1936.

Davenport, Charles Benedict. "Marriage Laws and Customs." In *Problems in Eugenics: Papers Communicated in 1st International Eugenics Conference*, 151–55. Eugenics Education Society, 1912.

Davenport, Charles Benedict, and Morris Steggerda. *Race Crossing in Jamaica.* Publication no. 395. Carnegie Institution of Washington, 1929.

Davenport, Charles Benedict, and David Weeks. "A First Study of Inheritance of Epilepsy." *Journal of Nervous and Mental Disease* 38, no. 11 (1911): 641–70.

De Vries, Ernest. "Description of a Young Human Anencephalic and Amyelic Embryo." *Anatomical Record* 36, no. 4 (1927): 293–317.

Down, Edwin Augustus. *The Sterilization of Degenerates*. N.p., 1910.

Downing, E. R. "The Inheritance of Human Characters, Physical and Mental." In Horatio Hackett Newman, *Readings in Evolution, Genetics, and Eugenics*, 459–72. University of Chicago Press, 1921.

Drysdale, T. M. "Transactions of the Obstetrical Society of Philadelphia." *American Journal of Obstetrics* 21, no. 6 (1888): 622–35.

Duncan, J. W. "Correspondence." *The Clinic* 2, no. 13 (1872): 150–52.

Duncan, T. C. "Cook County (Ill.,) Medical Society: Case of Monstrosity." *Medical Investigator* 4, no. 7 (1867): 76–77.

Edwards, J. "Case of Acephalous Monster." *Nashville Journal of Medicine and Surgery* 45, no. 6 (1890): 227–28.

Elliott, George T., Jr. "Difficult Obstetric Cases: Case LVI." *American Medical Times* 2, no. 12 (1861): 193.

Erwin, R. W. "Anencephalous Monster." *Missouri Medical and Surgical Journal* 10 (1873): 520–23.

Fackler, G. A. "Society Reports: Academy of Medicine." *Cincinnati Lancet and Clinic* (1885): 293–97.

Feuerlicht, Natalie. "Recurrent Anencephaly." *Journal of the American Medical Association* 143, no. 1 (1950): 23.

Fisher, George. "Does Maternal Mental Influence Have Any Constructive or Destructive Power in the Production of Malformations or Monstrosities at Any Stage of Embryonic Development?" *American Journal of Insanity* 26, no. 3 (1870): 241–95.

Fisher, George J. *Diploteratology: An Essay on Compound Human Monsters*. Van Benthuysen's Steam Printing House, 1866.

Flexner, Abraham. *Medical Education in the United States and Canada: A Report to the Carnegie Foundation for the Advancement of Teaching*. Carnegie Foundation for the Advancement of Teaching, 1910.

Frankenburger, J. M. "A Monstrosity." *Medical Record* 50, no. 15 (1896): 514–15.

Fraser, John. "A Sternopagous Monster." *American Journal of Obstetrics and Diseases of Women and Children* 23 (1890): 840–44.

Frazer, J. E. "Report on an Anencephalic Embryo." *Journal of Anatomy* 56 (1921): 12–19.

Freeborn, D. "Transactions of the New York Obstetrical Society: Formol or Formalin." *American Journal of Obstetrics and Diseases of Women and Children* 31, no. 2 (1895): 255–56.

French, J. M. "Society Reports." *Western and Southern Medical Recorder* 24 (1890): 539–45.

Galt, Francis L. "Medical Notes on a Trip Through the Pampa del Sacramento, Peru." *American Journal of the Medical Sciences* 134 (1874): 396–403.

Garland, G. "Acephalous Monster." *Western Journal of Medicine and Surgery* 7, no. 3 (1851): 212–14.

Garrett, J. W. B. "Singular Case of Monstrosity." *Western Journal of Medicine and Surgery* 6 (1850): 1–6.

Getchell, F. H. "Transactions of Societies: Summary of the Transactions of the College of Physicians of Philadelphia: Case of Monstrosity." *American Journal of the Medical Sciences* 106 (1867): 418.

Goddard, Henry. "The Height and Weight of Feeble-Minded Children in American Institutions." *Journal of Nervous and Mental Disease* 39, no. 4 (1912): 217–35.

Goddard, Henry. *The Kallikak Family: A Study in the Heredity of Feeble-Mindedness.* Macmillan, 1912.

Goode, B. P. "Anencephalic Foetus." *Cincinnati Lancet and Clinic* 6, no. 25 (1881): 566–67.

Gould, George. *An Illustrated Dictionary of Medicine, Biology, and Allied Sciences.* 4th ed. P. Blakiston's Son, 1899.

Gould, George M., and Walter Pyle. *Anomalies and Curiosities of Medicine.* W. B. Saunders, 1896.

Grandin, Egbert. "Transactions of the State Medical Society." *American Gynaecological and Obstetrical Journal* 3, no. 7 (1893): 633–42.

Grant, Madison. *The Passing of the Great Race; or, The Racial Basis of European History.* Scribner, 1916.

Green, Charles M. "The Care of Women in Pregnancy." *Boston Medical and Surgical Journal* 126, no. 8 (1892): 186–90.

Greene, F. "Clinical Memoranda." *Medical News* 56, no. 24 (1890): 653.

Guyer, Michael F., and Elizabeth A. Smith. "Studies on Cytolysins. I. Some Prenatal Effects of Lens Antibodies." *Journal of Experimental Zoology* 26, no. 1 (1918): 65–82.

Guyer, Michael F., and Elizabeth A. Smith. "Transmission of Eye-Defects Induced in Rabbits by Means of Lens-Sensitized Fowl-Serum." *Proceedings of the National Academy of Sciences of the United States of America* 6, no. 3 (1920): 134–36.

H. "Embryotic Influences—Acephalous Child." *Boston Medical and Surgical Journal* 22, no. 23 (1840): 362–63.

Hadlock, Dr. "Cincinnati Academy of Medicine: Acephalous Foetus." *Medical and Surgical Reporter* 21, no. 19 (1869): 280–81.

Haeckel, Ernst. *The Evolution of Man: A Popular Exposition of the Principal Points of Human Ontogeny and Phylogeny.* Trans. from German. D. Appleton, 1879.

Haeckel, Ernst. *Generelle Morphologie der Organismen. Allgemeine Grundzüge der Organischen Formen-Wissenschaft, mechanisch begründet durch die von Charles Darwin reformirte Descendenztheorie*. G. Reimer, 1866.

Haldemann, J. S. "Gleanings from Exchanges: Maternal Impressions and Acephalous Foetus." *Philadelphia Medical Times* 12, no. 22 (1882): 761–63.

Hamilton, Edward. "A Case of Exencephalus, with Specimen." *American Journal of Obstetrics and Diseases of Women and Children* 40, no. 4 (1899): 504–9.

Hamilton, Sadie Black. "Child Welfare Department." *National Notes* (1924): 7.

Hanks, H. T. "Specimen of Human Monstrosity Presented to the Society by Dr. H. J. Boldt." *American Journal of Obstetrics* 22, no. 12 (1889): 1292–97.

Hanks, H. T. "Transactions of the Obstetrical Society of New York: Fetal Monstrosity Without a Trace of Body." *American Journal of Obstetrics* 22, no. 4 (1889): 403–21.

Harrel, Sandy. "An Acephalous Monstrosity." *Nashville Journal of Medicine and Surgery* 75, no. 3 (1894): 103–5.

Harris, Robert P. "The Practice of Obstetrics Among the Chinese." *American Journal of Obstetrics and Diseases of Women and Children* 14, no. 3 (1881): 570–81.

Hasbrouck, Charles. "Notes of Country Obstetric Practice." *Transactions of the Medical Society of New Jersey* (1871): 189–219.

Hays, Isaac, ed. *The American Cyclopedia of Practical Medicine and Surgery; a Digest of Medical Literature*. Carey, Lea, and Blanchard, 1834.

Hestle, William. "Obstetrics." *American Gynaecological and Obstetrical Journal* 15 (1899): 386–93.

Hildreth, Charles T. "Art. I—Case of Notencephale." *Medical Magazine* 3 (1834): 3–16.

Hildreth, Charles T. *Case of Notencephale: With Engravings*. Published for the author, 1834.

Hilkowitz, William. "Society Reports: Academy of Medicine of Cincinnati, Anencephalus." *Cincinnati Lancet and Clinic* 37, no. 22 (1896): 565–72.

Hirst, Barton Cooke. "Clinical Notes." *American Journal of Obstetrics and Diseases of Women and Children* 35, no. 4 (1897): 536–40.

Hirst, Barton Cooke. "Teratologic Note." *Medical News* 64, no. 7 (1894): 184–85.

Hirst, Barton Cooke. "Two Recent Additions to the Teratological Collection in the Wistar and Horner Museum." *University of Pennsylvania Medical Magazine* 4, no. 10 (1892): 692–94.

Hirst, Barton Cooke, and George Piersol. *Human Monstrosities*. 4 vols. Lea Brothers, 1891–1893.

Hodge, Hugh Lenox. *The Principles and Practice of Obstetrics*. Henry C. Lea, 1866.

Hodge, Hugh Lenox. "Summary of the Proceedings of the Pathological Society of Philadelphia: Pseudencephalous Foetus." *American Journal of the Medical Sciences* 84 (1861): 435.

Hoffman, C. S. "A Peculiar Monstrosity." *American Journal of Obstetrics and Diseases of Women and Children* 29, no. 3 (1894): 367–68.

Holmes, Oliver Wendell. *The Complete Poetical Works of Oliver Wendell Holmes.* Cambridge ed. Houghton Mifflin, 1895.

Holmes, Oliver Wendell. *Medical Essays, 1842–1882.* Riverside ed. Vol. 9 of *The Writings of Oliver Wendell Holmes.* Houghton, Mifflin, 1891.

Holmes, Oliver Wendell. *The Poet at the Breakfast-Table: His Talks with His Fellow-Boarders and the Reader.* James R. Osgood, 1872.

Holton, H. D. "The Connecticut River Valley Medical Association." *American Medical Times* 4, no. 23 (1862): 325–26.

Horner, William Edmonds. *The United States Dissector: Or, Lessons in Practical Anatomy.* 4th ed. Lea & Blanchard, 1846.

"How These Problems Should Be Treated by Colored Club Women." *National Notes* (1931): 9.

Hudson, D. M. "Case of Monstrosity." *Medical Examiner* 114 (1854): 326.

Isaacs, C. E. "Extracts from the Report of the Proceedings of the New York Pathological Society: Cases of Anatomical Anomalies." *New York Journal of Medicine and Collateral Sciences* (1850): 331–32.

Jackson, J. B. S. "Case of Monstrosity, in Which the Brain, Heart, Lungs, Stomach, Liver, Spleen, Pancreas, and Right Kidney Were Wanting." *American Journal of the Medical Sciences* 42 (1838): 362–68.

Jackson, J .B. S. "Case of Monstrosity—(Siren)." *Boston Medical and Surgical Journal* 3, no. 3 (1869): 33–35.

Jackson, J. B. S. "Case of Monstrosity: Two Foetuses United." *Boston Society for Medical Improvement* 3 (1859): 147–50.

Jackson, J. B. S. *A Descriptive Catalogue of the Anatomical Museum of the Boston Society for Medical Improvement.* William D. Ticknor, 1847.

Jackson, J. B. S. *A Descriptive Catalogue of the Monstrosities in the Cabinet of the Boston Society for Medical Improvement.* Freeman and Bolles, 1847.

Jackson, J. B. S. *A Descriptive Catalogue of the Warren Anatomical Museum.* A. Williams, 1870.

Jackson, J. B. S. "Rhinencephalus and Some Allied Forms of Monstrosity." *Boston Medical and Surgical Journal* 98, no. 3 (1878): 66–73.

Jacobi, Abraham. "On the Etiological and Prognostic Importance of the Premature Closure of the Fontanels and Sutures of the Infantile Cranium." In *Contributions to Midwifery and Diseases of Women and Children, with a Report on the Progress of Obstetrics,* ed. E. Noeggerath and A. Jacobi, 70–105. Bailiere Brothers, 1859.

Jacobus, A. M. "Society Proceedings: Northwestern Medical and Surgical Society of New York." *Medical News* 73, no. 5 (1898): 155–59.

Jaggard, W. W. "Transactions of the Gynecological Society of Chicago: A Case of Fetal Aplasia." *American Journal of Obstetrics* 22, no. 1 (1889): 1209–22.
Jenkinson, John Wilfrid. *Experimental Embryology.* Clarendon Press, 1909.
Jewett, Charles. "Transactions of the New York Obstetrical Society: Dr. Coe." *American Gynaecological and Obstetric Journal* 4 (1894): 431.
Johnson, J. F. "Correspondence: A Double Monstrosity." *Atlanta Medical and Surgical Journal* 13, no. 4 (1896): 263.
Johnson, Otis. "Case of Monstrosity; Closure of Both Ears; Imperforate Anus; Double Fissure of the Palate." In *Extracts from the Records of the Boston Society for Medical Improvement,* 3:244. Printed for the Society for Medical Improvement, 1859.
Johnston, Christopher. "Description of a Pseudencephalic Monster (Genus 11, Thlipsencephalus, Isidore Geoff. St. Hilaire)." *American Journal of the Medical Sciences* 44, no. 87 (1862): 96–100.
Judkins, William. "Society Reports: Anencephalus Monstrosity (Dr. Withdrow)." *Cincinnati Lancet and Clinic* 24 (1890): 220.
Kellogg, John Harvey. *Tendencies Toward Race Degeneracy.* N.p., 1912. Reprinted from Senate Document no. 648. *New York Medical Journal* (1911). Digitized by the HathiTrust from a copy held by the University of Michigan. https://catalog.hathitrust.org/Record/005034851.
Keyes, Flint L. "Two Cases of Monstrosity." *Medical and Surgical Reporter* 12, no. 31 (1865): 501.
Knapp, Mark. "The Clinical History of an Anencephalous Monster." *Medical Record* 51, no. 15 (1897): 530–31.
Koogler, M. A. "A Report of Three Human Monstrosities." *American Journal of the Medical Sciences* 84 (1882): 129–32.
Lamb, Daniel S. "Transactions of the Medical Society of the District of Columbia." *National Medical Review* 8 (1898): 457–59.
Laughlin, Harry Hamilton. *Eugenical Sterilization in the United States.* Psychopathic Laboratory of the Municipal Court of Chicago, 1922.
Laughlin, Harry Hamilton. *Eugenical Sterilization: 1926; Historical, Legal, and Statistical Review of Eugenical Sterilization in the United States.* American Eugenics Society, 1926.
Leibman, G. "Another Case of Dropsy of the Amnion.—Tapping.—Deformed Foetus (Acephalon).—Version on the Head.—Recovery." *Medical and Surgical Reporter* 23, no. 7 (1870): 141.
Lewis, Henry F. "Iniencephalus." *American Journal of Obstetrics and Diseases of Women and Children* 34, no. 1 (1897): 11–39.
Lewis, Henry F. "On Iniencephalus." *Journal of the American Medical Association* 28, no. 9 (1897): 388–90.

Lichliter, D. "An Anencephalic Monster: Original Communications." *Cincinnati Lancet and Clinic* 6, no. 22 (1881): 493–95.

Lindsly, Harvey. *Medical Science and the Medical Profession in Europe and the United States: An Introductory Lecture.* P. Force, 1840.

Lowman, William. "Résumé on Maternal Impressions." *Medical Record* 36, no. 7 (1889): 176–79.

L. P. S. "Influence of Maternal Feelings—Acephalous Child, &c." *Boston Medical and Surgical Journal* 24, no. 5 (1841): 72–73.

Lucas and Pankake, Drs. "Anencephalous Monster." *Medical and Surgical Reporter* 63, no. 25 (1890): 716–17.

Lucas, R. O. "An Acephalus Babe." *Massachusetts Medical Journal* 4, no. 10 (1884): 447.

Lueck, A. W. "Acephalic Babe." *Medical and Surgical Reporter* 22, no. 8 (1870): 150.

Lusk, W. T. "A Case of Acardia." *Western Lancet* 3, no. 4 (1874): 200–201.

Mall, Franklin Paine. "A Study of the Causes Underlying the Origin of Human Monsters: Third Contribution to the Study of the Pathology of Human Embryos." *Journal of Morphology* 19, no. 1 (1908): 3–367.

Mall, Franklin Paine, and Arthur William Meyer. *Studies on Abortuses: A Survey of Pathologic Ova in the Carnegie Embryological Collection.* Carnegie Institution of Washington, 1921.

Manlove, J. "Remarks on a Case of an Acephalous Monster: Read Before the Medical Society of Tennessee at Its Annual Meeting." *Western Journal of Medicine and Surgery* 4, no. 5 (1845): 401–5.

Manouvrier, L., and George Grant MacCurdy. "On *Pithecanthropus Erectus.*" *American Journal of Science* 4, no. 21 (1897): 213–34.

Marcy, O. Henry, and R. H. Fitz. "A Case of Double Monstrosity—Union Upon the Anterior Median Line from Clavicle to Umbilicus." *Boston Medical and Surgical Journal* 8, no. 2 (1871): 17–20.

Mayer, Emil. "Acrania Monsters, with Report of a Case." *American Journal of the Medical Sciences* 83 (1882): 118–22.

McCassey, J. C. "Criminals and Defectives: How Best to Reduce Their Number." *Medical News* 79 (1901): 136–41.

McClendon, J. F. "An Attempt Toward the Physical Chemistry of the Production of One-Eyed Monstrosities." *American Journal of Physiology* 29, no. 3 (1912): 289–97.

Mead, Charles H. "A Quantitative Study in Human Teratology." *Human Biology* 2, no. 1 (1930): 1–33.

"Medical Items." *Medical Record* 30, no. 16 (1886): 444–48.

"Medical Items and News." *Medical Record* 4 (1869): 307–12.

"Medical Items and News." *Medical Record* 19, no. 20 (1881): 558–60.

Meigs, Charles D. "Case of a Monstrous Birth." *American Journal of the Medical Sciences* 30 (1855): 13–21.

Meigs, Charles D. *Obstetrics: The Science and the Art.* Lea & Blanchard, 1849.

Metcalf, John. "A Case of Monstrosity." *Boston Medical and Surgical Journal* 20, no. 22 (1839): 341–43.

Meyer, Adolf. "A Review of the Signs of Degeneration and of Methods of Registration." *American Journal of Insanity* 52, no. 3 (1896): 344–63.

"Microscopy." *American Naturalist* 19, no. 8 (1885): 828–32.

Middleton, M. "Cases of Malformation: With Reflections on Congenital Abnormities." *American Journal of the Medical Sciences* 55, no. 109 (1868): 69–76.

Millen, S. R. "Effects of Maternal Impressions on the Foetus." *Medical and Surgical Reporter* 49, no. 11 (1883): 305–6.

Minot, Francis. *Extracts from the Records of the Boston Society for Medical Improvement.* Vol. 4. Printed for the Society for Medical Improvement, 1862.

Minot, Francis. "Reports of Medical Societies: Extracts from the Records of the Boston Society for Medical Improvement: Anencephalous Foetus." *Boston Medical and Surgical Journal* 62 (1860): 160–66.

Moffat, R. U. "Medical Progress: Teratology." *Missouri Medical and Surgical Journal* 75, no. 6 (1898): 326–27.

Montgomery, E. "Cases of Monstrosity." *Missouri Medical and Surgical Journal* 19, no. 2 (1861): 232–34.

Moore, A. A. "Anencephalic Monster." *American Journal of the Medical Sciences* 54 (1867): 281–82.

Moore, A. A. "Anencephalic Monster." *Medical and Surgical Reporter* 47, no. 17 (1882): 461.

Morgan, Thomas Hunt. "The Relation Between Normal and Abnormal Development of the Embryo of the Frog." *Roux's Archives of Developmental Biology* 15 (1902): 238–313.

Morland, William. "Extracts from the Records of the Boston Society for Medical Improvement." *American Journal of the Medical Sciences* 50 (1853): 356–62. Reprinted in *Ohio Medical and Surgical Journal* 6, no. 1 (1853): 49–59.

Morse, John T. *Life and Letters of Oliver Wendell Holmes.* Standard Library ed. Houghton, Mifflin, 1896.

Mumford, James Gregory. *The Story of the Boston Society for Medical Improvement.* Darnell & Upham, 1901.

Munde, Paul F. "Transactions of the New York Obstetrical Society." *American Journal of Obstetrics and Diseases of Women and Children* 6, no. 4 (1874): 628–38.

Murphy, Douglas P. "Outcome of 625 Pregnancies in Women Subjected to Pelvic Radium or Roentgen Irradiation." *American Journal of Obstetrics and Gynecology* 18 (1929): 79.

Napheys, George Henry. *The Physical Life of Woman: Advice to the Maiden, Wife, and Mother.* George MacLean, 1870.

Neal, L. E. "Gynaecological and Obstetrical Society of Baltimore: Foetal Monstrosity, Placenta Praevia. Discussion." *Medical and Surgical Reporter of Philadelphia* 56, no. 15 (1887): 459–60.

Neil, J. D. "Brief of Current Literature, Obstetrics: An Anencephalus." *American Journal of Obstetrics and Diseases of Women and Children* 39, no. 4 (1899): 554.

Newbill, H. P. "Sirenomelian Monster (Sympus): An Anatomic Presentation." *American Journal of Diseases of Children* 62, no. 6 (1941): 1233–41.

Nicoll, Alexander Y., and Richard D. Arnold. "Account of an Anencephalus, or Human Monstrosity, Without a Brain and Spinal Marrow." *American Journal of the Medical Sciences* 22, no. 43 (1838): 253–57.

Nicoll, Alexander Y., and Richard D. Arnold. "Account of an Anencephalus, or Human Monstrosity Without a Brain and Spinal Marrow." *Southern Medical and Surgical Journal* 2, no. 1 (1837): 10–18.

Nicoll, Alexander Y., and Richard D. Arnold. "Account of a Human Monstrosity, Which Possessed Neither a Brain nor a Spinal Marrow." *Lancet* 29, no. 740 (1837): 202–4.

North, John. "A Lecture on Monstrosities." *American Medical Intelligencer* 4, no. 9 (1840): 130–37.

North, John. "A Lecture on Monstrosities: Part II." *American Medical Intelligencer* 4, no. 10 (1840): 150–58.

"Notes and Comments." *Atlanta Medical and Surgical Journal* 1, no. 2 (1884): 120–28.

Osborn, Henry Fairfield. *Present Problems in Evolution and Heredity.* Cartwright Lectures. Columbia College, 1892.

Oslin, S. S. "A Monstrosity." *Medical Review* 3 (1875): 197–200.

Overend, E. J. "Maternal Impressions." *Pacific Medical Journal* 33 (1890): 70–77.

Owen, W. G. "A Brownie Baby." *Medical News* 73, no. 11 (1898): 338–39.

Packard, D. "Anencephalous Monster, with Spina Bifida, and Failure of Development of the Anterior Abdominal Walls." *American Journal of the Medical Sciences* 84 (1861): 437–38.

Palmer, J. W. "Hermaphroditism, or Monstrosity." *Boston Medical and Surgical Journal* (1836): 377–78.

Pancoast, Seth. *The Ladies' New Medical Guide.* J. E. Potter, 1890.

Parsons, Usher. *Directions for Making Anatomical Preparations.* Carey & Lea, 1831.

Parvin, Theophilus. "The Influence of Maternal Impressions Upon the Foetus." *International Medical Magazine* 1, no. 5 (1892): 487–93.

Parvin, Theophilus. "Monsters." *Medical and Surgical Reporter* 77 (1897): 3–7.

Payne, F. R. "Abnormal Foetus." *Chicago Medical Examiner* 6, no. 7 (1865): 390–91.

Peck, George. "Bureau of Obstetrics: Abstract of Discussion." *Medical Advance* 17, no. 2 (1886): 117–23.

Pennell, W. W. "A Pseudocephaloid Infant." *Medical and Surgical Reporter* 62 (1890): 81.

Penney, Edward Winthrop. "A Case of Triplets, Hydramnion, and Monstrosity." *American Journal of Obstetrics* 22, no. 11 (1889): 1151–57.

Pepper, William. *Descriptive Catalogue of the Pathological Museum of the Pennsylvania Hospital.* Collins, 1869.

Perkins, J. "Anencephalous Monster." *Medical Record* 48, no. 14 (1895): 492.

"The Placards and Exhibitions of Freaks and Monstrosities." *Medical News* 59, no. 23 (1891): 665–66.

Pryor, W. R. "Society Meetings: New York Academy of Medicine, Section on Obstetrics and Gynecology." *American Medico-Surgical Bulletin* 10 (1896): 78.

Purdy, G. L. "Case of Monstrosity." *Western Medical Reformer* 1, no. 5 (1857): 204–6.

Purple, Samuel S. "A Literary, Historical, and Practical Sketch of Acrania, 'Brainless' or Pseudencephalus Monsters." *New York Journal of Medicine and Collateral Sciences* 5, no. 1 (1850): 40–58.

Ramsbotham, Francis H. *The Principles and Practice of Obstetric Medicine and Surgery: In Reference to the Process of Parturition.* 1st American ed. Lea & Blanchard, 1842.

Rankin, T. W. "Foetal Monstrosity." *Cincinnati Lancet and Clinic* 9 (1882): 529–30.

Ray, Robert, H. D. Bulkley, and John Watson. *A Catalogue of the Pathological Cabinet of the New York Hospital.* S. S. & W. Wood, 1860.

Rea, Charles. "Prolonged Gestation, Acrania Monstrosity, and Apparent Placenta Previa in One Obstetrical Case." *Journal of the American Medical Association* 30, no. 20 (1898): 1166–67.

Reamy, Thad. "Society Reports: Academy of Medicine, Discussion." *Cincinnati Lancet and Clinic* (1885): 293.

"Recent Literature: *Human Monstrosities.*" *Boston Medical and Surgical Journal* 128, no. 2 (1893): 45.

Reichler, Max. *Jewish Eugenics: A Paper Read Before the New York Board of Jewish Ministers.* Bloch, 1916.

"Remarkable Monstrosity." *Medical Surgical Report* 46 (1882): 350–51.

"Report of the Surgeon General." *Cincinnati Lancet and Clinic* 15, no. 25 (1885): 782–83.

"Reports of Societies: American Medical Institute." *Medical Investigator* 4, no. 11 (1867): 124–27.

Richards, J. "Maternal Impressions." *Philadelphia Medical Times* 19, no. 8 (1889): 340.

Riley, Henry A. "Medical Cases in the Courts." *Medical Record* 32, no. 14 (1887): 452–53.

Roberge, Joseph L. "Sympodia in Identical Twins: Report of a Case." *Journal of the American Medical Association* 186, no. 7 (1963): 728–29.

Rosedale, Raymond S. "Polygnathus Epignathus: A Case Report." *Archives of Otolaryngology* 74, no. 5 (1961): 529–31.

Ross, John, ed. *Globe Encyclopaedia*. Estes & Lauriat, 1877.

Russell, L. E. "Obstetrical Problems." *Western Medical Reformer* 59 (1899): 18–23.

Sabin, Florence Rena. *Franklin Paine Mall: The Story of a Mind*. Johns Hopkins Press, 1934.

Saint-Hilaire, Isidore Geoffroy. *Histoire générale et particulière des anomalies, de l'organisation chez l'homme et les animaux, ou, Traité de tératologie*. 3 vols. J-B. Baillière, 1832–1837.

Saur, Prudence B. *Maternity: A Book for Every Wife and Mother*. L. P. Miller, 1891.

Schumann, Edward. "Observations Upon the Formation of Terata." *American Journal of Obstetrics and Diseases of Women and Children* 67, no. 6 (1913): 1159–65.

Scovil, Elisabeth Robinson. *Preparation for Motherhood*. H. Altemus, 1896.

Shaller, John. "An Anencephalous Monster." *Cincinnati Lancet and Clinic* 27, no. 9 (1891): 264.

Shannon, T. "A Case of Monstrosity." *Medical and Surgical Report* 25 (1871): 180.

Shrader, I. M. "Some Incidents in the Practice of Obstetrics." *Western Medical Reformer* 57 (1897): 138–41.

Simpson, P. C., B. J. Trudinger, A. Walker, and P. J. Baird. "The Intrauterine Treatment of Fetal Cardiac Failure in a Twin Pregnancy with an Acardiac, Acephalic Monster." *American Journal of Obstetrics and Gynecology* 147, no. 7 (1983): 842–44.

Skinner, N. C. "A Singular Foetal Malformation." *Medical Examiner* 116 (1854): 461–66.

Smith, Allen J. "Apparent Fetal Substitution; Medico-Legal Note." *Medical News* 82, no. 11 (1903): 488–89.

Smith, David W. "Dysmorphology (Teratology)." *Journal of Pediatrics* 69, no. 6 (1966): 1150–69.

Smith, F. N. "A Case of Monstrosity." *American Medical Times* 2 (1861): 154.

Smith, George Ritter. "Report of a Case of Monstra per Defectum." *American Journal of Obstetrics and Diseases of Women and Children* 69, no. 4 (1914): 664–70.

Smith, Gould. "A Few Cases from My Experience in Obstetrics." *Cincinnati Lancet and Clinic* 28, no. 26 (1892): 840–44.

Smith, Robert Meade, and Andrew J. Parker. "Dissection of a Human Otocephalic Cyclops Monstrosity." *American Journal of the Medical Sciences* 84, no. 167 (1882): 132–40.

Snively, J. N. "Remarkable Case of Monstrosity." *Medical and Surgical Reporter* 24 (1871): 383.

Stahl, Frank. "Maternal Impressions and Their Significance: With Presentation of a Case of Anencephalia et Acrania." *American Journal of Obstetrics and Diseases of Women and Children* 33, no. 4 (1896): 501–17.

Stedman, Thomas L. "Influence of Maternal Impressions in the Etiology of Congenital Deformities." *Medical Record* 31, no. 1 (1887): A4–A9.

Stevenson, J. M. "Case of Monstrosity." *Medical and Surgical Reporter* 12 (1865): 223–24.

Stockard, Charles R. "The Artificial Production of One-Eyed Monsters and Other Defects, Which Occur in Nature, by the Use of Chemicals." *Anatomical Record* 3, no. 4 (1909): 167–73.

Stockard, Charles R. "The Artificial Production of Structural Arrests and Racial Degeneration." *Proceedings of Meetings of the New York Pathological Society* 13 (1913): 83–88.

Stockard, Charles R. "An Experimental Study of Racial Degeneration in Mammals Treated with Alcohol." *Archives of Internal Medicine* 10, no. 4 (1912): 369–98.

Stockard, Charles R. "The Influence of Alcohol and Other Anæsthetics on Embryonic Development." *American Journal of Anatomy* 10, no. 1 (1909): 369–92.

Stockard, Charles R. "Is the Control of Embryonic Development a Practical Problem?" *Proceedings of the American Philosophical Society* 51 (1912): 191–200.

Stokes, J. G. "Original Communications: Description of a Double Monster." *Medical Examiner* 15, no. 18 (1874): 433–35.

Stolz, Charles. "Some Common Monstrosities." *Transactions of the Indiana State Medical Society* (1898): 249–58.

Stout, H. R. "A Case of Placenta Praevia." *Medical Investigator* 9 (1874): 443–44.

Sweet, A. L. "An Interesting Obstetric Case." *Medical Record* 16, no. 19 (1879): 439.

Swinburne, John. "Acephalous Monstrosity (Dr. Boyce)." *Philadelphia Medical Times* 4, no. 23 (1874): 363–64.

Talbot, Eugene. "Degeneracy and Marriage." *Alienist and Neurologist* 20 (1899): 45–54.

Talbot, Eugene. "Heredity and Atavism." *Alienist and Neurologist* 19, no. 4 (1898): 628–57.

Talbot, Eugene S. *The Stigmata of Degeneracy.* Walter Scott, 1898.

Taylor, Alfred Swaine. *A Manual of Medical Jurisprudence.* 7th American ed. H. C. Lea, 1873.

Taylor, E. W. "The Spinal Cord in a Case of Anencephalus." *Journal of the Boston Society of Medical Sciences* 2, no. 4 (1897): 31–32.

Taylor, Julius. "Case of Monstrosity." *Western Lancet* 15, no. 7 (1854): 470–72.

Taylor, Thaddeus. "Report of Medical Societies: Medical Association of Louisiana (Dr. Taylor)." *Journal of the National Medical Association* 1, no. 3 (1909): 174–77.

Tebbets, James Allen. "Case of Premature Labor and Monstrosity." *Boston Medical and Surgical Journal* 28 (1843): 194–95.

"Teratology." *American Naturalist* 3, no. 3 (1869): 152–54.

Terry, C. "Remarks Upon Some Recently Reported Cases of Monstrosity." *American Journal of Obstetrics and Diseases of Women and Children* 2, no. 3 (1869): 369–98.

Thelander, H. E. "Use of the Term 'Monster.'" *Journal of the American Medical Association* 187, no. 8 (1964): 621.

Thomas, A. R. "Monstrosities." *American Journal of Homeopathic Materia Medica and Record of Medical Science* (1872): 389–94.

Thompson, H. K. "Anencephalic Monster; One of Twins." *Boston Medical and Surgical Journal* 193, no. 27 (1925): 1241–42.

Thompson, P. H. "Three Monstrosities." *Atlanta Medical and Surgical Journal* 2, no. 10 (1885): 592–95.

Thoms, Herbert. "Family Prevalence in Anencephaly: Report of Case." *Journal of the American Medical Association* 70, no. 1 (1918): 10–11.

Tiffany, L. McLane. "Surgical Disease of the White and Colored Races Compared." *Boston Medical and Surgical Journal* 116 (1887): 524–25.

Tingley, W. H. "Observations on the Above Case." *Missouri Medical and Surgical Journal* 14, no. 3 (1856): 219–36.

Tompkins, J. Edward. "An Anencephalous Monster." *Medical Record* 47, no. 22 (1895): 691.

Torbert, J. "An Unusual Monstrosity." *Boston Medical and Surgical Journal* 165, no. 7 (1911): 249–51.

Tuck, Henry, and J. B. S. Jackson. "Rare Form of Monstrosity; Case of Acephalus." *Boston Medical and Surgical Journal* 94, no. 16 (1876): 439–42.

"Tuskegee Institute Health Center Report Shows Improved Health Conditions in Macon County: Mother's Club Effective." *National Notes* (1928): 10.

Tyler, Samuel. "Case of Monstrosity." *American Journal of the Medical Sciences* 11, no. 22 (1846): 539.

Tyson, James. *Catalogue of the Specimens in the Pathological Museum of the Philadelphia Hospital*. Collins, 1874.

Underhill, J. W. "Transactions of the Obstetrical Society of Cincinnati: Maternal Impressions Affecting the Fetus in Utero." *American Journal of Obstetrics and Diseases of Women and Children* 11, no. 3 (1878): 626–40.

University of Texas. "Catalogue of the Department of Medicine." *Bulletin of the University of Texas* 118, Official Series no. 34 (1909): 11–181.

Velasquez, Pedro, John Stephens, and Barnum's American Museum. *Life of the Living Aztec Children*. Wynkoop, Hallenbeck & Thomas, 1860.

Waddel, Thomas. "Original Communications: Maternal Impressions." *Detroit Review of Medicine and Pharmacy* 11, no. 11 (1876): 723–42.

Walter, Herbert Eugene. *Genetics: An Introduction to the Study of Heredity.* Macmillan, 1913.

Werber, E. I. "Experimental Studies Aiming at the Control of Defective and Monstrous Development. A Survey of Recorded Monstrosities with Special Attention to the Ophthalmic Defects." *Anatomical Record* 9, no. 7 (1915): 529–62.

West, Francis. "An Account of an Anencephalous Foetus." *Medical Examiner* 1, no. 4 (1838): 60–61.

Williams, Stephen. "Case of Monstrosity, with Some Remarks Upon Moles, Marks, &c." *American Journal of Medical Sciences* (1835): 88–91.

Wilson, Robert T. "Original Communications: A Contribution to the History of Hydramnios." *American Journal of Obstetrics and Diseases of Women and Children* 20, no. 1 (1887): A1–A25.

Wistar Institute of Anatomy and Biology. *Catalogue of the Anatomical Museum of the University of Pennsylvania.* 1832. L. R. Bailey, 1850.

Wood Museum of Bellevue Hospital. *Catalogue of the Wood Museum of Bellevue Hospital, New York City, Comprising a Descriptive and Classified List of Anatomical and Pathological Specimens.* Dept. Press, 1880.

Wood, Richard. "An Anencephalous Monster." *Medical Record* 48, no. 25 (1895): 893.

Woodruff, L. "Anencephalic Monsters." *Cincinnati Lancet and Clinic* 37, no. 24 (1896): 622–23.

Woodward, A. "A Case of Melancholia." *Medical Investigator* 9, no. 103 (1872): 319–20.

Woodward, J. J. *Catalogue of the Medical Section of the United States Army Medical Museum.* US Government Printing Office, 1867.

W. W. "Monstrosities." *Western Medical and Physical Journal* 3, no. 3 (1835): 413–42.

Wyman, Jeffries. "Description of an Anencephalous Foetus with Unusual Malformation." *Boston Medical and Surgical Journal* 71, no. 3 (1864): 49–52.

Wyman, Jeffries. "On the Measurement of Crania." *Anthropological Review* 6, no. 23 (1868): 345–49.

Wythe, W. T. "Proceedings of the San Francisco Medical Society: Acephalous Fetus (Dr. Blach)." *Pacific Medical and Surgical Journal* 7, no. 6 (1873): 288–93.

SECONDARY SOURCES

Ahmed, Sara. "Affective Economies." *Social Text* 22, no. 2 (2004): 117–39.

Ahmed, Sara. *The Cultural Politics of Emotion.* Edinburgh University Press, 2014.

Allen, Garland. "The Eugenics Record Office at Cold Spring Harbor, 1910–1940: An Essay in Institutional History." *Osiris* 2, no. 1 (1986): 225–64.

Amirault, Chris. "Posing the Subject of Early Medical Photography." *Discourse: Journal for Theoretical Studies in Media and Culture* 16, no. 2 (1993): 51–76.

Anderson, Warwick. *Collectors of Lost Souls: Turning Kuru Scientists Into Whitemen*. Johns Hopkins University Press, 2008.

Anderson, Warwick. *Colonial Pathologies: American Tropical Medicine, Race, and Hygiene in the Philippines*. Duke University Press, 2006.

Appel, Toby A. *The Cuvier–Geoffroy Debate: French Biology in the Decades Before Darwin*. Oxford University Press, 1987.

Apple, Rima D. *Perfect Motherhood: Science and Childrearing in America*. Rutgers University Press, 2006.

Arni, Caroline. "Traversing Birth: Continuity and Contingency in Research on Development in Nineteenth-Century Life and Human Sciences." *History and Philosophy of the Life Sciences* 37, no. 1 (2015): 50–67.

Asma, Stephen T. *On Monsters: An Unnatural History of Our Worst Fears*. Oxford University Press, 2009.

Barclay, Jenifer. "Bad Breeders and Monstrosities: Racializing Childlessness and Congenital Disabilities in Slavery and Freedom." *Slavery and Abolition* 38, no. 2 (2017): 287–302.

Barclay, Jenifer. *The Mark of Slavery: Disability, Race, and Gender in Antebellum America*. University of Illinois Press, 2021.

Baynton, Douglas. *Defectives in the Land: Disability and Immigration in the Age of Eugenics*. University of Chicago Press, 2016.

Baynton, Douglas. "Disability and the Justification of Inequality in American History." In *The New Disability History: American Perspectives*, ed. Paul K. Longmore and Lauri Umansky, 33–57. New York University Press, 2001.

Bederman, Gail. *Manliness and Civilization: A Cultural History of Gender and Race in the United States, 1880–1917*. University of Chicago Press, 1996.

Berry, Daina Ramey. *The Price for Their Pound of Flesh: The Value of the Enslaved, from Womb to Grave, in the Building of a Nation*. Beacon, 2017.

Berry, S. N., B. Severtsen, A. Davis, L. Nelson, M. H. Hutti, and G. Oneal. "The Impact of Anencephaly on Parents: A Mixed-Methods Study." *Death Studies* 46, no. 9 (2022): 2198–207.

Bogdan, Robert. *Freak Show: Presenting Human Oddities for Amusement and Profit*. University of Chicago Press, 1988.

Bogdan, Robert, Douglas Biklen, Arthur Shapiro, and David Spelkomen. "The Disabled: Media's Monster." *Social Policy* 13, no. 2 (1982): 32–35.

Bolker, Jessica A. "Model Species in Evo-Devo: A Philosophical Perspective." *Evolution & Development* 16, no. 1 (2014): 49–56.

Bonanno, Mark A. "The Case of Baby K: Exploring the Concept of Medical Futility." *Annals of Health Law* 4 (1995): 151–72.

Borst, Charlotte G. *Catching Babies: The Professionalization of Childbirth, 1870–1920*. Harvard University Press, 1995.

Boster, Dea. *African American Slavery and Disability: Bodies, Property, and Power in the Antebellum South, 1800–1860*. Routledge, 2013.

Braidotti, Rosi. "Signs of Wonder and Traces of Doubt: On Teratology and Embodied Differences." In *Feminist Theory and the Body: A Reader*, ed. Janet Price and Margrit Shildrick, 290–301. Routledge, 1999.

Brammall, Kathryn. "Monstrous Metamorphosis: Nature, Morality, and the Rhetoric of Monstrosity in Tudor England." *Sixteenth Century Journal* 27, no. 1 (1996): 3–21.

Brandt, Allan. *No Magic Bullet: A Social History of Venereal Disease in the United States Since 1880*. 35th anniv. ed. Oxford University Press, 2020.

Braun, Lundy. *Breathing Race Into the Machine: The Surprising Career of the Spirometer from Plantation to Genetics*. University of Minnesota Press, 2014.

Briggs, Laura. "The Race of Hysteria: 'Overcivilization' and the 'Savage' Woman in Late Nineteenth-Century Obstetrics and Gynecology." *American Quarterly* 52, no. 2 (2000): 246–73.

Briggs, Laura. *Reproducing Empire: Race, Sex, Science, and U.S. Imperialism in Puerto Rico*. University of California Press, 2002.

Brown, Kathleen. *Foul Bodies: Cleanliness in Early America*. Yale University Press, 2009.

Brown, P., S. Zavestoski, S. McCormick, B. Mayer, R. Morello-Frosch, and R. Gasior Altman. "Embodied Health Movements: New Approaches to Social Movements in Health." *Sociology of Health & Illness* 26, no. 1 (2004): 50–80.

Browne-Marshall, Gloria J. *Race, Law, and American Society: 1607–Present*. 2nd ed. Routledge, 2013.

Bruchac, Margaret M. "A Pragmatic Approach to Reconciliation: Thoughts on Transforming Repatriation Practice." In *Pragmatism and the New Museum Anthropology*, ed. Christina J. Hodge and Christina Kreps, 120–34. Bloomsbury Press, 2024.

Butler, Judith. *Bodies That Matter: On the Discursive Limits of "Sex."* Routledge, 1993.

Butler, Judith. *Gender Trouble: Feminism and the Subversion of Identity*. Routledge, 1990.

Cadden, Joan. *Meanings of Sex Difference in the Middle Ages: Medicine, Science, and Culture*. Cambridge University Press, 1993.

Canguilhem, Georges. "Monstrosity and the Monstrous." Trans. Therese Jaeger. *Diogenes* 10, no. 40 (1962): 27–42. Retranslated in *Knowledge of Life*, ed. Paola

Marrati and Todd Meyers, trans. Stefanos Geroulanos and Daniela Ginsburg, 134–48. Fordham University Press, 2008.

Carby, Hazel. *Reconstructing Womanhood: The Emergence of the Afro-American Woman Novelist.* Oxford University Press, 1987.

Cecil, Rosanne, ed. *The Anthropology of Pregnancy Loss: Comparative Studies in Miscarriage, Stillbirth, and Neonatal Death.* Berg, 1996.

Centers for Disease Control and Prevention. "Updated Estimates of Neural Tube Defects Prevented by Mandatory Folic Acid Fortification—United States, 1995–2011." *Morbidity and Mortality Weekly Report* 64, no. 1 (2015): 1–5.

Chávez-García, Miroslava. *States of Delinquency: Race and Science in the Making of California's Juvenile Justice System.* University of California Press, 2012.

Chen, Mel Y. *Animacies: Biopolitics, Racial Mattering, and Queer Affect.* Duke University Press, 2012.

Chen, Mel Y. " 'The Stuff of Slow Constitution': Reading Down Syndrome for Race, Disability, and the Timing That Makes Them So." *Somatechnics* 6, no. 2 (2016): 235–48.

Churchill, F. B. *August Weismann: Development, Heredity, and Evolution.* Harvard University Press, 2015.

Claes, Tinne, and Veronique Deblon. "When Nothing Remains: Anatomical Collections, the Ethics of Stewardship, and the Meanings of Absence." *Journal of the History of Collections* 30, no. 2 (2018): 351–62.

Cohen, Jeffrey Jerome, ed. *Monster Theory: Reading Culture.* University of Minnesota Press, 1996.

Cooper Owens, Deirdre Benia. *Medical Bondage: Race, Gender, and the Origins of American Gynecology.* University of Georgia Press, 2017.

Cott, Nancy. *The Bonds of Womanhood: "Woman's Sphere" in New England, 1780–1835.* With a new preface. 2nd ed. Yale University Press, 1997.

Crawford, Julie. *Marvelous Protestantism: Monstrous Births in Post-Reformation England.* Johns Hopkins University Press, 2005.

Crowther, Kathleen. *Policing Pregnant Bodies: From Ancient Greece to Post-Roe America.* Johns Hopkins University Press, 2023.

Cryle, Peter, and Elizabeth Stephens. *Normality: A Critical Genealogy.* University of Chicago Press, 2017.

Dain, Bruce R. *A Hideous Monster of the Mind: American Race Theory in the Early Republic.* Harvard University Press, 2002.

Daston, Lorraine. "Type Specimens and Scientific Memory." *Critical Inquiry* 31, no. 1 (2004): 153–82.

Daston, Lorraine. "What Can Be a Scientific Object? Reflections on Monsters and Meteors." *Bulletin of the Academy of Arts and Sciences* 52, no. 2 (1998): 35–50.

Daston, Lorraine, and Peter Galison. *Objectivity.* Zone, 2007.

Daston, Lorraine, and Katharine Park. *Wonders and the Order of Nature, 1150–1750*. Zone, 1998.

Davies, Surekha. *Renaissance Ethnography and the Invention of the Human: New Worlds, Maps, and Monsters*. Cambridge University Press, 2016.

Desmond, Jane C. "Postmortem Exhibitions: Taxidermied Animals and Plastinated Corpses in the Theaters of the Dead." In *Displaying Death and Animating Life: Human–Animal Relations in Art, Science, and Everyday Life*, 347–77. University of Chicago Press, 2016.

Diaz, Francisco. "Morton, the Maya, and Me: Reflections from a Yucatec Maya Graduate Student." In "The Morton Cranial Collection and Legacies of Scientific Racism in Museums," ed. Paul Wolff Mitchell. Special issue, *History of Anthropology Review* 45 (2021). https://histanthro.org/news/observations/morton-the-maya-and-me.

Dietrich, Michael R. "From Hopeful Monsters to Homeotic Effects: Richard Goldschmidt's Integration of Development, Evolution, and Genetics." *American Zoologist* 40, no. 5 (2000): 738–47.

Doyle, Nora. "'The Highest Pleasure of Which Woman's Nature Is Capable': Breast-Feeding and the Sentimental Maternal Ideal in America, 1750–1860." *Journal of American History* 97, no. 4 (2011): 958–73.

Doyle, Nora. *Maternal Bodies: Redefining Motherhood in Early America*. University of North Carolina Press, 2018.

Dron, Heather. "Teratology Transformed: Uncertainty, Knowledge, and Conflict Over Birth Defects in Midcentury America." PhD diss., University of California, San Francisco, 2016.

Dubow, Sara. *Ourselves Unborn: A History of the Fetus in Modern America*. Oxford University Press, 2010.

Duden, Barbara. *The Woman Beneath the Skin*. Harvard University Press, 1991.

Durbach, Nadja. *Spectacle of Deformity: Freak Shows and Modern British Culture*. University of California Press, 2010.

Edwards, Elizabeth. "Photographic 'Types': The Pursuit of Method." *Visual Anthropology* 3, nos. 2–3 (1990): 235–58.

Edwards, Elizabeth. "Photography and Anthropological Intention in Nineteenth Century Britain." *Revista de dialectología y tradiciones populares* 53, no. 2 (1998): 23–48.

Engel, Trevor. "A 'Most Remarkable Trait': 'Flathead' Skulls, Indigenous Pathologization, and Transinstitutionalization." *Osiris* 39, no. 1 (2024): 117–34.

Epstein, Steven. *Impure Science: AIDS, Activism, and the Politics of Knowledge*. University of California Press, 1996.

Erevelles, Nirmala. *Difference and Disability in Global Contexts: Enabling a Transformative Body Politic*. Palgrave Macmillan, 2011.

Erevelles, Nirmala, and Michael Gill. "The Absent Presence of Elsie Lacks: Hauntings at the Intersection of Race, Class, Gender, and Disability." *African American Review* 50, no. 2 (2017): 123–37.

Eze, Emmanuel Chukwudi. Introduction to *Race and the Enlightenment: A Reader*, ed. Emmanuel Chukwudi Eze, 1–9. Blackwell, 1997.

Fabian, Ann. *The Skull Collectors: Race, Science, and America's Unburied Dead.* University of Chicago Press, 2010.

Fett, Sharla M. *Working Cures: Healing, Health, and Power on Southern Slave Plantations.* University of North Carolina Press, 2000.

Few, Martha. "Atlantic World Monsters: Monstrous Births and the Politics of Pregnancy in Colonial Guatemala." In *Women, Religion, and the Atlantic World*, ed. Lisa Vollendorf and Daniella J. Kostroun, 205–22. University of Toronto Press, 2009.

Fields, Karen E., and Barbara Fields. *Racecraft: The Soul of Inequality in American Life.* Verso, 2014.

Fissell, Mary. *Vernacular Bodies: The Politics of Reproduction in Early Modern England.* Oxford University Press, 2004.

Flores-Villalobos, Joan. *The Silver Women: How Black Women's Labor Made the Panama Canal.* University of Pennsylvania Press, 2023.

Foucault, Michel. *Abnormal: Lectures at the Collège de France, 1974–1975.* Picador, 2003.

Foucault, Michel. *Birth of the Clinic: An Archaeology of Medical Perception.* Pantheon, 1973.

Fraser, Gertrude Jacinta. *African American Midwifery in the South: Dialogues of Birth, Race, and Memory.* Harvard University Press, 1998.

Fredrickson, George. *The Black Image in the White Mind: The Debate on Afro-American Character and Destiny, 1817–1914.* Wesleyan University Press, 1987.

Freidenfelds, Lara. *The Myth of the Perfect Pregnancy: A History of Miscarriage in America.* Oxford University Press, 2020.

Fuentes, Marisa. *Dispossessed Lives: Enslaved Women, Violence, and the Archive.* University of Pennsylvania Press, 2016.

Gailani, Salim Samar Al-. "Teratology and the Clinic: Monsters, Obstetrics, and the Making of Antenatal Life in Edinburgh, c. 1900." PhD diss., University of Cambridge, 2010.

Gamble, Vanessa Northington. *Making a Place for Ourselves: The Black Hospital Movement, 1920–1945.* Oxford University Press, 1995.

Garland-Thomson, Rosemarie. "Disability." In *Keywords in Health Humanities*, ed. Sari Altschuler, Jonathan Metzl, and Priscilla Wald, 58–61. New York University Press, 2023.

Garland-Thomson, Rosemarie. "Disability Studies: A Field Emerged." *American Quarterly* 65, no. 4 (2013): 915–26.

Garland-Thomson, Rosemarie. *Extraordinary Bodies: Figuring Physical Disability in American Culture and Literature.* Columbia University Press, 1997.

Garland-Thomson, Rosemarie. "Feminist Disability Studies." *Signs* 30, no. 2 (2005): 1557–87.

Garland-Thomson, Rosemarie, ed. *Freakery: Cultural Spectacles of the Extraordinary Body.* New York University Press, 1996.

Garland-Thomson, Rosemarie, Michael Mark Chemers, and Analola Santana. "Introduction: Step Right Up! A New Introduction to the Old Freak Show." In *Freak Inheritance: Eugenics and Extraordinary Bodies in Performance,* ed. Rosemarie Garland-Thomson, Michael Mark Chemers, and Analola Santana, xv–xxii. Oxford University Press, 2024.

Gilbert, Scott F. *Developmental Biology.* 10th ed. Sinauer, 2014.

Gilbert, Scott F. "The Generation of Novelty: The Province of Developmental Biology." *Biological Theory* 1, no. 2 (2006): 209–12.

Gilbert, Scott F., and David Epel. *Ecological Developmental Biology: The Environmental Regulation of Development, Health, and Evolution.* 2nd ed. Oxford University Press, 2015.

Gilman, Sander. *Inscribing the Other.* University of Nebraska Press, 1991.

Golden, Janet. *Message in a Bottle: The Making of Fetal Alcohol Syndrome.* Harvard University Press, 2005.

Gómez, Pablo. *The Experiential Caribbean: Creating Knowledge and Healing in the Early Modern Atlantic.* University of North Carolina Press, 2017.

Goodwin, Michele. *Policing the Womb: Invisible Women and the Criminalization of Motherhood.* Cambridge University Press, 2020.

Gorbach, Frida. "Teratology in Mexico. 19th Century." *Medicina nei secoli* 26, no. 1 (2014): 245–67.

Gould, Stephen Jay. *The Mismeasure of Man.* Norton, 1996.

Gowing, Laura. *Common Bodies: Women, Touch, and Power in Seventeenth-Century England.* Yale University Press, 2003.

Hagner, Michael. "Enlightened Monsters." In *The Sciences in Enlightened Europe,* ed. William Clark, Jan Golinski, and Simon Schaffer, 175–218. University of Chicago Press, 1999.

Haller, John S. *Outcasts from Evolution: Scientific Attitudes of Racial Inferiority, 1859–1900.* University of Illinois Press, 1971.

Halttunen, Karen. "Humanitarianism and the Pornography of Pain in Anglo-American Culture." *American Historical Review* 100 (1995): 303–34.

Hammonds, Evelynn. "Black (W)Holes and the Geometry of Black Female Sexuality." *differences: A Journal of Feminist Cultural Studies* 6, nos. 2–3 (1994): 126–45.

Hammonds, Evelynn. "Straw Men and Their Followers: The Return of Biological Race." Social Science Research Council, 2006. http://raceandgenomics.ssrc.org/Hammonds.

Hammonds, Evelynn. "Toward a Genealogy of Black Female Sexuality: The Problematic of Silence." In *Feminist Theory and the Body*, ed. Janet Price and Margrit Shildrick, 93–104. Routledge, 1999.

Hammonds, Evelynn, and Rebecca Herzig. *The Nature of Difference: Sciences of Race in the United States from Jefferson to Genomics*. MIT Press, 2008.

Haney-López, Ian. *White by Law: The Legal Construction of Race*. New York University Press, 2006.

Haraway, Donna. "A Cyborg Manifesto: Science, Technology, and Socialist-Feminism in the Late Twentieth Century." In *Simians, Cyborgs, and Women: The Reinvention of Nature*, 149–81. Routledge, 1991.

Harding, Sandra G., ed. *The "Racial" Economy of Science: Toward a Democratic Future*. Indiana University Press, 1993.

Hartman, Saidiya. *Scenes of Subjection: Terror, Slavery, and Self-Making in Nineteenth-Century America*. Oxford University Press, 1997.

Hartman, Saidiya. *Wayward Lives, Beautiful Experiments*. Norton, 2019.

Henry, Kelsey, Anna Hinton, and Sony Coráñez Bolton. "Origins, Objects, Orientations: New Histories and Theories of Race and Disability." *Disability Studies Quarterly* 43, no. 1 (2023). https://doi.org/10.18061/dsq.v43i1.9719.

Higginbotham, Evelyn Brooks. "African-American Women's History and the Metalanguage of Race." *Signs* 17 (1992): 251–74.

Hine, Darlene Clark. "Co-Laborers in the Work of the Lord: Black Women Physicians in the Nineteenth Century." In *Hine Sight: Black Women and the Re-Construction of American History*, 147–62. Carlson, 1994.

Hodes, Martha. "The Mercurial Nature and Abiding Power of Race: A Transnational Family Story." *American Historical Review* 108 (2003): 84–118.

Hogarth, Rana A. *Medicalizing Blackness: Making Racial Differences in the Atlantic World, 1780–1840*. University of North Carolina Press, 2017.

Hopwood, Nick. *Haeckel's Embryos: Images, Evolution, and Fraud*. University of Chicago Press, 2015.

Huet, Marie-Hélène. *Monstrous Imagination*. Harvard University Press, 1993.

Hunt-Kennedy, Stefanie. *Between Fitness and Death: Disability and Slavery in the Caribbean*. University of Illinois Press, 2020.

Imada, Adria L. *An Archive of Skin, an Archive of Kin: Disability and Life-Making During Medical Incarceration*. University of California Press, 2022.

Jackson, Zakiyyah Iman. *Becoming Human: Matter and Meaning in an Antiblack World*. New York University Press, 2021.

Jacobson, Matthew Frye. *Barbarian Virtues: The United States Encounters Foreign Peoples at Home and Abroad, 1876–1917.* Hill and Wang, 2000.

Jaffary, Nora E. "The Monstrous Nation: The 1895 *Salon de Anomalías* in Mexico's National Museum, 1895." *Journal of Women's History* 34, no. 2 (2022): 11–30.

Jaffary, Nora E. *Reproduction and Its Discontents in Mexico: Childbirth and Contraception from 1750 to 1905.* University of North Carolina Press, 2016.

Jewson, Norman. "The Disappearance of the Sick-Man from Medical Cosmology, 1770–1870." *Sociology* 10 (1976): 225–44.

Johnson, Walter. *Soul by Soul: Life Inside the Antebellum Slave Market.* Harvard University Press, 1999.

Jones, David S. *Rationalizing Epidemics: Meanings and Uses of American Indian Mortality Since 1600.* Harvard University Press, 2004.

Jordanova, Ludmilla. "The Art and Science of Seeing in Medicine: Physiognomy 1780–1820." In *Medicine and the Five Senses*, ed. W. F. Bynum and Roy Porter, 122–33. Cambridge University Press, 1993.

Juzda, Elise. "Skulls, Science, and the Spoils of War: Craniological Studies at the United States Army Medical Museum, 1868–1900." *Studies in History and Philosophy of Science Part C: Studies in History and Philosophy of Biological and Biomedical Sciences* 40, no. 3 (2009): 156–67.

Karschay, Stephan. *Degeneration, Normativity, and the Gothic at the Fin de Siècle.* Palgrave Macmillan, 2015.

Keel, Terence. *Divine Variations: How Christian Thought Became Racial Science.* Stanford University Press, 2018.

Kemp, Martin. "A Perfect and Faithful Record: Mind and Body in Medical Photography Before 1900." In *Beauty of Another Order: Photography in Science*, ed. Ann Thomas, 120–49. Yale University Press, 1997.

Kemp, Martin. "Style and Non-Style in Anatomical Illustration: From Renaissance Humanism to Henry Gray." *Journal of Anatomy* 216, no. 2 (2010): 192–208.

Kenny, Stephen C. "The Development of Medical Museums in the Antebellum American South: Slave Bodies in Networks of Anatomical Exchange." *Bulletin of the History of Medicine* 87, no. 1 (2013): 32–62.

Kershner, R. B. "Degeneration: The Explanatory Nightmare." *Georgia Review* 40, no. 2 (1986): 416–44.

Kevles, Daniel J. *In the Name of Eugenics: Genetics and the Uses of Human Heredity.* University of California Press, 1985.

Khater, Micah. "No Use to the State: Phrasing Escape and a Black Radical Epistolary of Disability in Early Twentieth-Century Alabama Prisons." *Disability Studies Quarterly* 43, no. 1 (2023). https://doi.org/10.18061/dsq.v43i1.9662.

Kim, Jina B. "Disability in an Age of Fascism." *American Quarterly* 72, no. 1 (2020): 265–76.

Kline, Wendy. *Building a Better Race: Gender, Sexuality, and Eugenics from the Turn of the Century to the Baby Boom*. University of California Press, 2001.

Kline, Wendy. "Eugenics in the United States." In *Oxford Handbook of the History of Eugenics*, ed. Alison Bashford and Philippa Levine, 511–22. Oxford University Press, 2010.

Kool, Simeon. *Intimate Subjects: Touch and Tangibility in Britain's Cerebral Age*. University of Chicago Press, 2024.

Krieger, Nancy, and Elizabeth Fee. "Man-Made Medicine and Women's Health: The Biopolitics of Sex/Gender and Race/Ethnicity." *International Journal of Health Services* 24, no. 2 (1994): 265–83.

Kudlick, Catherine. "Disability History: Why We Need Another 'Other.'" *American Historical Review* 108 (2003): 763–79.

Ladd-Taylor, Molly. *Fixing the Poor: Eugenical Sterilization and Child Welfare in the Twentieth Century*. Johns Hopkins University Press, 2017.

Laqueur, Thomas. *Making Sex: Body and Gender from the Greeks to Freud*. Harvard University Press, 1992.

Lawrence, Susan, and Susan E. Lederer. "Medical Specimens and the Erasure of Racial Violence: The Case of Harriet Cole." *Medical Humanities* 49, no. 3 (2023): 457–67.

Leavitt, Judith Walzer. *Brought to Bed: Childbearing in America, 1750 to 1950*. 30th anniv. ed. Oxford University Press, 2016.

Leavitt, Judith Walzer. "The Growth of Medical Authority: Technology and Morals in Turn-of-the-Century Obstetrics." In *Women and Health in America: Historical Readings*, 2nd ed., ed. Judith Walzer Leavitt, 636–58. University of Wisconsin Press, 1999.

Lewis, Jan. "Mother's Love: The Construction of an Emotion in Nineteenth-Century America." In *Mothers and Motherhood: Readings in American History*, ed. Rima D. Apple and Janet Lynne Golden, 52–71. Ohio State University Press, 1997.

Lindquist, Wendi A. "Stealing from the Dead: Scientists, Settlers, and Indian Burial Sites in Early-Nineteenth-Century Oregon." *Oregon Historical Quarterly* 115, no. 3 (2014): 324–43.

Linton, Simi. *Claiming Disability: Knowledge and Identity*. New York University Press, 1998.

Lira, Natalie. *Laboratory of Deficiency: Sterilization and Confinement in California, 1910s–1950s*. University of California Press, 2021.

Livingston, Julie. "Comment: On the Borderland of Medical and Disability History." *Bulletin of History of Medicine* 87 (2013): 560–64.

Long, Gretchen. *Doctoring Freedom: The Politics of African American Medical Care in Slavery and Emancipation*. University of North Carolina Press, 2012.

Longmore, Paul. "A Note on Language and the Social Identity of Disabled People." *American Behavioral Scientist* 28, no. 3 (1985): 419–24.

Longmore, Paul. "Screening Stereotypes: Images of Disabled People in Television and Motion Picture." In *Why I Burned My Book and Other Essays on Disability*, 131–46. Temple University Press, 2003.

Lovejoy, Arthur O. *The Great Chain of Being: A Study of the History of an Idea*. 1936. Harvard University Press, 2001.

Löwy, Ilana. *Tangled Diagnoses: Prenatal Testing, Women, and Risk*. University of Chicago Press, 2016.

Mach, Stephanie. "Affective Responses to Normalized Violence in Museums." In "The Morton Cranial Collection and Legacies of Scientific Racism in Museums," ed. Paul Wolff Mitchell. Special issue, *History of Anthropology Review* 45 (2021). https://histanthro.org/news/observations/affective-responses.

Maienschein, Jane. "Heredity/Development in the United States, Circa 1900." *History and Philosophy of Life Sciences* 9 (1987): 79–83.

Maienschein, Jane. "Shifting Assumptions in American Biology: Embryology, 1890–1910." *Journal of the History of Biology* 14, no. 1 (1981): 89–113.

Marsella, Jamie. "'Better Babies, Better Mothers, Better City': Eugenic Maternalism, the Babies Welfare Association, and the Urban Better Baby Contest." *Bulletin of the History of Medicine* 98, no. 3 (2024): 370–93.

Martin, Aryn, and Kelly Holloway. "'Something There Is That Doesn't Love a Wall': Histories of the Placental Barrier." *Studies in History and Philosophy of Science Part C: Studies in History and Philosophy of Biological and Biomedical Sciences* 47, Part B (2014): 300–310.

Mason, Jennifer. *Civilized Creatures: Urban Animals, Sentimental Culture, and American Literature, 1850–1900*. Johns Hopkins University Press, 2005.

McGuinness, Aims. *Path of Empire: Panama and the California Gold Rush*. Cornell University Press, 2008.

McLeary, Erin. "Science in a Bottle: The Medical Museum in North America, 1860–1940." PhD diss., University of Pennsylvania, 2001.

McMahon, Lucia. "'So Truly Afflicting and Distressing to Me His Sorrowing Mother': Expressions of Maternal Grief in Eighteenth-Century Philadelphia." *Journal of the Early Republic* 32, no. 1 (2012): 27–60.

Mitchell, Michele. *Righteous Propagation: African Americans and the Politics of Racial Destiny After Reconstruction*. University of North Carolina Press, 2004.

Mitchell, Paul Wolff. "Editor's Introduction: The Morton Cranial Collection and Legacies of Scientific Racism in Museums." Special issue, *History of Anthropology Review* 45 (2021). https://histanthro.org/news/observations/editors-introduction-morton.

Mittman, Asa Simon, and Peter J. Dendle, eds. *The Ashgate Research Companion to Monsters and the Monstrous*. Routledge, 2012.

Molina, Natalia. *Fit to Be Citizens? Public Health and Race in Los Angeles, 1879–1939*. University of California Press, 2006.

Monroe, Rachel. "A Medical-History Museum Contends with Its Collection of Human Remains." *The New Yorker*, June 23, 2025.

Morantz-Sanchez, Regina Markell. *Sympathy & Science: Women Physicians in American Medicine*. 2nd ed. University of North Carolina Press, 2000.

Morgan, Jennifer L. *Laboring Women: Reproduction and Gender in New World Slavery*. University of Pennsylvania Press, 2004.

Morgan, Jennifer L. "Partus sequitur ventrem: Law, Race, and Reproduction in Colonial Slavery." *Small Axe: A Caribbean Journal of Criticism* 22, no. 1 (2018): 1–17.

Morgan, Jennifer L. *Reckoning with Slavery: Gender, Kinship, and Capitalism in the Early Black Atlantic*. Duke University Press, 2021.

Morgan, Jennifer L. "'Some Could Suckle Over Their Shoulder': Male Travelers, Female Bodies, and the Gendering of Racial Ideology, 1500–1770." *William and Mary Quarterly* 54, no. 1 (1997): 167–92.

Morgan, Lynn. *Icons of Life: A Cultural History of Human Embryos*. University of California Press, 2009.

Muigai, Wangui. "'Something Wasn't Clean': Black Midwifery, Birth, and Postwar Medical Education in *All My Babies*." *Bulletin of the History of Medicine* 93, no. 1 (2019): 82–113.

Nouailles, Bertrand. *Le monstre, la vie, l'écart: La tératologie d'Étienne et d'Isidore Geoffroy Saint-Hilaire*. Classiques Garnier, 2017.

Nuriddin, Ayah. "Engineering Uplift: Black Eugenics as Black Liberation." In *Nature Remade: Engineering Life, Envisioning Worlds*, ed. Luis A. Campos, Michael R. Dietrich, Tiago Saraiva, and Christian C. Young, 186–202. University of Chicago Press, 2021.

O'Brien, Elizabeth. *Surgery and Salvation: The Roots of Reproductive Injustice in Mexico, 1770–1940*. University of North Carolina Press, 2023.

Omi, Michael, and Howard Winant. *Racial Formation in the United States*. Routledge, 1994.

Oppenheimer, Jane M. "Some Historical Relationships Between Teratology and Experimental Embryology." *Bulletin of the History of Medicine* 42, no. 2 (1968): 145–59.

Park, Katharine. *Secrets of Women: Gender, Generation, and the Origins of Human Dissection*. Zone, 2006.

Patterson, Lindsey. "The Disability Rights Movement in the United States." In *The Oxford Handbook of Disability History*, ed. Michael Rembis, Catherine J. Kudlick, and Kim Nielsen, 439–57. Oxford University Press, 2018.

Paugh, Katherine. *The Politics of Reproduction: Race, Disease, and Fertility in the Age of Abolition*. Oxford University Press, 2017.

Paul, Diane B. "Reflections on the Historiography of American Eugenics: Trends, Fractures, Tensions." *Journal of the History of Biology* 49, no. 4 (2016): 641–58.

Pauly, Philip. *Biologists and the Promise of American Life: From Meriwether Lewis to Alfred Kinsey*. Princeton University Press, 2000.

Pauly, Philip. "How Did the Effects of Alcohol on Reproduction Become Scientifically Uninteresting?" *Journal of the History of Biology* 29, no. 1 (1996): 1–28.

Pernick, Martin S. *The Black Stork: Eugenics and the Death of "Defective" Babies in American Medicine and Motion Pictures Since 1915*. Oxford University Press, 1996.

Petryna, Adriana. *Life Exposed: Biological Citizens After Chernobyl*. Princeton University Press, 2002.

Picart, Caroline Joan, and John Edgar Browning, eds. *Speaking of Monsters: A Teratological Anthology*. Palgrave Macmillan, 2012.

Pomata, Gianna. *Contracting a Cure: Patients, Healers, and the Law in Early Modern Bologna*. Johns Hopkins University Press, 1998.

Ponce, Rachel N. "'They Increase in Beauty and Elegance': Transforming Cadavers and the Epistemology of Dissection in Early Nineteenth-Century American Medical Education." *Journal of the History of Medicine and Allied Sciences* 68, no. 3 (2013): 331–76.

Poovey, Mary. "Anatomical Realism and Social Investigation in Early Nineteenth-Century Manchester." In *Making a Social Body: British Cultural Formation, 1830–1864*, 73–97. University of Chicago Press, 1995.

Preston, Samuel H., and Michael R. Haines. *Fatal Years: Child Mortality in Late Nineteenth-Century America*. Princeton University Press, 1991.

Puar, Jasbir. *The Right to Maim: Debility, Capacity, Disability*. Duke University Press, 2017.

Qureshi, Sadiah. *Peoples on Parade: Exhibitions, Empire, and Anthropology in Nineteenth Century Britain*. University of Chicago Press, 2011.

Ragab, Ahmed. "Monsters and Patients: An Archaeology of Medicine, Islam, and Modernity." *History and Theory* 55, no. 4 (2016): 112–30.

Rapp, Rayna. *Testing Women, Testing the Fetus: The Social Impact of Amniocentesis in America*. Routledge, 1999.

Ray, Sara. "From Monsters to Malformations: Anatomical Preparations as Objects of Evidence for a Developmental Paradigm of Embryology, 1770–1850." *Journal of the History of Biology* 55, no. 1 (2022): 35–57.

Reagan, Leslie J. *Dangerous Pregnancies: Mothers, Disabilities, and Abortion in Modern America*. University of California Press, 2010.

Reagan, Leslie J. *When Abortion Was a Crime: Women, Medicine, and Law in the United States, 1867–1973*. University of California Press, 1997.

Redman, Samuel J. *Bone Rooms: From Scientific Racism to Human Prehistory in Museums*. Harvard University Press, 2016.

Rembis, Michael. *Defining Deviance: Sex, Science, and Delinquent Girls: 1890–1960*. University of Illinois Press, 2013.

Reverby, Susan. "Ethical Failures and History Lessons: The U.S. Public Health Service Research Studies in Tuskegee and Guatemala." *Public Health Reviews* 34, no. 1 (2012): 1–18.

Rich, Miriam. "The Curse of Civilised Woman: Race, Gender, and the Pain of Childbirth in Nineteenth-Century American Medicine." *Gender & History* 28 (2016): 57–76.

Rich, Miriam. "Monstrosity in Medical Science: Race-Making and Teratology in the Nineteenth-Century United States." *Isis* 114, no. 3 (2023): 513–36.

Richards, Evelleen. "A Political Anatomy of Monsters, Hopeful and Otherwise: Teratogeny, Transcendentalism, and Evolutionary Theorizing." *Isis* 85, no. 3 (1994): 377–411.

Richardson, Sarah. *The Maternal Imprint: The Contested Science of Maternal–Fetal Effects*. University of Chicago Press, 2021.

Roberts, Carolyn. "Pharmaceutical Captivity, Epistemological Rupture, and the Business Archive of the British Slave Trade." *Business History Review* 97, no. 2 (2023): 283–305.

Roberts, Dorothy E. *Fatal Invention: How Science, Politics, and Big Business Re-Create Race in the Twenty-First Century*. New Press, 2011.

Roberts, Dorothy E. *Killing the Black Body: Race, Reproduction, and the Meaning of Liberty*. Pantheon, 1997.

Roberts, Dorothy E. "Unshackling Black Motherhood." *Michigan Law Review* 95, no. 4 (1997): 938–64.

Roberts, Samuel Kelton. *Infectious Fear: Politics, Disease, and the Health Effects of Segregation*. University of North Carolina Press, 2009.

Roe, Shirley A. *Matter, Life, and Generation: Eighteenth-Century Embryology and the Haller–Wolff Debate*. Cambridge University Press, 2003.

Rooks, Noliwe. *Ladies' Pages: African American Women's Magazines and the Culture That Made Them*. Rutgers University Press, 2004.

Roque, Ricardo. "Authorised Histories: Human Remains and the Economies of Credibility in the Science of Race." *Kronos*, no. 44 (2018): 69–85.

Rose, Sarah F. *No Right to Be Idle: The Invention of Disability, 1840s–1930s*. University of North Carolina Press, 2017.

Rosen, Jeff. "Of Monsters and Fossils: The Making of Racial Difference in Malvina Hoffman's Hall of the Races of Mankind." *History and Anthropology* 12, no. 2 (2001): 101–58.

Rosenberg, Charles E. "The Bitter Fruit: Heredity, Disease, and Social Thought in Nineteenth- Century America." *Perspectives in American History* 8 (1974): 189–95.

Rosenberg, Charles E. *The Care of Strangers: The Rise of America's Hospital System.* Johns Hopkins University Press, 1995.

Rosenberg, Charles E. *Explaining Epidemics, and Other Studies in the History of Medicine.* Cambridge University Press, 1992.

Rosenberg, Charles E. *No Other Gods: On Science and American Social Thought.* Rev. and exp. ed. John Hopkins University Press, 1997.

Rosenberg, Charles E. "Social Class and Medical Care in Nineteenth-Century America: The Rise and Fall of the Dispensary." *Journal of the History of Medicine and Allied Sciences* 29, no. 1 (1974): 32–54.

Rosenberg, Charles E. "The Therapeutic Revolution: Medicine, Meaning, and Social Change in Nineteenth-Century America." *Perspectives in Biology and Medicine* 20, no. 4 (1977): 485–506.

Roth, Cassia. "The Degenerating Sex: Female Sterilisation, Medical Authority, and Racial Purity in Catholic Brazil." *Medical History* 64, no. 2 (2020): 173–94.

Roth, Cassia. *A Miscarriage of Justice: Women's Reproductive Lives and the Law in Early Twentieth-Century Brazil.* Stanford University Press, 2020.

Samuels, Ellen. "Examining Millie and Christine McKoy: Where Enslavement and Enfreakment Meet." *Signs* 37, no. 1 (2011): 53–81.

Samuels, Ellen. *Fantasies of Identification: Disability, Gender, Race.* New York University Press, 2014.

Savitt, Todd L. *Race and Medicine in Nineteenth- and Early-Twentieth-Century America.* Kent State University Press, 2007.

Schalk, Sami. *Bodyminds Reimagined: (Dis)ability, Race, and Gender in Black Women's Speculative Fiction.* Duke University Press, 2018.

Schalk, Sami, and Jina B. Kim. "Integrating Race, Transforming Feminist Disability Studies." *Signs* 46, no. 1 (2020): 31–55.

Schiebinger, Londa. *Nature's Body: Gender in the Making of Modern Science.* Beacon, 1993.

Schlich, Thomas. *The Origins of Organ Transplantation: Surgery and Laboratory Science, 1880–1930.* University of Rochester Press, 2010.

Schuller, Kyla. *The Biopolitics of Feeling: Race, Sex, and Science in the Nineteenth Century.* Duke University Press, 2018.

Schwalm, Leslie A. *Medicine, Science, and Making Race in Civil War America.* University of North Carolina Press, 2023.

Schwartz, Marie Jenkins. *Birthing a Slave: Motherhood and Medicine in the Antebellum South.* Harvard University Press, 2010.

Schweik, Susan. "Archaeology of the 'Feebleminded': In the Archives with Lee Swearengin." *Osiris* 39 (2024): 135–49.

Scotch, Richard K. "'Nothing About Us Without Us': Disability Rights in America." *OAH Magazine of History* 23, no. 3 (2009): 17–22.

Shah, Nayan. *Contagious Divides: Epidemics and Race in San Francisco's Chinatown*. University of California Press, 2001.

Sharpe, Christina. *Monstrous Intimacies: Making Post-Slavery Subjects*. Duke University Press, 2010.

Sheldon, Myrna Perez. "Sexual Selection as Race Making." *British Journal for the History of Science* 6 (2021): 9–23.

Shildrick, Margrit. *Dangerous Discourses of Disability, Subjectivity, and Sexuality*. Palgrave Macmillan, 2009.

Shildrick, Margrit. *Embodying the Monster: Encounters with the Vulnerable Self*. Sage, 2002.

Smedley, Audrey. *Race in North America: Origin and Evolution of a Worldview*. 4th ed. Routledge, 2011.

Smith, Pamela, Amy Meyers, and Harold Cook, eds. *Ways of Making and Knowing: The Material Culture of Empirical Knowledge*. University of Chicago Press, 2017.

Smith-Ruiu, Justin. *Nature, Human Nature, and Human Difference: Race in Early Modern Philosophy*. Princeton University Press, 2015.

Spencer, Frank. "Some Notes on the Attempt to Apply Photography to Anthropometry During the Second Half of the Nineteenth Century." In *Anthropology and Photography, 1860–1920*, ed. Elizabeth Edwards, 99–107. Yale University Press, 1992.

Spillers, Hortense J. "Mama's Baby, Papa's Maybe: An American Grammar Book." *Diacritics* 17, no. 2 (1987): 65–81.

Starr, Paul. *The Social Transformation of American Medicine*. Basic, 1982.

Stepan, Nancy Leys. "Biology and Degeneration: Races and Proper Places." In *Degeneration: The Dark Side of Progress*, ed. J. Edward Chamberlin and Sander L. Gilman, 97–120. Columbia University Press, 1985.

Stepan, Nancy Leys. *"The Hour of Eugenics": Race, Gender, and Nation in Latin America*. Cornell University Press, 1996.

Stepan, Nancy Leys. *The Idea of Race in Science: Great Britain, 1800–1960*. Archon, 1982.

Stepan, Nancy Leys. "Race and Gender: The Role of Analogy in Science." *Isis* 77, no. 2 (1986): 261–77.

Stepan, Nancy Leys. "Race, Gender, Science, and Citizenship." *Gender & History* 10, no. 1 (1998): 26–52.

Stern, Alexandra Minna. *Eugenic Nation: Faults and Frontiers of Better Breeding in Modern America*. University of California Press, 2005.

Stocking, George W. "The Turn-of-the Century Concept of Race." *Modernism/Modernity* 1, no. 1 (1994): 4–16.

Stocking, George W. *Victorian Anthropology*. Collier Macmillan, Free Press, 1987.

Subramaniam, Banu. *Ghost Stories for Darwin: The Science of Variation and the Politics of Diversity*. University of Illinois Press, 2014.

Theobald, Brianna. *Reproduction on the Reservation: Pregnancy, Childbirth, and Colonialism in the Long Twentieth Century*. University of North Carolina Press, 2019.

Tromp, Marlene, ed. *Victorian Freaks: The Social Context of Freakery in Britain*. Ohio State University Press, 2008.

Turner, Felicity. *Proving Pregnancy: Gender, Law, and Medical Knowledge in Nineteenth-Century America*. University of North Carolina Press, 2022.

Turner, Sasha. *Contested Bodies: Pregnancy, Childrearing, and Slavery in Jamaica*. University of Pennsylvania Press, 2017.

Turner, Sasha. "The Nameless and the Forgotten: Maternal Grief, Sacred Protection, and the Archive of Slavery." *Slavery & Abolition* 38 (2017): 232–50.

Ulrich, Laurel Thatcher. *A Midwife's Tale: The Life of Martha Ballard, Based on Her Diary, 1785–1812*. Knopf, 1990.

Vásquez, Lorenah, Miriam Rich, and Lisa Campo-Engelstein. "Beyond Policing Bodies: A Broader Conception of Fairness in Women's Sports." *American Journal of Bioethics* 24, no. 11 (2024): 29–30.

Veatch, Robert M. "Abandon the Dead Donor Rule or Change the Definition of Death?" *Kennedy Institute of Ethics Journal* 14, no. 3 (2004): 261–76.

Velocci, Beans. *Sex Isn't Real: The Invention of an Incoherent Binary*. Duke University Press, 2026.

Vyas, Darshali A., Leo G. Eisenstein, and David S. Jones. "Hidden in Plain Sight: Reconsidering the Use of Race Correction in Clinical Algorithms." *New England Journal of Medicine* 383, no. 9 (2020): 874–82.

Wailoo, Keith. *Dying in the City of the Blues: Sickle Cell Anemia and the Politics of Race and Health*. University of North Carolina Press, 2001.

Wailoo, Keith, Alondra Nelson, and Catherine Lee, eds. *Genetics and the Unsettled Past: The Collision of DNA, Race, and History*. Rutgers University Press, 2012.

Warkany, Josef. "The Medical Profession and Congenital Malformations." *Teratology* 20, no. 2 (1979): 201–4.

Warner, John Harley. *Against the Spirit of System: The French Impulse in Nineteenth-Century American Medicine*. Princeton University Press, 1998.

Warner, John Harley. *The Therapeutic Perspective: Medical Practice, Knowledge, and Identity in America, 1820–1885*. Princeton University Press, 1997.

Warner, John Harley. "Witnessing Dissection: Photography, Medicine, and American Culture." In John Harley Warner and James M. Edmonson, *Dissection: Photographs of a Rite of Passage in American Medicine, 1880–1930*, 7–29. Blast, 2009.

Weiner, Marli F., with Mayzie Hough. *Sex, Sickness, and Slavery: Illness in the Antebellum South*. University of Illinois Press, 2012.

Welter, Barbara. "The Cult of True Womanhood: 1820–1860." *American Quarterly* 18, no. 2 (1966): 151–74.

Whatcott, Jess. *A Menace to the Future: A Disability and Queer History of Carceral Eugenics*. Duke University Press, 2024.

White, Deborah Gray. *Ar'n't I a Woman? Female Slaves in the Plantation South*. Norton, 1999.

Willoughby, Christopher. *Masters of Health: Racial Science and Slavery in U.S. Medical Schools*. University of North Carolina Press, 2022.

Willoughby, Christopher. "Professors of Racial Medicine: Imperialism and Race in Nineteenth-Century United States Medical Schools." *Medical History* 68, no. 2 (2024): 146–61.

Wilson, Dudley Butler. *Signs and Portents: Monstrous Births from the Middle Ages to the Enlightenment*. Routledge, 1993.

Withycombe, Shannon. "From Women's Expectations to Scientific Specimens: The Fate of Miscarriage Materials in Nineteenth-Century America." *Social History of Medicine* 28, no. 2 (2015): 245–62.

Withycombe, Shannon. *Lost: Miscarriage in Nineteenth-Century America*. Rutgers University Press, 2018.

Wolf, Jacqueline. *Deliver Me from Pain: Anesthesia and Birth in America*. Johns Hopkins University Press, 2009.

Wu, Cynthia. *Chang and Eng Reconnected: The Original Siamese Twins in American Culture*. Temple University Press, 2012.

Yudell, Michael. *Race Unmasked: Biology and Race in the Twentieth Century*. Columbia University Press, 2014.

Index

Printed and bound by CPI Group (UK) Ltd, Croydon, CR0 4YY

16/09/2026

14963453-0001